FORENSIC PSYCHIATRY
An Indian Perspective

FORENSIC PSYCHIATRY
An Indian Perspective

RC Jiloha MBBS MD
Professor and Head
Department of Psychiatry and
Rehabilitation Science
Hamdard Institute of Medical Sciences and Research
Jamia Hamdard, New Delhi, India

Prerna Kukreti MBBS MD IDMHLHR
Assistant Professor
Department of Psychiatry
Lady Hardinge Medical College
New Delhi, India

Dinesh Kataria MBBS MD PhD MHA MPhil
Professor and Head
Department of Psychiatry
Lady Hardinge Medical College
New Delhi, India

Foreword
Amita Dhanda

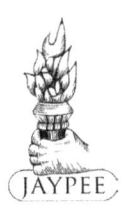

The Health Sciences Publisher
New Delhi | London | Panama

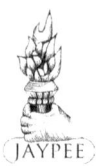

Jaypee Brothers Medical Publishers (P) Ltd

Headquarters
Jaypee Brothers Medical Publishers (P) Ltd
4838/24, Ansari Road, Daryaganj
New Delhi 110 002, India
Phone: +91-11-43574357
Fax: +91-11-43574314
Email: jaypee@jaypeebrothers.com

Overseas Offices

J.P. Medical Ltd
83 Victoria Street, London
SW1H 0HW (UK)
Phone: +44 20 3170 8910
Fax: +44 (0)20 3008 6180
Email: info@jpmedpub.com

Jaypee-Highlights Medical Publishers Inc
City of Knowledge, Bld. 235, 2nd Floor, Clayton
Panama City, Panama
Phone: +1 507-301-0496
Fax: +1 507-301-0499
Email: cservice@jphmedical.com

Jaypee Brothers Medical Publishers (P) Ltd
17/1-B Babar Road, Block-B, Shyamoli
Mohammadpur, Dhaka-1207
Bangladesh
Mobile: +08801912003485
Email: jaypeedhaka@gmail.com

Jaypee Brothers Medical Publishers (P) Ltd
Bhotahity, Kathmandu
Nepal
Phone: +977-9741283608
Email: kathmandu@jaypeebrothers.com

Website: www.jaypeebrothers.com
Website: www.jaypeedigital.com

© 2019, Jaypee Brothers Medical Publishers

The views and opinions expressed in this book are solely those of the original contributor(s)/author(s) and do not necessarily represent those of editor(s) of the book.

All rights reserved. No part of this publication may be reproduced, stored or transmitted in any form or by any means, electronic, mechanical, photocopying, recording or otherwise, without the prior permission in writing of the publishers.

All brand names and product names used in this book are trade names, service marks, trademarks or registered trademarks of their respective owners. The publisher is not associated with any product or vendor mentioned in this book.

Medical knowledge and practice change constantly. This book is designed to provide accurate, authoritative information about the subject matter in question. However, readers are advised to check the most current information available on procedures included and check information from the manufacturer of each product to be administered, to verify the recommended dose, formula, method and duration of administration, adverse effects and contraindications. It is the responsibility of the practitioner to take all appropriate safety precautions. Neither the publisher nor the author(s)/editor(s) assume any liability for any injury and/or damage to persons or property arising from or related to use of material in this book.

This book is sold on the understanding that the publisher is not engaged in providing professional medical services. If such advice or services are required, the services of a competent medical professional should be sought.

Every effort has been made where necessary to contact holders of copyright to obtain permission to reproduce copyright material. If any have been inadvertently overlooked, the publisher will be pleased to make the necessary arrangements at the first opportunity. The **CD/DVD-ROM** (if any) provided in the sealed envelope with this book is complimentary and free of cost. **Not meant for sale.**

Inquiries for bulk sales may be solicited at: jaypee@jaypeebrothers.com

Forensic Psychiatry: An Indian Perspective

First Edition: 2019

ISBN: 978-93-5270-498-9

Dedicated to

Professor N N Wig who taught us
"Protective privilege ends where the public peril begins……"

Foreword

The Convergence of Law and Psychiatry

This textbook on *Forensic Psychiatry: An Indian Perspective* by RC Jiloha, Prerna Kukreti and Dinesh Kataria is an effort to comprehensively map out the various sectors in which law and psychiatry intersect with each other in a democratic polity. It is important to place this caveat of democracy as evidently legal norms would operate differently in an authoritarian system. The former allows difference and dissent whereas the latter demands total conformity.

The authors have tried to render the task manageable and the information accessible by dividing the book into eight sections focussing on different dimensions of forensic psychiatry. Thus, if section II is focusing attention on medicolegal responsibilities in doctor-patient relationship; section VIII examines a range of issues such as organ transplantation and euthanasia which have a relevance to mental health. I am taking a page out of their book and providing some generic categories to assist in understanding this relationship between law and psychiatry. Before doing so, I think it is apposite to reflect upon the commonalities and differences of the two disciplines. Both law and psychiatry require humans to conform to social norms. The law sees such conformity as necessary for the orderly functioning of society. And psychiatry views it as needed for humans to live in harmony and peace with the world around them. The law attempts to reach this goal through a system of incentives and disincentives which impel people to keep their behavior within the contours of the legal. Psychiatry has put in place a range of therapeutic interventions which are aimed to assist conformity. Other than these metaobjectives, both disciplines attempt to both regulate and facilitate human relations.

Even as compliance to legal norms is encouraged, total observance is not expected. Rather a democratic polity allows for a modicum of disagreement and dissent. Special interventions are planned when the disagreement comes to be viewed as deviance or a disorder. If the non-conforming behavior is perceived as deviance, managing the individual is allocated to the criminal justice system; the therapeutic system takes over if the conduct is diagnosed as a disorder. The very fact that the behavior could be seen as one or the other brings home the cheek by jowl existence of the two disciplines. Psychiatry aspires to be part of the healing professions and to that extent claims a more benevolent visage,[1] however, considering the force and compulsory care is an integral part of its practice, this claim of benevolence does not obtain a universal endorsement.[2] This anomalous position adopted by mainstream psychiatry makes its position problematic as it seems to be speaking for both the controller and the controlled. It aligns with social controllers when it allows for compulsory treatment

---

[1] Section II of the book focusses attention on the obligations surrounding this doctor-patient relationship
[2] See for example chapter 5 of section II where exceptions to informed consent are addressed as a part of the psychiatric doctor-patient relationship.

and for the controlled when it asks for therapy to prevail over punishment. Insofar as this book comprehensively documents the various sites at which, and modes and procedures through which, law and psychiatry interact, it therefore provides an opportunity to assess the pulls and pressures of this relationship. In this foreword, I provide a template which generically classifies the multiple contexts addressed in the book and thereby make my contribution to seeing the interconnections between various areas of law and psychiatry.

Psychiatry in Law

In this first part I deal with those contexts wherein the law is either proactively seeking psychiatric expertise or psychiatric opinion is viewed as relevant and even proves to be determinative for some judges and courts.[3]

To Adjudge the Authenticity of The Guilty Intention
A wrongful act is determined to be a crime if the wrongful act is accompanied by a wrongful intention. This core principle of criminal culpability has been compromised by many statutory provisions which make the doing of a wrongful act sufficient to impose criminal culpability. Except for these strict liability offenses, a guilty intention is a necessary ingredient of criminal liability. Evidence or expert testimony which questions or supports the presence of such guilty intention is one of the sites where psychiatric expertise has been accorded legal recognition. The Indian Penal Code, 1860 makes unsoundness of mind which prevents the person from knowing the nature of an act or that it is wrongful and contrary to law as a defense against criminal culpability. To decide whether such defense can be availed by the accused or not, psychiatric evidence is again relevant.[4] As in principle, psychiatric evidence is relevant not determinative, there is a large body of case law which distinguishes medical from legal insanity. Even so, medical insanity being the threshold condition, psychiatric evidence is accorded high probity in criminal culpability trials and in practice for some judges it is virtually conclusive evidence.[5]

Since the adoption of the United Nations Convention on the Rights of Persons with Disabilities (UNCRPD) the inclusion of the defense of insanity in the general defenses has been controversial. Persons with disabilities who have been agitating for universal legal capacity are also demanding parity in criminal responsibility and hence have been seeking the abolition of the defense. Other law reformers believe that the state of mind should only be considered for purposes of sentencing and not to determine culpability. If sanity and insanity are not seen as dichotomous conditions, but part of a continuum, then evidence on the state of mind evidence should be perceived as relevant for all accused persons. Such use of psychiatric evidence means that psychiatry is then being used for customising sentencing for all and not just singling out and excluding some. The law as it stands, does not use psychiatry so. This book in chapter 22 speaks of the existing law and present practices. A lot of psychiatric experts have expressed

---

[3]See especially chapter 11 of section III which addresses the matter of expert testimony in Court.
[4]Chapter 18 of section V of the book examines the defence of insanity.
[5]See Amita Dhanda Legal Order and Mental Disorder (Sage Publications New Delhi 2000). Also see chapter 21 of this book.

dissatisfaction in the way in which their expertise is used in courts. Such like treatment occurs causing the expertise is rarely offered as assistance to the courts, but is proffered to buttress the case of a party. It may be worth considering whether both the equity of the proceedings and the status of the advice would be enhanced if the expertise is only proffered as advice to the court and not in some selected cases but to individuate sentencing in all cases. This question needs to be specially raised because the defense of insanity may allow for acquittal, but the acquittal alone does not result in discharge. For such discharge to happen a different kind of advice is needed from psychiatry.

To Predict Future Wrongful Behavior

Section 335 of the Code of Criminal Procedure does not allow for discharge to follow upon acquittal on grounds of insanity. Instead the Court concerned is required to record whether the accused had done the alleged act and special procedures must be followed before a decision to discharge the accused can be made. A psychiatric prediction on the dangerousness of the accused in the future is one such protocol. And such prediction continues to be demanded even as numerous studies question the scientific status of such prediction. Be that as it may, a psychiatric prediction of dangerousness has a direct bearing on the restoration of the liberty of the accused.

Capacity to Stand Trial

The questions of criminal culpability are considered by the Courts only after the accused is found competent to stand trial. Or to say it differently, if the accused is not considered to be incapable of standing trial by reason of unsoundness of mind. The Code of Criminal Procedure does not compel psychiatric evidence, and the opinion of a medical practitioner in the service of the government is considered sufficient. However, psychiatric evidence wherever provided is accorded greater weightage, especially as there is greater deference to medical opinion in this context, in comparison to the 'defense of insanity' trials.[6]

Maintenance of order is one of the primary functions of law and the above recount shows how psychiatry has been implicated in supporting the enforcers of the law. What is the bearing of this involvement on the therapeutic aspirations of psychiatry needs discussion. Can psychiatry perform both policing and healing functions that are both look out of society and the patient population? A question I will return to when I move to the second part of this foreword.

To Support the Victims of Wrongful Behavior

Psychiatric expertise is not just sought out for determining criminal culpability, it has also seen to be relevant to decide upon the mental distress suffered by adult and child victims of violence and abuse. Such expert opinion is often sought to devise a compensation and rehabilitation package for the victim independent of what sanctions may be imposed upon the perpetrator of the abuse or violence. Since women are disproportionately present as victims of abuse and violence, it is important that oppressive patriarchal practices are not normalized,

---

[6]Chapter 20 of the book

and the distress of the individual woman diagnosed as maladjustment rather than abuse. I am drawing attention to this fact because it is often found that the trauma experienced by individual persons against routinized maltreatment is often dismissed as the over-sensitivity of the individual person and the wrongfulness of the behavior or practice is not questioned. An inability to adjust to unjust social expectations often socially marks out a person. This individual protest and hurt need to be so recognized as dissent and not disorder in order that the bar of acceptable social behavior is raised. The changed social perceptions of domestic violence and sexual harassment started with individual women finding such behavior objectionable. Insofar as psychiatric opinion influences legal decisions and public policy, it is important that the complained wrongful behavior is perceived as the consequence of an iniquitous social structure and not the reaction of an overly sensitive mind.

To Evaluate the Capacity to Act

Psychiatric expertise has not only been sought to determine issues surrounding culpability in criminal law; it has also been drawn upon to decide questions of competence in civil law.[7] Such a need occurs because unsoundness of mind has been almost routinely incorporated in the law as a condition, which deprives individuals of the right to exercise their legal capacity. Whilst in some legal contexts just the fact of unsoundness of mind or psychiatric diagnosis is considered sufficient to deny the right to act (for example the right to adopt) in most others the law requires the psychiatric diagnosis to be of a kind which prevents the person with the diagnosis from performing a specific function. In principle, the psychiatric diagnosis is not determinative, but in practice since the psychiatric diagnosis is the reason for the inquiry on competence, its presence is often seen by both judge and psychiatrist as conclusive of the matter of legal capacity. A psychiatric diagnosis in a health setting plays out differently than in a civil rights situation. In the health context, it is ostensibly intended to provide treatment and care to the person who is diagnosed as ill. In the legal context, however, the information is being largely obtained to decide whether the person who has been diagnosed as psychiatrically ill can continue to exercise his or her legal capacity. It may be the same diagnosis, but the use of which has been put changes and this changed use need to be understood by both judge and psychiatrist. Till psychiatric care is voluntarily sought and provided, the matter is between therapist and client. However, if the voluntary care can be made compulsory, and the diagnosis used to deny the diagnosed person of their civil rights, then the bonafides of the therapeutic reasoning becomes questionable.

Law in Psychiatry

To provide Therapeutic Support Both Voluntarily and Involuntarily
When psychiatrists provide therapeutic support on demand they are at par with other medical and healing professions who are providing aid to people who are seeking it. The law will come into the professional-patient equation, only if there are complaints of negligence, malpractice

---

[7]Section IV of the book

or unsatisfactory quality of service. However, psychiatric interventions, unlike other medical services are also provided against the will and preference of the patient. Or when the patient is unable to consent. The therapeutic rationale behind such compulsory care is that the illness clouds the patient's judgment, which prevents the seeking out of the care, which otherwise would have been voluntarily accessed. Without getting into the rightness or wrongness of the belief, it is important to note that such involuntary care cannot be provided without explicit permission of the law. In India, the Constitution of India recognizes that no person shall be deprived of life and liberty except according to procedure established by law. By reason of this right, compulsory care can be provided only if there is a legislation, which provides a procedure through which such compulsory care can be provided. Thus, till such time, psychiatry and psychiatrists believe that compulsory care and treatment can go hand in hand, the relationship between law and the practice of psychiatry will remain. Rather psychiatrists would not be able to compulsorily provide treatment without legal sanction.[8]

After the adoption of the CRPD, the provisioning of compulsory psychiatric care has been majorly questioned. Such care it has been contended was against the form and the spirit of the Convention, which at no point permits the use of force.[9] And if no mental health laws are made then the practice of legal compulsory care would die. The absence of a law allowing compulsion may not at once cause coercive practices to cease. However, the process of decay would begin as professionals would not be comfortable providing services in a manner which is not permitted by the law. The recent judgments of the Delhi High Court[10] addressing the matter of compulsory admission in a private nursing home and a state psychiatric facility show that if a power is conferred by the law, then it must be either exercised in accordance with the law or not at all. And this would be the case irrespective of the number of times the alleged illegal procedure has been followed without being challenged. Safeguards are provided in a law for a purpose and professionals cannot exercise the power in neglect of the safeguards. Such neglect would invite sanctions as good intentions do not constitute an adequate defense against the failure to follow the procedure prescribed by the law.

The fact of compulsion would not only impact upon admission, but all other dimensions of the admission procedure and the treatment regimen. The Delhi High Court required some kind of preliminary inquiry and satisfaction before a private ambulance can be deployed to compulsorily transport a person with psychiatric illness to a psychiatric hospital.[11] Insofar as an advance directive incorporates the will of the person seeking treatment, despite the statute permitting doctors to ignore the directive where they deem fit,[12] the courts may read down this permission and accord greater significance to the preference of the person seeking

---

[8] See Dhanda supra note 4
[9] Amita Dhanda " From Duality to Indivisibility: Mental health and Human Rights" South African Journal of Human Rights (2016) Vol 32 No 3 pp 438-56.
[10] Dr Sanghamitra Acharya vs State of Delhi http://lobis.nic.in/ddir/dhc/SMD/judgement/18-04-2018/SMD18042018CRLW18042017.pdf Ravinder vs Government of Delhi https://mail.google.com/mail/u/0/#search/amitgeorge%40outlook.com/163028c61f3169cf?projector=1&messagePartId=0.1
[11] See Sanghamitra supra note 10
[12] Sections 9 and 11 allow for the directives to be bypassed.

treatment. The category of nominated representative under the Mental Health Care Act of 2017 is an amalgam of persons nominated by the person with psychiatric illness and persons nominated by statute. In terms of the powers of the nominated representative, the statute does not distinguish between the two kinds of representatives. If like the Delhi High Court, other courts in the country accord preference to the principle of least restrictive alternative, then it can be anticipated that a distinction may be introduced between representatives nominated by the person and the statutorily created list. The opinion of the representative nominated by the person being accorded greater deference than the statutorily created list. Be that as it may, it would be important to appreciate that a therapeutic practice which is not solely grounded in the consent of the patient will at all times be treated differently than those fields of treatment where the therapist cannot act, if the patient does not provide consent.

The Competing Obligations of Confidentiality and Social Control
In the first section of this foreword I had referred to statutory contexts which seek psychiatric opinion on the future behavior of a detenu? Only if a person is certified as not likely to commit any act which causes danger to others, can the release of such detenu be ordered. These demands of prediction are not just made by the executive; psychiatrists are impelled to make such predictions themselves when patients disclose the intention to cause harm. The imminence of the disclosed threat needs to be considered by the psychiatrist, to determine whether there was a case for waiving the duty of confidentiality? Psychiatrists are thus required to choose between competing obligations. Evidently, the choices are also influenced by the kind of reporting obligations. Courts have placed on psychiatrists in situations where the patient had gone and acted on the disclosures and either caused harm to self or another. Defensive social control, psychiatry flourishes whenever the threshold for breaching the obligation of confidentiality is low. For psychiatry to operate as a healing profession, it would need to extricate itself from the social control obligations placed on it by the law. Without eschewing these policing duties, the profession cannot escape the scepticism and suspicion to which it is exposed.

With the United Nations Convention on the Rights of Persons with Disabilities completing a decade, the paradigm of disability rights has been gaining momentum in all parts of the world. The Committee on Disability Rights has kept the pressure going on State parties with its concluding observations and general comments. Of special interest is General Comment[13] wherein the Committee has shared its jurisprudence on the matter of legal capacity (Article 12 of the Convention). Insofar as the UNCRPD takes persons with psychosocial disabilities, both the provisions of the Convention and the jurisprudence of the Committee are of special significance in settling some of the critical questions raised by persons with disabilities before both disciplines that is law and psychiatry. The book in your hand comprehensively documents the relationship between law and psychiatry and thereby provides authoritative information on what is the current legal position? This book should be perused not only to know what

---

[13] https://documents-dds-ny.un.org/doc/UNDOC/GEN/G14/031/20/PDF/G1403120.pdf?OpenElement

the law is but also to reflect upon what it ought to be. The authors have put out the invitation, which I hope will be accepted by all those who are interested in this challenging field of law and psychiatry.

Amita Dhanda
Professor and Head
Centre for Disability Studies
Centre for Legal Philosophy and Justice Education
NALSAR University of Law
Justice City Hyderabad, Telangana, India

Preface

"Psychiatrist is the only expert witness who is asked to form opinion as to man's responsibility and man's punishability, which is not an easy task."

Seymour L Halleck

In recent years, the focus of forensic psychiatry has increasingly moved from institutions to the community. One of the many demands made on clinicians today is keeping up to date with the ever-increasing pace of developments in forensic psychiatry knowledge in the biological and psychosocial spheres, including criminology and clinical and forensic psychology. The developments taking place in law, ethics and the criminal justice system are also relevant to the practicing psychiatrists. As forensic psychiatry involves the interface between the law and psychiatry, forensic psychiatrists have particular expertise in the assessment and management of patients with mental disorders who have been, or have the potential to be, violent and offensive. Forensic psychiatrists work in a myriad range of settings such as prisons, psychiatric hospitals and the community, in general. There are specialized services and teams within forensic psychiatry including adolescent forensic psychiatry, forensic learning disability and psychotherapy.

The emerging neurobiology of behavior elucidates mechanisms of psychiatric disorders, which are relevant for legal concepts such as the propensity toward violent behavior or the susceptibility to the development of a mental disorder.

The primary role of a forensic psychiatrist is the treatment of mentally ill offenders. These are patients who have committed crimes when mentally ill or who have become unwell while in prison. Such patients can receive an order for hospital treatment instead of a prison sentence or can be transferred from prison to hospital for the required treatment. Due to their offending behavior, these patients need to be treated in the secure environment of a psychiatric hospital. Services are available depending upon the nature and extent of the risks.

My (first author) liking for forensic psychiatry began with my joining as a house-physician in Psychiatry ward at Medical College, Rohtak in January, 1976 where all psycho-criminal cases in the jurisdiction of Haryana state were referred for evaluation and management. Under the experienced guidance of Professor Vidyasagar, I discovered the subject and studied it extensively. Evaluation and treatment of complex criminal patients and the ethical issues involved in their management were indeed quite challenging. It was a stimulating and encouraging experience for a beginner like me to observe how Professor Vidyasagar had to defend and explain his diagnostic skills and management decisions in a courtroom full of lawyers, presided over by a judge. It required courage and talent to face the opposite party knowing they were set out to challenge the very basis of opinions. As a professional expert, one needs to be clear and precise in what one does and says because each spoken word carries importance. Well-maintained records written in a legible handwriting go a long way in a professional's defense. Facts not recorded, how-so-ever evident they may be, carry no value. Anything not recorded, translates to not acknowledged. I found all these challenges quite fascinating and engrossing. As time passed, I developed an intense interest in the subject.

Later, as a postgraduate student of Psychiatry at PGI Chandigarh, I managed to further continue with my interest by completing a placement in forensic psychiatry at the National Institute of Mental Health and Neurosciences in Bengaluru in a secure psychiatric hospital ward with severe and enduring mentally ill offenders.

Now forty years later, as a mental health expert, I have a wide gamut of work, which also encompasses assessment of medicolegal cases referred by the courts or police for admission to hospital, writing case reports, liaising with local community mental health teams. We offer sound advice on risk assessment and management, and ongoing management of both inpatients and outpatients.

The common comorbidities of serious mental illnesses, personality disorder and substance misuse, combined with complex social issues such as rape, murder, separation, broken homes, child custody, etc. make forensic patients challenging to manage. I enjoy and value working in a multidisciplinary team and have found this work to be the most effective and rewarding in the forensic setting. There is little debate that issues surrounding the practice of psychiatry bring researchers and clinicians squarely into the territory of law, and usually the criminal law. In perhaps no other domains are the approaches of the medical and legal professions so divergent.

In our effort of writing this book, our goal is not only to inform the students and clinicians about the increasing use of their work in the judicial context, but also to prepare them for the ethical and practical issues that will arise when their work enters the legal area. While the field of 'Forensic Psychiatry' is vast, we have chosen only the crucial areas in which the importance of scientific concepts is occurring at a particularly rapid rate and the application of these concepts in day-to-day clinical practice is of paramount significance.

Though this book is limited in its scope and depth, it is 'user friendly' within the mental health and legal contexts for which it is written. It is meant for students of forensic psychiatry to acquire basic skills in the subspecialty of forensic psychiatry and apply those skills in their day-to-day clinical practice.

To facilitate this aim, the book is divided into major sections and chapters in a carefully considered order. While the book strives to provide an integrated overview of current knowledge, chapters are also designed to stand alone and independently which may imply some overlap in content between them. However, despite it being a first accredited attempt we hope that it has been kept to an acceptable minimum.

The book carries the professional experience of all the three authors gathered while working in different forensic settings, while the second author is formally trained in the subject. We have reverence for the law and its potential to benefit from the responsible and accurate translation of psychiatric concepts. We hope that this document will help clinicians and students to understand their significant role in the process and to prepare them to venture into this novel terrain in furtherance of both mental health and justice.

We believe this book will achieve wide acceptance through its succinct, user-friendly and practical approach. While a textbook alone does not make a good forensic psychiatrist, we hope this book will provide a sound foundation of theoretical knowledge required for competent practice by clinicians. Students of Modern medicine, Homeopathy, Ayurveda, Unani, Siddha, Alternative medicine, Dentistry, Para/Allied medical students, Nursing, Physiotherapy, Occupational therapy, Medicine., Psychology, Postgraduate students in Psychiatry, Family medicine, Doctoral scholars, all will find the content of the book relevant for their academic needs and curriculum requirements.

RC Jiloha

Acknowledgments

When clinicians and researchers discover and implement advances in the diagnosis and treatment of mental disorders, they rarely do with the legal system in mind. Nonetheless, the discoveries that clarify the neurobiological underpinning of human behavior are centrally relevant to the law, which often concerns itself with, and places great emphasis and importance on, mental state. This emphasis and importance carry great significance for our trainees in mental health, who in the future, are responsible for ensuring sound scientific evidence in the delivery of justice as forensic psychiatrists.

An opportunity befell my way last year when I (the first author of the book) was entrusted the task of organizing the PG development program of IPS (NZ) for the year 2018. I decided to have 'forensic psychiatry' as the theme of the program as it would give ample opportunity to the postgraduate students to discuss law in relation to psychiatry otherwise not given much importance.

In an informal chat during the World Federation of Mental Health meet held at New Delhi in November 2017, Professor Dinesh Kataria of Lady Hardinge Medical College suggested me to write a book on forensic psychiatry for the postgraduate students when I shared my intention of holding PG development program in July 2018 on the subject of law and mental health. No doubt, his suggestion was quite appealing left merely with six months for such a huge task, it appeared almost impossible.

Despite of my own tormenting personal preoccupations, I nodded in affirmation to work on the project when he promised to make all possible reference material on the subject available and help in preparing the manuscript. He also took the responsibility of getting the manuscript published. Both his promises, he carried out honestly and sincerely.

Perhaps the biggest contribution Dr Kataria made in this project is not only accept the co-authorship, but allow one of the most learned faculty members of his department, Dr Prerna Kukreti also for the co-authorship. Her being the part of the project has indeed added academic dignity to the book with her scholarly inputs, making it readers' friendly. We have worked together to achieve our goal of disseminating information to the budding psychiatrists about the basics of forensic psychiatry.

Other members of Dr Kataria's team, including Dr Ankit Goel, Dr Sucheta Tiwari, Dr Sneha Sharma, Dr Harita Mathur and Dr Deeksha Kalra have contributed immensely in editing the manuscript. Tables and Flowcharts contributed by Dr Ankit Goel have made the book lucid to read. We also thank all the faculty members of Department of Psychiatry, Lady Hardinge Medical College for sharing the clinical work and cooperating the authors during writing of book. I along with Prerna Kukreti and Dinesh Kataria express our thanks to them and all others who were associated with this project.

All three authors also extend their heartfelt gratitude to all the teachers at their respective centers of teaching and training namely Pt BD Sharma Postgraduate Institute of Medical Sciences, Rohtak, PGIMER, Chandigarh, GB Pant Hospital and IHBAS, New Delhi whose teachings have been instrumental in shaping vision of authors for the book.

Finally, my own family mainly drove me crazy, but according to Freud, as it will be learnt during the course of reading this book, passion is what fuels the writer, so you played your part perfectly. My wife, Krishna and my loving daughter Raahat, you both make me a better person. Thank you. I love you both in the whole wide universe.

My sincere gratitude to Shri Jitendar P Vij (Group Chairman), Mr Ankit Vij (Managing Director), Ms Chetna Malhotra Vohra (Associate Director—Content Strategy) and Ms Moumita Roy Das (Development Editor) of M/s Jaypee Brothers Medical Publishers (P) Ltd, New Delhi, India, in publishing the book.

RC Jiloha

Contents

SECTION I: INTRODUCTION

Chapter 1: History of Forensic Psychiatry — 3
- Physician 5
- Lunatic Asylum Superintendent 6
- Expert Witness 6
- Forensic Psychiatrist 6

Chapter 2: Introduction to Forensic Psychiatry — 10
- Clinical Forensic Psychiatry 10
- Legal Psychiatry 11
- Relation between Law and Psychiatry 11
- Current Issues in Forensic Psychiatry 12
- Forensic Psychiatry in India 13
- Research in Forensic Psychiatry in India 14
- Future Directions 14

Chapter 3: Law and Psychiatry in India — 17
- Law and Psychiatry in India 17
- Legal Statutes Concerning Mental Health Establishments and Deaddiction 20
- Mental Healthcare Reforms in India 28

SECTION II: MEDICOLEGAL RESPONSIBILITIES IN DOCTOR-PATIENT RELATIONSHIP

Chapter 4: Medical Jurisprudence and Medical Negligence — 33
- Indian Medical Degrees Act, 1916 34
- The Indian Medical Council (IMC) Act, 1956 34
- Medical Council of India (MCI) 34
- Duties of a Doctor 37
- Professional Misconduct 45
- Rights and Privileges of Registered Medical Practitioners 47
- Privileges and Rights of Patients 47
- Duties of a Patient 48
- Doctor-patient Relationship 48
- Medical Negligence 49

Chapter 5: Consent and Capacity Assessment — 56
- Legal Relevance of Obtaining Consent 56
- Types of Consent 57
- Important Elements of Consent 57
- Invalid Consent 62
- Cautions to Exercise while Taking Consent 63

| Chapter | 6: | Psychiatry Case Records and Right to Access Records | 66 |

- *General Principles Concerning Importance of Medical Records* 66
- *Privacy, Confidentiality and Psychiatry Case Records* 67
- *Fiduciary Relationship as Applied in Healthcare Setting* 69
- *Principles of Confidentiality Specific for Mental Health Settings* 69

SECTION III: GENERAL PRINCIPLES OF FORENSIC PSYCHIATRY EVALUATION

| Chapter | 7: | Approach to a Forensic Psychiatry Interview and Case Taking | 81 |

- *Context of Forensic Psychiatry Interview* 81
- *Indications of Forensic Interview in India* 81

| Chapter | 8: | Special Investigative Techniques in Forensic Psychiatry | 87 |

- *Polygraph Testing* 87
- *Brain Mapping and Brain Fingerprinting* 88
- *Narco-analysis* 90
- *National Human Rights Guidelines for Use of DDT* 91

| Chapter | 9: | Ethical Issues in Forensic Psychiatry | 93 |

- *Ethics and Psychiatry* 93
- *Legal and Moral Responsibility* 95
- *Personal Beliefs and Professional Opinion* 95
- *Ethics and Forensic Psychiatry* 95
- *Ethical Issues in Forensic Psychiatry Research* 98
- *Ethics in Research Involving Prisoners* 98

| Chapter | 10: | Ethnicity, Culture and Forensic Psychiatry | 102 |

- *What is Culture?* 102
- *Impact of Culture on Distress* 104
- *Cultural Explanations* 105
- *Pathways into Care* 106
- *Epidemiological Problems* 107
- *Management Issues* 108
- *Race and Ethnicity* 109
- *Ethnicity in Forensic Psychiatry* 109

| Chapter | 11: | Report Writing in Forensic Psychiatry: General Principles | 113 |

- *Structure of a Forensic Report* 113
- *Characteristics of a Good Report* 115
- *What not to Include in a Forensic Psychiatry Report* 115
- *Issues to be Aware of while Reporting* 116

| Chapter | 12: | Psychiatrist as an Expert Witness in Court | 117 |

- *Role of Psychiatrist as an Expert Witness* 117
- *Oral Evidence (Court Appearances) vs Documentary Evidence (Reports Submitted)* 117
- *Types of Oral Evidence* 118
- *Role of Expert Witness* 118
- *Courtroom Behavior* 119

Chapter 13:	**Malingering**	121
	• *Malingering and Psychiatry 121*	
	• *Assessment of Malingering in Psychiatry Settings 123*	
	• *Psychological Assessment of Malingering 125*	
	• *Differential Diagnosis 127*	

SECTION IV: INTERSECTION OF MENTAL HEALTH AND CIVIL LAW

Chapter 14:	**Testamentary Capacity**	133
	• *Law of Succession 133*	
	• *Codicil 135*	
	• *Essentials of Will Making 135*	
	• *Testamentary Capacity 137*	
	• *Important Elements of Testamentary Capacity 138*	
	• *Factors Affecting Testamentary Capacity 139*	
	• *Symptoms of Testamentary Incapacity 142*	
	• *Law and Testamentary Capacity 143*	
	• *Assessment of Testamentary Capacity 143*	
	• *Common Cognitive Screening Tests 145*	
	• *Retrospective Assessment 146*	
	• *Documentation for Assessment of Testamentary Capacity and Undue Influence 147*	
Chapter 15:	**Marriage and Divorce-related Issues with Regard to Mental Illnesses**	150
	• *Indian Laws Concerning Marriage and Divorce 151*	
	• *Discriminatory Practices for Persons with Mental Illness: Amendment is Needed 153*	
	• *Legal Aspects of Impotence 156*	
	• *Examination of a Person with Impotence 156*	

SECTION V: INTERSECTION OF MENTAL HEALTH AND CRIMINAL LAW

Chapter 16:	**Courts in India and Judicial Process**	161
	• *Courts in India 161*	
	• *Procedures in Criminal Courts 165*	
Chapter 17:	**Principles and Procedures of Trial of Cases in India**	169
	• *Types of trials 169*	
	• *Rights of Accused during Stages of Trial 171*	
	• *Role of Psychiatrist during Different Stages of Trials 172*	
Chapter 18:	**Role of Forensic Psychiatrist during Different Stages of Trial**	174
	• *Violation of Rights of Persons with Mental Illness during Trial 174*	
	• *Relevance of Performing these Forensic Psychiatry Assessment by Mental Health Professionals 175*	
Chapter 19:	**Pretrial Assessment: Fitness for Interview by Police**	177
	• *Need of Assessment 177*	
	• *Aims of Assessment 177*	
	• *Forensic Psychiatry Assessment of Fitness to be Interviewed by Police 178*	
	• *Assessing Suggestibility and Reliability of Confessions 179*	

Chapter 20: **During Trial Assessment: Fitness to Stand Trial** — 181
- *Need of Assessment of Fitness to Stand Trial* 181
- *Historical Evolution of Fitness to Stand Trial Construct* 182
- *Report Writing for Courts* 187

Chapter 21: **Prisoners with Mental Illness not Fit to Stand Trial** — 189

Chapter 22: **During Trial Assessments: Assessment for Insanity Defense** — 197
- *Substantive Law Concerning Insanity and Criminal Responsibility in India* 198
- *Important Case Laws from Indian Courts* 202

SECTION VI: MEDICOLEGAL RESPONSIBILITIES CONCERNING MANAGEMENT OF CASES OF SEXUAL OFFENCE

Chapter 23: **Medicolegal Approach for Management of Adult Victims of Sexual Violence** — 209
- *Magnitude of the Problem* 209
- *Health Consequences of Sexual Assault* 210
- *Understanding Legal Provisions Concerning Sexual Offences* 211
- *Role of Health Professionals (Based on Guidelines Issued by the Ministry of Health and Family Welfare)* 213
- *Legal Responsibilities of Health Professionals* 215
- *Medical Examination and Reporting of Sexual Assault* 216
- *Treatment Guidelines and Psychosocial Support* 218
- *Documentation* 221
- *Patient Information* 221
- *Role of Family, Friends and Community* 222
- *Interface with Legal Agencies* 222
- *Interface with Social Welfare Agencies* 225

Chapter 24: **Medicolegal Approach for Management of Victims of Child Sexual Abuse** — 227
- *Epidemiology* 227
- *Psychological Effects of Child Sexual Abuse* 228
- *Understanding Childhood Sexual Offences through Legal Perspective in India* 228
- *Victim Perpetrator Dynamics: Understanding CSA through Psychological Perspective* 231
- *Effects of Child Sexual Abuse* 231
- *Medicolegal Approach to a Case of CSA (Based on Guidelines Issued by Ministry of Women and Child Welfare)* 232
- *Capacity Assessment as Asked by Court Regarding Victims of Sexual Violence* 242
- *Management* 243

SECTION VII: LEGAL STATUTES OF RELEVANCE TO MENTAL HEALTH

Chapter 25: Mental Healthcare Act, 2017 — 247
- *Need for Legislation in Mental Health: Challenges and Special Issues Concerning Mentally Ill* 247
- *Implications of Mental Healthcare Act (MHCA), 2017 in Clinical Practice* 250
- *Certain New Concepts of Clinical Relevance in MHCA* 251
- *Monitoring and Regulatory Agencies in MHCA* 254
- *Specifics of Establishing or Maintaining a Mental Health Establishment* 256
- *Rights of Persons with Mental Illness that Mental Health Establishments must Safeguard* 258
- *What Constitutes Basic Medical Record* 261
- *Modifications in Approach in Assessment, Admission, Treatment, Discharge* 265
- *Other Important Concepts for Inpatient Care* 271
- *Offences: Contravention of Provisions of Act* 274
- *Interaction with Judiciary* 274

Chapter 26: Legislation Related to Addiction Psychiatry in India — 276
- *What is a Drug?* 276
- *The Drugs and Cosmetics Act, 1940; The Drugs and Cosmetics Rules, 1945* 288

Chapter 27: Rights of Persons with Disabilities Act, 2016 — 291
- *Disability Conditions of Relevance for Mental Health* 292
- *Critical Appraisal of Rights of Persons with Disabilities Act, 2016* 295
- *Certification Guidelines for Mental Disabilities as Mentioned in Rights of Persons with Disability Rule, 2018 as per Rights of Persons with Disabilities Rules, 2017* 295
- *Guidelines for Individual Disability Certification* 296
- *Critical Appraisal of Rights of Persons with Disabilities Rules, 2017* 298

SECTION VIII: OTHER MEDICOLEGAL ISSUES OF RELEVANCE FOR MENTAL HEALTH PROFESSIONALS

Chapter 28: Human Rights of Persons with Mental Illness — 303
- *Right to Health* 304
- *Global Developments and Rights of Persons with Mental Illness* 304
- *Indian Perspective of Human Rights of Persons with Mental Illness* 306
- *Post-UNCRPD Era: Legislative Reforms in India* 308
- *Rights and Privileges of Persons with Mental Illness* 309
- *Concordance of Mental Healthcare Act with MI Principles for Treatment of Persons with Mental Illness* 315
- *Implementation of Human Rights in India* 322
- *The Role of the Legislation* 322

Chapter 29: Medicolegal Issues in Suicide Risk Assessment and Management — 325
- *Prevalence and Risk Factors* 326
- *Attempted Suicide* 327
- *Risk Factors for Suicide* 328
- *Methods of Suicide* 330
- *Laws Concerning Suicide* 331

- *Medicolegal Provisions Pertaining to Complete Suicide in a Healthcare Setting 333*
- *Psychological Autopsy 336*
- *Malpractice Suits Following Complete Suicide 337*
- *Indian Psychiatric Society Guidelines for Responsible Reporting of Suicide in Media 339*

Chapter 30: Violence, Crime and Mental Disorders — 344
- *Violence 344*
- *What is Aggression? 345*
- *What is Violence? 345*
- *Types of Violence 346*
- *Victims of Violence 348*
- *Biopsychosocial Model of Violence 348*
- *Philosophy of Violence 348*
- *Genetics and Violence 349*
- *Psychological Theories of Violence 349*
- *Mental Illness and Violence 350*
- *Are the Public at Risk? 363*
- *Crime in Social Context 363*
- *Social Factors in Crime 367*
- *Social Factors in Crime Prevention 368*
- *Forensic Psychiatry and Crime 369*

Chapter 31: Homicide and Mental Disorders — 373
- *Culpable Homicide 373*
- *Mental Disorders and Homicide 374*
- *Infanticide and Related Behaviors 375*
- *Honor Killing 376*
- *Murder-Suicide 378*
- *Nonfatal Assaults 378*
- *Neurobiology of Criminal Behavior 379*
- *Crime and Violence from Developmental Perspective 380*

Chapter 32: Medicolegal Responsibilities in Management of Victims of Domestic Violence — 384
- *Prevalence 384*
- *Dynamics of Violence 386*
- *Mental Illness and Increased Vulnerability 388*
- *Risk Factors for Domestic Violence 389*
- *Identification of Domestic Violence Experienced by Psychiatric Patients 389*
- *Interventions for Psychiatric Patients Experiencing Domestic Violence 392*

Chapter 33: Medicolegal Responsibilities in Management of Homeless Persons with Mental Illness — 395
- *Concept of Homelessness 395*
- *Legal Provisions of Relevance to Homeless Persons with Mental Illness 400*
- *Medicolegal Approach to a Case of Homeless Person with Mental Illness 401*
- *Some Unique Initiatives for Homeless Persons with Mental Illness 402*
- *Strategies for Community-based Interventions for Homeless Persons with Mental Illness 403*

Chapter 34:	**Clinical Legal and Ethical Issues Concerning Gender Dysphoria and Sex Reassignment Interventions**	406

- *Normal Human Sexuality* 406
- *What is Gender Dysphoria?* 407
- *Gender Dysphoria: Nosological Construct* 408
- *Identifying Gender Dysphoria: Tools and Strategies* 408
- *Role of Psychiatrists* 410
- *Different Treatment Strategies* 410
- *Role of Mental Health Professional in Sex Reassignment Interventions* 411
- *Components of Psychiatry Evaluation* 412
- *Post-treatment Ethical Legal Difficulties Faced in India* 412

Chapter 35:	**Legal Responsibility of Psychiatrist in Organ Transplantation**	415

- *Laws and Rules Governing Organ Transplantation in India* 415
- *Role of Mental Health Professional in Transplantation Process* 418

Chapter 36:	**Childhood Bullying and Forensic Psychiatry**	421

- *Bullying and Chronic Stress* 422
- *Bullying and Risk of Mental Illness* 422
- *Bullying and Somatic Symptoms* 422
- *Stress Responses and Allostatic Load* 423
- *Bullying, Inflammation and Metabolic Dysfunction* 423
- *Forensic Aspects of Bullying* 424

Chapter 37:	**Forensic Psychiatry and Psychiatry Subspecialties**	427

- *General Hospital Psychiatry* 427
- *Geriatric Mental Health* 430
- *Addiction Psychiatry* 434

Chapter 38:	**Euthanasia and Living Wills**	444

- *Conceptual Controversies* 444
- *Religious Views on Euthanasia* 448
- *Living Will* 450
- *Passive Euthanasia: Supreme Court Guidelines on Advance Directives* 450
- *The Medical Treatment of Terminally Ill Patients (Protection of Patients and Medical Practitioners) Bill* 451
- *Misuse in Psychiatry and Position Statement of APA for Psychiatrists* 452

Chapter 39:	**Legal Issues Concerning Treatment of Foreign Nationals with Mental Health Problems**	455

- *Travel and Mental Illnesses* 455
- *Context of Presentation of Foreign Nationals* 456
- *Indian Laws Governing Entry, Stay and Exit of Foreign Nationals* 456
- *Legal Responsibilities of Health Professionals during Treatment of Foreign Nationals* 457
- *Fitness for Air Travel* 458

Index   461

SECTION I
Introduction

CHAPTER

History of Forensic Psychiatry

> **LEARNING OBJECTIVES**
> - History: Interplay of mental illness and civil and criminal laws
> - Evolution of forensic psychiatry
> - Status of forensic psychiatry in India
> - Overview of Indian Acts and laws of significance to psychiatry

▪ INTRODUCTION

As a medical specialty, psychiatry did not really exist before late 18th century, but issues involving legal and social problems go back as far as civilization itself. In ancient Babylonia legal system, intention was considered important in judging actions, known as the Code of Hammurabi. In ancient Hebrew Law, an act, was determined by intent, would keep safe someone who had killed by accident, preventing from being captured by avenging relatives.[1] In India, insanity was seen as ground for leniency. Around 880 BC, laws in India permitted special consideration to retarded individuals and children younger than 15 years of age.[2] Greek philosopher Plato differentiated rational and irrational behaviors and said that humans are free to choose their actions. He further said that harsher punishments should come to those who committed harms with a calculation.[3] The writings of Macer in 180 AD, during the time of Marcus Aurelius, reveal that a lunatic, if escaped from the custody of his relatives and caused harm to others made the relatives liable for execution. A curious form of kinship malpractice, with a very harsh penalty was established because of this format.[4] In England in the pre-Norman times, there was no separate criminal code – family of an insane murderer's was expected to pay compensation and look after the victim's family. In Norman times, insanity was no defense but a special circumstance for referral to the king for pardon.[5] Ancient Jewish Talmud recommended execution of the murderer who committed the crime under intoxication of alcohol.[6] In Islamic law, murder by a mentally ill person or minor is considered as involuntary homicide and subject is only to compensate for the loss.[2] While the legal code of Draco (for harshness of the code "draconian" is derived) in Greece distinguished murder from involuntary homicide.[3]

Aristotle held a person morally responsible if, he knowing the circumstances and without external compulsion, deliberately chose to commit an act.[6] In 5th century AD Europe, an insane was considered as *compos mentis non est* (not having control in mind and unable to understand consequences of his act), like infant or a four-footed animal. Henry Bracton, Chief

Justice of England believed that crime was not committed unless 'will to harm' is present and such an intent lacked in young children and mad people. In 1265, he devised a test to identify insane known as "Wild beast test".[5] However, the medieval period in Europe and other parts of the world was dominated by 'witch-craft' and super-natural beliefs and the mentally ill were thought to be in league with the devil.[7] The subjects of forensic attention, in the public language, were "madman, stupid, crazy, raving, insane, demented" etc.[8]

Since 14th century, the defense of insanity has been well recognized in English courts, when complete madness was considered as a defense to a criminal charge. By 1518, it was fully established that the lack of guilty mind and intellect meant a lack of criminal responsibility.[9]

In 17th century, Sir Mathew Hale opined that mere presence of insanity was not enough to remove criminal responsibility[10] as insanity could be partial or limited and allowed two kinds of verdicts:
1. Not guilty
2. Committed act was *non compos mentis*.

In the 18th century, monomania became an immensely popular term in France[11] and people used this term in their usual conversation for erratic behavior. In Europe, from 1760 to 1845, 350 criminal defendants used insanity in their defense. They alleged a mental disturbance for their crime and the claim came from their own statements, neighbors or the relatives who had observed their condition. However, about 25% of them also produced medical evidence in favor of their defense.[12] During 1790s, Immanuel Kant used the terms like, accountability, freedom and proper use of mental faculties, while pleading. He distinguished four types of psychosis relevant to forensic psychiatry: (a) amentia (chaotic thinking), (b) dementia (delusions of reference), (c) insania (disturbed judgment) and (d) vesania (disorder of reason). In 1800, he suggested courts for opinion of psychologists and not physicians for, understanding capacity and insanity status in cases of criminal responsibility. Case of Hadfield in 1800 is an illustration, who after severe brain damage started having bizarre delusions, ".... going to destroy the world so he has to sacrifice his life to prevent it." He tried to shoot at King George III and was held not guilty as his insanity was proved.[13] Before the 19th century, law did not see any requisite for psychiatric testimony, as the judges only set the standards but it was in the 19th century that the psychiatric witness came into existence.

The independent medical witness started replacing the judges as expert witness after 1825. The beginning of 19th century saw Thomas Percival in England describing expert testimony in his book *Medical Ethics* and Gold emphasizing the need for co-evolution of general and forensic psychiatry.[14] *Treatise on the Medical Jurisprudence of Insanity* written in 1838 by Isaac Ray became an international classic[15] and during the same time, Morton Birnbaum, a general practitioner advocated for the right to treatment.[16] In 1843, warden of the prison was murdered by a man named Abner Rogers who pleaded "not guilty by reason of insanity" based on the chloroform overdose which he was given during a previous surgery. He was acquitted of the act and sent to the Illinois Asylum.[17]

The same year, M'Naughten of Scotland claimed "voice of God" had instructed him to kill Mr Robert Peel the then Prime Minister. But mistakenly he killed prime minister's private secretary. He was declared not guilty by reason of insanity. The House of Lords developed the insanity test: "To establish a defense on the ground of insanity, it must be clearly proved that, at the time of committing the act, the party accused was laboring under such a defect of reason, from disease of the mind, as not to know the nature and quality of the act he was doing; or, if he did know it, that he did not know he was doing what was wrong."

In the 1870s and 1880s came the organic versus functional distinction, the distinction between disease of the brain and the disease of the mind. In US in 1881, occurred an important case involving a presidential assassination. The 20th president of the USA, President James A Garfield, was assassinated by person named Charles Guiteau within 200 days of his election. Guiteau was obviously insane but he was still found guilty and subsequently was hanged. His brain autopsy displayed "fairly good evidence for syphilis".[18] At the trial, a vital issue had been whether there was mind or brain disease present.

In the later part of 19th century, Emil Kraepelin advocated theories of context and naturalistic dependence of mental events relevant in forensic perspective. The forensic field and in fact the society as a whole, tussles with the problem of the psychopaths who are often referred as suffering from "moral insanity" and the phrase '*manie sans délire*' in the French literature, suggests disturbance without cognitive impairment in such people.[19]

Many medicolegal societies have evolved with the more recent developments, such as the American Academy of Psychiatry and the Law (AAPL), which attempt to fill the gaps between the drastically different disciplines of psychiatry and law. The AAPL currently has about 2000 members, moreover a number of other organizations around the world inhabit this clinical-law interface.[20]

On the basis of these developmental facts, the modern forensic psychiatry can be conveniently described as the combination of three historic roles psychiatrists have performed: the *physician* tending the mentally ill; the *superintendent* of lunatic asylum; and the *expert witness* to the court. All three have their own origin.[21]

PHYSICIAN

The physician applies his specialized knowledge in order to treat the sick. The theme across many cultures, including India, China, Europe and the Islamic world, is that physicians deal only with physical health; mental ill-health was not seen as a medical problem, but as a personal, or family one, mostly dealt with by socioreligious rituals.

The 18th century witnessed industrial revolution, leading on to dislocation of families and disruption of kinship network; as a by-product, mentally ill confined to boundaries of home, reached on to roads as homeless or landed up in jails unfortunately. Mental illness became more a cause of social concern than medical attention. Intolerant approach of the society lead to establishment of lunatic asylums in outskirts of city to provide relief to the society from the nuisance created by the mentally ill and segregate them from mainstream society rather than to treat.[22]

The European traders who encroached upon the Indian subcontinent brought asylum culture to this part of the world where kinship network was still very strong and institutionalization of the mentally ill was unknown before their arrival to this part of the world.

LUNATIC ASYLUM SUPERINTENDENT

When mentally ill became a recognized social problem and the mentally ill were committed to the lunatic asylums, which were non-medical institutions till the beginning of 20th century, asylums offered a human sanctuary to the distressed, in the over-crowded 'bins' whose sole purpose was removal of the obviously mentally ill from the streets and to provide only the custodial care. Each asylum had a superintendent as its in-charge who was a non-medical person who merely oversaw the unqualified 'lunatic attendants' in the service of lunatics. Nineteenth century asylums included those developed specially-to-deal with the 'criminally insane.'

EXPERT WITNESS

The importance of an expert witness is traceable back to the Roman Empire with courts accepting evidence from physicians, amongst others. In case of mentally ill, it was not yet seen as part of medicine; therefore, juries and judges regarded themselves as competent to decide the question of insanity. With the proliferation of asylums in the late 19th century, the asylum administrators came to be recognized as expert witnesses.

With the new scientific developments of early 20th century, such as Kraepelin's identification and classification of psychotic disorders, Charcot's research on hypnosis and hysteria, and Freud's establishment of psychoanalysis, the practitioners of psychiatry, who now had an institutional home in the asylums, were recognized as a single profession with a specialized body of knowledge. Psychiatrists, now so-called edged out office-based neurologists from the treatment of mentally ill.

Psychiatry consolidated its professional position during the 20th century, with armies turning to it after the World Wars (I and II) for treatment of their shell-shocked soldiers and that led to development of group therapy. With the discovery of antipsychotics—which presaged the ascendency of Biological Psychiatry and side-lining of psychoanalysis, medical model of psychiatry was affirmed renew. During the latter half of the 20th century, psychiatry subspecialties developed such as Child Psychiatry, Liaison Psychiatry and Community Psychiatry.

FORENSIC PSYCHIATRIST

This specialty was a relatively late entrant and separated from mainstream general psychiatry because of institutional and ethical reasons. From 1980s onwards, a group of psychiatrists in Europe established themselves with a distinctively different job–caring for patients detained in a secure hospital environment, or in prison who were adequate in number to develop their own sub-professional identity.

Many psychiatrists in the United States who had traditionally concentrated on assessment of defendants or litigants for the courts, rather than treating patients, re-designated themselves as 'forensicists' and sought separate recognition in the American Academy of Psychiatry and Law (AAPL). Thus somewhat, divergent ethical and clinical traditions of forensic psychiatry were established in US and Europe, where the doctor's duty primarily was to facilitate justice for state than formal doctor-patient therapeutic relationship.[20]

Forensic Psychiatry is considered a poorly defined specialty and there is little structured training in most countries including India (WHO working group).[23] A working knowledge of law regulating the psychiatry practice assists clinicians in providing patients a good care. It is difficult to expect psychiatrists to be as knowledgeable of the law as lawyers, but they should have understanding of how the psychiatry and law interact in various common clinical situations.[17] Pollack[20] interpreted forensic psychiatry being limited to psychiatric evaluation for legal purposes and described it as broader general field in which psychiatric principles, theories, practices and concepts are applied to legal issues. The history of forensic psychiatry is perceived as "entrance of medicine into court".[21]

India has very few qualified forensic psychiatrists at present, who are largely working in general psychiatry setting.[24] Over the years, concerns in psychiatry in India have changed and the discipline has moved from the concept of the colonial period "Mad Doctor" who attempted to treat florid psychoses, to "Superintendents" who ran lunatic asylums, to "Alienists" whose concern was a careful examination, description, and classification, of mental illness,[25] and then to the new field of psychoanalysis, or inquiry into individual psychic pain and suffering caused by unconscious drives and neurotic conflicts. Stalwarts like Girindersekhar Bose and David Satyanand, with an emphasis on psychoanalytic techniques and in-depth therapy over long periods of time, during the 4th and 5th decades of 20th century dominated the scene of psychiatry in India.[26,27] The present-day psychiatry increasingly places more emphasis on behavior, and has moved away from theories of neurotic conflict or lengthy analytic treatment. Emphasis has shifted to modification of behavior in the present, rather than primarily formulating an understanding of how such behavior may have developed in the past. Human Rights Activists and Judicial interventions[28,29] have brought both structural and functional change to deliver mental health services in the country. Change is visible on what used to be a mental hospital or a Department of Psychiatry at a medical college is variously called Institute of Human Behavior or a Department of Human Behavior, Department of Behavioral Science, or the Department of Behavioral Health. Forensic Psychology is an emerging field in the country during the recent years.[30] Psychological skills have been used in certain high profile criminal cases in recent past to assess the criminal behavior of the accused. To name, some of these cases are, Poetess Madhumita Shukla murder case of 2003, Nithari serial killing case 2006, Aarushi-Hemraj murder case 2008 and Sunanda Pushkar case 2017.[31] Global trend of deinstitutionalization of the mentally ill and the introduction of Mental Healthcare Act 2017 has resulted in the need to establish a sophisticated forensic mental health system,[32,33] and thus has enhanced the scope for Forensic Psychiatry to develop in the country.

REFERENCES

1. Prince JD. Review: The Code of Hammurabi. Am J Theol. 2004;8(3):601-15.
2. Magherini G, Biotti V. Madness in Florence in the 14th–18th centuries: judicial inquiry and medical diagnosis, care and custody. Int J Law Psychiatry. 1998;21(4):335-68.

3. Taylor CCW, Hare RM, Barnes J. Greek Philosophers, Socrates, Plato, and Aristotle. Oxford: Oxford University Press; 1999.pp.103-89.
4. Spruitt JE. The penal conceptions of the Emperor Marcus Aurelius in respect of lunatics: reflections on D. 1,18,14. Int J Law Psychiatry. 1998;21:315-34.
5. Methuen N. A History of English Law. 4. London: Crime and insanity in England: The historical perspective. Edinburgh University Press, 1922.
6. Campbell M. Behind the Name: Meaning, Origin and History of the Name "Aristotle". Behind the Name: The Etymology and History of First Names. www.behindthename.com Retrieved 6 April, 2018.
7. Gutheoil TG. The history of psychiatry. J Am Acad Psychiatry Law. 2005;33:259-62.
8. Hardwicke's Annual biography, Google Books. Books.google.com Retrieved 3 June, 2017.
9. Roy C. Plea of insanity in India as a defence in criminal; trial: A critical overview. Mental Health Law in the Criminal Justice System: An Expert Training Workshop. Delhi Judicial Academy, New Delhi, 2018.
10. Eigen JP, Andoll G. From mad doctor to forensic witness: the evolution of early English court psychiatry. Int J Law Psychiatry. 1986;9:159-70.
11. Goldstein J. Professional knowledge and professional self-interest: the rise and fall of monomania in 19th century France. Int. J Law Psychiatry. 1998;21:385-96.
12. Kant MA. On criminal law and psychiatry. Int J Law Psychiatry. 1998;21:335-42.
13. Mendelson D. English medical experts and the claims for shock occasioned by railway collisions in the 1860's: issues of law, ethics and medicine. Int J Law Psychiatry. 2002;25:303-30.
14. American Academy of Psychiatry and the Law: Ethics Guidelines for the Practice of Forensic Psychiatry, Section IV, Revised 1995.
15. Gold LH. Rediscovering forensic psychiatry. In: Simon RI, Gold LH (Eds). Textbook of Forensic Psychiatry. Washington, DC: American Psychiatric Press; 2004.pp.3-36.
16. Cornish W, Clarke G. Law and Society in England 1750-1950. London: Sweet & Maxwell; 1989.pp. 603-4.
17. https://en.wikipedia.org/wiki/USS_Rogers_(DD-876) visited on 17.12.2017.
18. Unsworth C. Law and lunacy in psychiatry's golden age. Oxford Journal of Legal Studies. 1993;13(4):7-9.
19. Hoff P. Emil Kraepelin and forensic psychiatry. Int J Law Psychiatry. 1998;21:343-54.
20. Pollack S. The American Board of Forensic Psychiatry. Bull Am Acad Psychiatry Law. 1985;13(2):173.
21. Eastman N, Adshead G, Fox S, et al. Forensic Psychiatry. Oxford University Press; 2012 .p. 712.
22. Sharma SD. Mental health: the pre-independence scenario. In: Agarwal SP(Ed). Mental Health: An Indian Perspective. Directorate General of Health Services. Ministry of Health and Family Welfare, Government of India, 2005.
23. Brody EB. The World Federation for Mental Health: its origins and contemporary relevance to WHO and WPA policies. World Psychiatry. 2008;3:54-5.
24. Asokan TV. Forensic psychiatry in India: the road ahead. Indian Journal of Psychiatry. 2014;56(2):121-7.
25. Wig NN, Avasthi A. Origin and growth of general hospital psychiatry. In: Agarwal SP (Ed). Mental Health: An Indian Perspective. Directorate General of Health Services. Ministry of Health and Family Welfare, Government of India, 2005.
26. Neki JS. Psychotherapy in India: The Presidential address. Indian Journal of Psychiatry. 1977;19:145.
27. Jain S, Murthy P, Sarin A. The story of Satyanand. Indian Journal of Psychiatry. 2015;57:419-22.

28. Bar Council of India. Available from: http://www.barcouncilofindia. org. [Last accessed 2017 Jun 21].
29. Nambi S. Legal Aspects of Psychiatry: Indian Perspective. Manashanti Publications; 2008.
30. Shorter E. A History of Psychiatry: From an Era of the Asylum to the Age of Prozac. New York: Wiley, 1997.
31. The Forensic Psychology Test. The Times of India, January 19 New Delhi, 2018.
32. Bursztajn HJ, Scherr AE, Brodsky A. The rebirth of forensic psychiatry in light of recent historical trends in criminal responsibility. Psychiatric Clinics of North America. 1994;17:611-35.
33. Mental Healthcare Act, 2017. Ministry of Health and Family Welfare, Government of India Publication, New Delhi.

CHAPTER 2

Introduction to Forensic Psychiatry

> **LEARNING OBJECTIVES**
> - Clinical forensic psychiatry vs legal psychiatry
> - Relation between law and psychiatry
> - Forensic psychiatry in India
> - Forensic psychiatry research in India

The word *forensic* is derived from Latin adjective *forensics*, which means *"of or before the forum"*—courts or public debate. Pollack[1] defines forensic psychiatry as a "broad general field in which psychiatric theories, concepts, principles and practices are applied to any and all legal issues." The American Academy of Psychiatry and Law (AAPL) recommends the definition of Forensic Psychiatry adopted by the American Board of Forensic Psychiatry, "forensic psychiatry is a subspecialty of psychiatry in which scientific and clinical expertise is applied to legal issues in legal contexts embracing civil, criminal, and correctional or legislative matters; forensic psychiatry should be practiced in accordance with guidelines and ethical principles enunciated by the profession of psychiatry."[2]

All psychiatric activity by definition may contain some element of forensics because there is close association of clinical forensic psychiatry with the law. Therefore, all psychiatrists must be familiar with those areas of law that bear directly on treatment and managing their patients. These include mental health laws, mental capacity law, the law and procedure related to public protection and report writing for hospital medical boards, mental health boards and for courts. Psychiatrists are not required to become quasi-lawyers, but have to understand how lawyers and courts reason and make decisions particularly at the interface with psychiatry.

CLINICAL FORENSIC PSYCHIATRY

Clinical forensic psychiatry refers to the practice of psychiatry where assessment and treatment of psychiatric patients associated with offending behavior is done, the patient may or may not have been convicted. Since forensic clinical psychiatry is closely associated with legal aspects of clinical practice, a clear understanding of law is necessary to practice clinically. It is not viable to negotiate the patient out of mental health care and criminal justice system without proper knowledge of appropriate law. Only if it is based on substantial knowledge of law and legal process, clinical forensic psychiatry can be pursued ethically and effectively.

Traditional concept of forensic psychiatry mainly concerned with criminal responsibility and fitness to stand trial has long been dissipated, and now several civil aspects of mental health as well as issues related to treatment of mental illness come under the domain of forensic psychiatry.

LEGAL PSYCHIATRY

It consists of all the laws related to various mental disorders, treatment and care of those suffering from these disorders. Psychiatry and law have a relationship, which is bilateral in nature, which comprises giving of psychiatric evidence in a variety of civil and criminal legal context at one end and the use of law for clinical purposes and for regulation of clinical practice at the other. The relationship between the two is at the center of forensic psychiatry, within which it is strongly represented by comparison with other psychiatry branches.[3]

RELATION BETWEEN LAW AND PSYCHIATRY

The objective of a specialty and the interest of its practitioners determine the constructs it utilizes. The constructs, in the specialty of psychiatry are often determined by pursuit of human welfare through proper understanding the illness in order to inverse it or its effects. On the other hand, law follows abstract justice. This at times involves balancing welfare of various parties against each other or against welfare of society. Even in the same discipline, various branches may lead to different approaches in determining the constructs.[4]

As criminal law at trial is associated with responsibility, its definition of mental disorders is characteristically constricted, and it mainly addresses justice rather than human welfare. In sentencing, the constructs utilized are without reference to the welfare of the individual concerned.

Within every clinical domain, the constructs are entirely different from biological and psychological constructs embraced in medicine, psychiatry and clinical psychology, and are concerned mainly with the diagnosis and treatment of the person.

Different constructs in mental disorders for different legal purposes include, fitness to stand trial, insanity defense, diminished responsibility, automatism and reliability of confession or mitigation of sentence on grounds of mental illness primarily for public protection. Here the patient welfare is not the construct under consideration but delivery of justice in a fair manner.

In civil laws, there are constructs for damage in relation to nervous shock or personal injury and broader notions such as fitness for childcare, fitness to make a will, fitness to carry on with a marriage and so on.

The purpose of mental health and all its allied sciences is the prosperity of the patients, who should get health benefits. The law deals with justice for all, which includes concern for the rights of both the victims as well as the defendant. The way to strike out a balance between pursuit of patient welfare and public protection is inevitably different for mental healthcare experts and legal agencies. Both law and psychiatry address concerns, which are related and are with possibly different values. Thus negotiating the interface between them is legally and ethically, crucial yet difficult.[5] Forensic psychiatrist has to strike a balance.[5]

CURRENT ISSUES IN FORENSIC PSYCHIATRY

Forensic psychiatrists are endowed with a crucial task, in words of Halleck, "The psychiatrist is the only expert witness who is asked to form opinion as to man's responsibility and man's punishability, which is not an easy task."[6]

In a study, 79% of the potential jurors believe that the insanity defense is abused.[7] The public perception of insanity defense is not favorable as the public thinks that insanity as defense is raised 40 times more common than its actual situation.[7,8] According to the public opinion, some diagnoses may unjustly get the criminals off. Some of them include:
- Post-traumatic stress disorder (PTSD)
- Temporal lobe epilepsy (TLE)
- Dissociative reaction
- Premenstrual syndrome (PMS)
- Pathological gambling.

The public opinion is outraged by insanity acquittals more often when the defendant is closer to normality. People become unwilling to excuse any conduct, which hints of a rational criminal motive. According to the common public view of a mental illness any evidence of the ability to organize and premeditate a criminal act, should not be the basis of acquittal.[9] In reality, a psychotic person is quite capable of rational planning based on a delusional belief.

If the defense is contested, proving insanity is not an easy task; it is always an uphill fight. Juror stereotypes of the criminally insane are drooling, raving maniacs or manipulative and malevolent. Eighty percent of successful insanity defenses occur when the defense and prosecution experts come to an understanding that the offender was legally insane. The public has long been concerned about malingered insanity defenses. After the Hinckley verdict in 1982, columnist Carl Rowan stated, "It is about time we faced the truth that the 'insanity' defense is mostly last gasp legal maneuvering, often hoaxes, in cases where a person obviously has done something terrible".[10] Concern about defendants' successfully faking mental illness to avoid responsibility dates back to at least the 10th century.[11-14] Even though we have more accurate tests for evaluating malingering today, the public remains sceptical about everyone claiming to be insane. Defendants who raise a legitimate insanity defense have a difficult time succeeding if their case goes to trial. Only 21% of jurors actually listen carefully to the jury instructions and apply the correct test for insanity rather than allowing their own preconceptions to determine their insanity opinion (A jury is a body of people under oath who are convened to render an impartial verdict legitimately given to them by a court, or for setting a penalty or judgment. Jurors refer to group of juries, it can be a body of legal representatives alone or mix of civilians and legal representatives as per law of the land prevailing in different countries. This system has been abolished from Indian legal statutes).[7] Most jurors believe that if a defendant has refused psychiatric medication that he is blameworthy rather than insane.[11] Prosecutors are reluctant to concede an insanity defense in high profile cases even when the evidence is overwhelming. In one Texas filicide case, the prosecution would not agree to an insanity verdict even when his own psychiatric expert, two defense experts, and two court-appointed experts all concurred due to insanity as defense the defendant was not guilty. The prosecutor went to considerable expense in trying the case, although the county did not have sufficient money in their budget to repair the roof of the courthouse. Based on e-mail posts to newspaper articles, the prosecutor was correct in concluding that the public would have been upset with him if he had conceded an insanity verdict. Contrary to the expert evidence, the prosecutor went ahead in his judgment with giving due respect to the public sentiments.[15]

FORENSIC PSYCHIATRY IN INDIA

In India, the beginning of Forensic Psychiatry dates back to drafting of the Indian Penal Code (IPC) by Thomas Babington Macaulay during the mid-19th century. During the same time, the M'Naughten's rules were incorporated into the IPC, (Section 84, and 85 are the basis for the insanity defense), which are continuing even today. In cases of crime, the intention to commit crime is an important parameter, which a forensic expert ought to know. *Mens rea*, a Latin word used for guilty mind, is the mental element consist of:
- An intent of committing a crime
- Knowledge about one's action or lack of an action could cause commitment of a crime.

Actus reus nob facit reum nis mens sit rea. It means, the "act is not culpable unless the mind is guilty". Both *actus rea* (guilty act) and *mens rea* (guilty mind) should be there for a crime. Someone acting without mental fault is not accountable in criminal law.

Diminished responsibility is a potential defense for the defendant to argue that–even though the law is broken by the accused, he ought not to be held criminally liable for it owing to diminishing or impairing of his mental functions at the time of committing the crime. In India, the doctrine of diminished responsibility is used only in murder cases to reduce the charges to manslaughter. There have been many landmark judgments with regard to Section 84, IPC, 1860.[16]

Civil responsibility of mentally ill is relevant across diverse areas of human interaction. For example, issues such as marriage, divorce, testamentary capacity, contract, voting, consent for treatment and other activities like fitness for holding and continuing jobs, succession of property rights, guardianship, and social welfare benefits have reference to mental health and illness either directly or indirectly. All these have been elaborately documented in Indian legal system and will be discussed in the following chapters of the book. The provisions in the Mental Healthcare Act, 2017,[17] and the Rights of Persons with Disabilities Act, 2016[18] bring a paradigm shift in the conceptualization of care of the psychiatric disorders wherein the care related activities center around the patient's capacity to decide.

In India, there is very little infrastructure and organized training in forensic psychiatry at present. Most psychiatric units do not have a dedicated forensic psychiatry ward unit. Most forensic evaluations are done by the treating psychiatrists having little or no formal training in forensic psychiatry. Thus, in many cases, decisions occur by trial and error or in good faith, rather than being based in skill and competence.[19] There are no specialized training programs in forensic psychiatry in India. Countries like UK offer a 3-year advanced structured training program in forensic psychiatry, which can be taken after 3 years of core psychiatry training. There are a few centers in the country where training in Forensic Psychology has been initiated.[20]

RESEARCH IN FORENSIC PSYCHIATRY IN INDIA

Research on areas such as negligence, informed consent, confidentiality, certification, seclusion, suicide, homicide, and the complication of various therapies, is grossly inadequate in India.[21] A recent survey conducted on prison inmates by a premier mental health institute of the country[22] showed that 79.6% prisoners had either mental illness or substance use disorder. After excluding substance use, 27.6% had diagnosable mental disorder. There were high rates of tobacco use within the prison and in fact a 4-time increase in tobacco consumption after getting into prison. On conducting a random urine drug screen, 61.3% tested positive for one or the other drug. About 12.7% has life-time history of major depression and 9.1% had current episode of major depression. Nearly 2.2% of prisoners had psychosis. Another study on prisoners revealed the prevalence of 3-4% psychiatric morbidity with depression and schizophrenia as the most common diagnosis in patients who are involved in major criminal acts and majority of patients with schizophrenia were linked in cases of homicide.[22] These studies highlight the need for mental health care in prisons.

Forensic psychiatric administration supervision and teaching requires participation in training programs of law and medicine together. Liaison with lawyers, police, courts and correctional systems is highly relevant. Working in a forensic psychiatry multidisciplinary team offers forensic psychiatric expertise to the trainees. Training in ethics and human rights with skills in interacting with the media on medicolegal issues will strengthen the discipline of forensic psychiatry in India.[23]

FUTURE DIRECTIONS

More accurately structured instruments need to be developed to assess violence risk, suicide risk, and malingering. Some courts have already indicated that mere opinion in the absence of some scientific data has little evidentiary value.[15] Forensic psychologists who routinely use objective testing will have an advantage. The field of forensic psychology is growing faster than forensic psychiatry.

The role of computers in forensic psychiatry is likely to expand, which will make it easier to index and manage extensive data. Courts are beginning to require that all filings be done electronically. Because of de-institutionalization, the practice of psychiatry will continue to shift to jails and prisons. Paucity of psychiatrists for mentally ill prisoners, class action lawsuits have mandated that the services are made available.

Today, many academic departments of psychiatry want to establish a forensic fellowship along with their geriatric and psychosomatic fellowships. Academic department chairs now value consultation with forensic psychiatrists regarding the legal regulation of psychiatry. They appreciate the opportunity to talk about legal aspects of confidentiality, civil commitment, and informed consent. Overall, the future of forensic psychiatry is bright.[24]

Forensic psychiatry remains a neglected area in India and other countries in South-East Asia. This is unlike many of the developed settings where it has become an established subspecialty with a focus on clinical services, training, and research. Academic centers need to actively engage in developing this area. They need to consider the fast growing need of developing this specialty, recognize the vast scope of the field, and device curricula that cater to the diverse needs of the country. Dedicated clinical services need to be started for this vulnerable patient population. Apart from the training of students of mental health disciplines courses catering to the different mental health disciplines, students in other branches of medicine and law also need to be trained in the forensic aspects of mental health care. Various other stakeholders who need regular sensitization and training in issues relating to mental health include law enforcement agencies, judiciary, advocates, and women and child welfare departments, and the commissions related to the mental health. Government should take initiatives to establish centers in forensic psychiatry on the lines of NIMHANS, Bengaluru, where postdoctoral fellowship in forensic psychiatry has been started since 2016. The institute also proposes Center for Human Rights, Ethics, Law and Mental Health.[23]

Though forensic psychiatry has emerged as an important subspecialty of psychiatry in the developed world, psychiatrists do not have one opinion on their role in the criminal justice system. Some believe their role is to diagnose and treat mentally ill such as psychotic patients without addressing the risk of offending except insofar as it is functionally linked to mental disorder. Others argue that their role is to assist in psychological explanation of serious crimes, and if possible reduce the risk of repetition of crime.

Both the groups have their own problems for the profession and the individual practitioners, because association between mental illness and violence is not straight forward, nor can violence be managed by addressing mental disorder alone. Forensic psychiatrists are expected to contribute to public protection and at the same time, there are unavoidable role conflicts between being a doctor and working with the criminal justice system. Both these aspects need to be accommodated by forensic psychiatry.

REFERENCES

1. Pollack S. Forensic psychiatry-a specialty. Bull Am Acad Psychiatry Law. 1974:2:1-6.
2. American Academy of Psychiatry and the Law Ethics Guidelines for the Practice of Forensic Psychiatry Adopted May, 2005. Available at: http://www.aapl.org/ethics.htm. Last accessed on 12 June 2018.
3. Gutheil TG. Forensic psychiatry as a specialty. Psychiatric Times. 2004:21.
4. Glenn HP. Legal Traditions of the World: Oxford University Press; 2000 .pp. 255-76.
5. Alfredo Calcedo-Barba. The ethical implications of forensic psychiatry practice. World Psychiatry. 2006;5(2):93-4.
6. Halleck SL. A critique of current psychiatric roles in the legal process. Wisc Law Rev. 1966;379.
7. Skeem JL, Golding SL. Describing juror's personal conceptions of insanity and their relationship to case judgments. Psych Pub Pol L. 2001;7:561.
8. Pasewark R, Seidenzahl D. Opinions concerning the insanity plea and criminality among patients. Bull Am Acad Psychiatry Law. 1979;7:199-202.
9. Resnick PJ. Perceptions of psychiatric testimony: a historical perspective on the hysterical invective. Bull Am Acad Psychiatry Law. 1986;14(3):203-19.
10. Rowan C. Cleveland Plain Dealer, 1982.
11. Brittain RP. The history of legal medicine: the assizes of Jerusalem. Medicolegal J. 1966;34:72-3.
12. Collinson GD. A Treatise on the Law Concerning Idiots, Lunatics, and Other Persons Non Compotes Mentis. London: W. Reed, 1812.

13. The New York Times, December 5, 1881 .p. 4.
14. Finkel N. Commonsense Justice: Jurors' Notions of the Law. Cambridge, MA: Harvard University Press, 1995.
15. Coble V. State. Texas Ct. of Criminal Appeals, 330 S.W. 3d 253 (2010).
16. The Indian Penal Code (Act No XLV of 1860), 1860. Allahbad, Ram Narain Lal, Beni Prasad, Law Publishers. 1980.
17. Mental Healthcare Act 2017. Government of India Publication, New Delhi, 2017.
18. Rights of Persons with Disabilities Act 2016, Government of India Publication, New Delhi, 2016.
19. Math SB, Kumar CN, Moirangthem S. Insanity defense: Past, present, and future. Indian J Psychol Med. 2015;37:381-7.
20. [https://targetstudy.com/colleges/post-graduate-diploma-in-forensic-psychology-diploma-colleges-in-india.html. Last accessed on 10 February 2018.
21. Math SB, Murthy P, Parthasarathy R, et al. Mental health and substance use problems in prisons. Bangalore: NIMHANS; 2011.
22. Chadda RK, Amarjeet. Clinical profile of patients attending a prison psychiatric clinic. Indian J Psychiatry. 1998;40:260-5.
23. Murthy P, Malathesh BC, Kumar CN, et al. Mental health and the law: an overview and need to develop and strengthen the discipline of forensic psychiatry in India. Indian J Psychiatry. 2016;58:S181-6.
24. Eastman N, Adshead G, Fox S, et al. Forensic Psychiatry. Oxford University Press, 2012.

CHAPTER

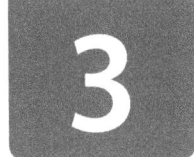

Law and Psychiatry in India

> **LEARNING OBJECTIVES**
> - Indian Medical Council Act, 1956
> - Narcotic Drugs and Psychotropic Substances Act (NDPSA), 1985
> - Consumer Protection Act, 1986
> - Mental Health Act (MHA), 1987
> - Rehabilitation Council of India Act (RCI Act), 1992
> - Protection of Human Rights Act (PHR Act), 1993
> - Persons with Disability (Equal Opportunities, Protection of Rights and Full Participation) Act (PWD), 1995
> - National Trust for the Welfare of the Persons with Autism, Cerebral Palsy, Mental Retardation, and Multiple Disabilities Act (NTA), 1999
> - Cigarette and Other Tobacco Products Act (COTPA), 2003
> - Right to information Act (RTI Act) 2005
> - Protection of Women from Domestic Violence Act (PWDVA), 2005
> - United Nations Convention for Rights of Persons with Disabilities (UNCRPD), 2006
> - Protection of Children from Sexual Offences Act (POCSO Act), 2012
> - Transplantation of Human Organ Act, 2014
> - Rights of Persons with Disabilities Act (RPWD Act), 2016
> - Mental Healthcare Act (MHCA), 2017
> - Marriage and divorce related Acts
> - Indian contract laws
> - Laws concerning criminal responsibility

LAW AND PSYCHIATRY IN INDIA

Law in India refers to the legal system operative in the country. If we look back at the ancient times, there was a discrete tradition of law having an autonomous school with legal theory and practice. In India, there is an illustrious history of law as a part of religious prescriptions and philosophical sermon.[1] The legal system was broadly based on explicitly defined and elaborately practiced social institution of caste-system established by a divine ordinance or at least with divine approval according to Hindu religious scriptures.[2] Legitimizing the caste-system, Lord Krishna says, "I myself have created the arrangement known as *Chaturvarna* assigning them different occupations in accordance with their deeds of previous lives." (Gita IV, 13). Bhagwad Gita, the most revered holy book for an ordinary Hindu describes one's social and legal status on the basis of law of *karma* based on the deeds of the previous lives. This concept presupposes a series of birth, *Karma* and rebirth justifying every social and legal inequality in the country. The *Arthashastra* which dates back to 400 BC and the *Manusmriti* to 100 AD were significant treatises in the past, texts that were once considered to be influential legal documents.[3] Manu's essential philosophy comprised of tolerance and pluralism and provided differential penalty for the offenders in accordance with their caste hierarchy. Brahmins enjoyed immunity against capital punishment; *brahm-hatya* (killing of a Brahmin) being a sinful act. [Manusmriti VIII, 89] If a *shudra* offended a Brahmin, the punishment accorded was severest [Manusmriti VIII, 267] in comparison to others for the same crime.

In the Islamic regime, *Sharia* law approached India, but was made applicable mostly to the Muslim population. But later, as India became part of the British Empire, there was a disruption in this tradition, Hindu and Islamic laws were replaced by the common law. Thus, the present judicial system of India is derived largely from the British system and while having little correlation to the institutions in the Pre-British era.[3] Much of the modern Indian Laws are based on English Common Law with a considerable influence of Europe and America. Several legislations introduced by British are still operational in independent India. Thus, the roots of most of the legislations related to mentally ill can be drawn back to the British period. There is a dynamic association between the concept of mental illness, their treatment and the law.[4,5] Psychiatrists are largely concerned with dangerousness, competency determination, diminished responsibility and/or the welfare of society,[6] most of the earlier legislations for mentally ill were concerned with these aspects.

Historically, the relationship between law and psychiatry comes at the time of management of the mentally ill which often involves limiting personal liberty of the patient. Most countries in the world have laws which regulate treatment of patients with psychiatric illlness. Although there are intricate descriptions of several forms of mental disorders in Ayurveda, an Indian system of medicine,[7] Britishers invented the care of mentally ill in the asylums in India.[8] After the English began to exercise their political power in India, a chain of lunatic asylums came along the coast-line of Indian peninsula governed by the English Lunacy Acts. After the First War of Independence in 1857, numerous laws were introduced in rapid succession for establishing and regulating the asylums and providing custodial care for the mentally ill.[9] These laws are:
1. The Lunacy (Supreme Courts) Act, 1858
2. The Lunacy (District Courts) Act, 1858
3. The Indian Lunatic Asylum Act, 1858 (with amendments in 1886 and 1889)
4. The Military Lunatic Act, 1877.

These Acts reflect the legalistic casing for the custodial management of the person with mentally illness without protecting the interest of the inmates.[10] In first decade of the 20th century, awareness in public about the terrible conditions of the asylums heightened the enactment of Indian Lunacy Act 1912 (Act 4), which has guided the destiny of Psychiatry in India.[11] This act clearly defined the procedure of admission and certification. The provision for voluntary admission was added with emphasis on preventing the society from dangerousness of mentally ill. In 1920, Lunatic asylums were re-named as mental hospitals with central supervision. The same year, the control of administration of these hospitals was given from passed prison authorities to the medical personnel. The Act also provided provisions of judicial inquisitions for mentally ill persons.[12]

During the early part of the 20th century, several significant developments in mental health branch took place which brought a paradigm shift in care of mentally ill. Psychiatry began to move out of the traditional mental hospital confines to the general hospitals with improved treatment modalities in the form of electroconvulsive therapy and anti-psychotic medication making it conceivable to effectively treat the persons with mentally illness.[13] After World War II took place, UN General Assembly in 1948 adopted the Universal Declaration of Human Rights (UDHRs). Article 1 of the UDHRs provides that "all people are free and equal in rights and dignity, establishing that people with mental disabilities are protected by human rights law by virtue of their basic humanity".[14] Indian Psychiatric Society, founded in 1947, submitted a draft in 1949 called Mental Health Bill which was to substitute the outdated ILA-1912 as it had outlived its utility in the light of ongoing developments in the mental health care. After several efforts, Mental Health Act (MHA-1987) came into existence 1987.[15]

Legislations drafted in 1980s onwards emphasize on the rights of person mentally ill. People with mental illness have historically been victimized by family members, caregivers, professionals, law enforcing agencies, friends and institutions mostly because of their susceptibility to abuse and violation of their basic human rights. Subsequent Acts set an imperative for a mechanism that protects and ensure appropriate, suitable, timely, and humane services to health care. These mechanisms include legislative provisions and policies to ensure protection of the rights of the vulnerable group.[16] National Mental Health Programme (NMHP, along with its functional arm, the District Mental Health Programme, DMHP) was launched in 1982 to bring the mental healthcare services at patients' door-step.[17,18] Following are the mental health related Acts introduced in 1980s and later:

Legal statutes concerning mental health establishments and deaddiction:
- Narcotic Drugs and Psychotropic Substances Act (NDPSA), 1985.
- Mental Health Act (MHA), 1987
- Mental Healthcare Act (MHCA) 2017

Legal statutes concerning substance of abuse:
- Narcotic Drugs and Psychotropic Substances Act (NDPSA), 1985
- Cigarette and Other Tobacco Products Act (COTPA), 2003

Legal statutes concerning medical jurisprudence:
- Indian Medical Council Act, 1956
- Consumer Protection Act, 1986

Legal statutes concerning protection and promotion of rights of persons with disability:
- Protection of Human Rights Act (PHR Act), 1993
- Persons with Disability (Equal Opportunities, Protection of Rights and Full Participation) Act (PWD), 1995
- National Trust for the Welfare of the Persons with Autism, Cerebral Palsy, Mental Retardation, and Multiple Disabilities Act (NTA), 1999
- Right to Information Act (RTI Act), 2005

- United Nations Convention for Rights of Persons with Disabilities (UNCRPD), 2006
- Rights of Persons with Disabilities Act (RPWD Act), 2016

Legal statutes concerning interface of civil law and mental health:
- Marriage and divorce related Acts
- Indian contract laws
- Protection of Women from Domestic Violence Act (PWDVA), 2005
- Transplantation of Human Organ Act

Legal statutes concerning interface of criminal law and mental health:
- Protection of Children from Sexual Offences Act (POCSO Act), 2012
- Laws concerning criminal responsibility

Legal statutes concerning mental health professional training:
- Rehabilitation Council of India Act (RCI Act), 1992

LEGAL STATUTES CONCERNING MENTAL HEALTH ESTABLISHMENTS AND DEADDICTION

1. *The Narcotic Drugs and Psychotropic Substances Act (NDPSA), 1985:* This Act consolidates and amends the various provisions for controlling and regulating operation related to narcotic drugs and psychotropic substances under the Opium Act, 1878 and the Dangerous Drugs Act, 1930. The Act was amended in 1989, 2001 while the latest amendment in 2014. The last amendment was aimed at ensuring essential opioid medicines for medical use, which was tragically difficult in the previous Acts. Spread in eight chapters, the Act enlists punishments for production, possession, transportation, trading, purchase and use of any of the listed substances. It also provides immunity form punishment to persons using small quantity for personal consumption by giving them option for availing for deaddiction services at nearest designated mental health facility.[19]

2. *Mental Health Act 1987:* This Act came after 40 years of independence of the country repealing the Indian Lunacy Act of 1912. In the definition of mental illness the act excludes mental retardation and stresses upon treatment rather than just custodial care. However, the Act continues with the practice of admission under reception order and the tradition of custodial care. It empowers the central and state governments for the establishing of Mental Health Authority for the regulation and supervision of the psychiatric hospitals/nursing homes and for advising Central/State Governments on matters related to mental health. There is a provision of admission under certain special circumstances in a psychiatric hospital/nursing home which is included (Section 19) in addition to admission on the reception orders and voluntary admission. Emphasis is also made on the protection of human rights of the mentally ill in this Act[18] without addressing the fundamental rights of the patients. [20]

    The Act mainly concentrates on the various legal procedures related to licensing, regulation of admissions and matters related to guardianship of the mentally ill.

    Considering its relevance in current context, the MHA, 1987 suffers from glaring omissions which included:

- It does not address the fundamental right "right to life and liberty" enshrined in constitution under article 21. It provides that no one should be deprived of these basic rights except according to procedures established by law. Thus, arbitrarily keeping persons with mental illness in closed ward in mental hospitals without any review mechanism under perview of Mental Health Act is unconstitutional.
- The Act excluded mental retardation with the good will of preventing undue institutionalization of such persons, but persons with mental retardation with significant behavioral problems requiring admission were kept out of the therapeutic benefits offered under this Act.
- The Act only covered psychiatric hospitals/nursing homes and excluded other places like persons with mental illness are kept on name of deaddiction, rehabilitation or religious healing, leaving them to follow unstandardized practices.
- The Act just focused on hospital-based custodial care, ignoring community care.
- The Act failed to give prominence to choices of persons with mental illness as individual or regarding range of treatment.
- The Supreme Court of India has stated that all doctors, whether in a government hospital or otherwise have a professional responsibility for rendering medical services when required during emergency situations with due expertise for protecting life, but this Act fails to provide provision for emergency care for helping families of mentally ill.
- The Act has many good principles, but even after decades of enactment, many states did not make rules for implementation and some states did not constitute state mental health authorities.

  Human rights activists have questioned about the MHA (1987) regarding its constitutional validity and the Act was repealed by Mental Healthcare Act, 2017.[21]

3. *Mental Healthcare Act (MHCA), 2017:* In compliance with the international instruments United Nations Convention on Rights of Persons with Disabilities (UNCRPD), the Indian parliament enacted Mental Health Care Act, 2017 which came on 7th April 2017 to deliver mental healthcare and services for the mentally ill. The Act provides to guard, promote and fulfill the rights of persons with mental illness during delivery of mental health care and services and for all matters connected therewith or incidental thereto.

- Act defines mental illness and mandates practitioners to make diagnosis only in harmony with nationally and internationally acknowledged medical standards (including latest edition of International Classification of Disease (ICD) of the World Health Organization, WHO).
- It talks about fundamental rights of persons with mental illness and makes it duty of government and healthcare providing agencies to ensure they are delivered and adequate safeguard mechanism are in place to prevent its abuse.
- It brings under its ambit all mental health establishments, whether government or non-government, being used for therapeutic or rehabilitative purpose of all modalities of healing (medicianal like allopathic, ayurvedic, unani, homeopathy, siddha or religious). All such organizations keeping mentally ill persons will have to follow the standard prescribed regulations for licensing.

- The Act aims for decriminalizing the attempt to commit suicide by seeking to warrant that the persons who have attempted suicide are offered opportunities for rehabilitation from the law in contrast of being tried or punished for the same.
- It empowers mentally ill persons with a variety of rights, permitting them to make decisions in relation to their health, given that they have the capacity to make decision about treatment and care.
- It brings in mechanism of review boards for safeguard of any violation of rights of persons with mental illness,
- Insurers now inevitably have to make provisions for medical insurance for treatment of mentally ill on the basis similar to what is available for treatment of physical ailments.[22,23]

Legal statutes concerning substance of abuse

4. *Narcotic Drugs and Psychotropic Substances Act (NDPSA), 1985. (already discussed)*
5. *The Cigarettes and Other Tobacco Products (Prohibition of Advertisement and Regulation of Trade and Commerce, Production, Supply and Distribution) COTP Act, 2003:* This Act repealed The Cigarettes (Regulation of Production, Supply and Distribution) Act, 1975 in compliance with the Resolution which was passed by the 39th World Health Assembly, advising the member states to implement the various measures for providing non-smokers a protection from involuntary exposure to tobacco smoke.[24]

- It prohibits advertisement of cigarette and other tobacco products and provides for the regulation of trade and commerce in, and production, supply and distribution of cigarettes and other tobacco products in India.[25]
- It prohibits smoking of tobacco in public places, except in special smoking zones assigned for the purpose.
- It prohibits advertisement of tobacco products including cigarettes. No person shall participate in advertisement of tobacco product, or allow a medium of publication to be used for advertisement of tobacco products.
- No person shall sell video-film of such advertisement, distribute leaflets, documents, or give space for erection of advertisement of tobacco products. However, restricted advertisement is allowed on packages of tobacco products, entrances of places where tobacco products are sold. Surrogate advertisement is prohibited as well under the Act.

Legal statutes concerning medical jurisprudence

6. *The Indian Medical Council (IMC) Act, 1956:* The Act provides for the constitution of the Medical Council of India (MCI). The MCI regulates standards of medical education, permission to start new medical colleges, medical courses or increase the number of seats, registration of doctors, standards of professional conduct of medical practitioners. The Medical Council of India was established in 1934 under the Indian Medical Council Act, 1933. In 1956, the old Act was repealed and a new one was enacted. This was further modified in 1964, 1993 and 2001. The government superseded the MCI by issuing an ordinance in May 2010. The Central Government constituted the board of governors (BoG), comprising of not more than 7 members with one of them as chairperson till the new council was to be elected (time frame given was of 2 years). The government was liable to get the ordinance converted into a bill within 6 weeks from the date of the commencement of Parliament.

Since then, the health ministry sought extension of the tenure of BoGs many times. It is planned to replace it with national medical council.[10]

7. *The Consumer Protection Act (CPA), 1986:* The Consumer Protection Act was passed on 24th December, 1986 for the better protection of the interest of consumers and to make provisions for the establishment of consumer councils and other authorities for the settlement of consumer's dispute and for matters connected therewith.[25] Till 1995, even courts were not clear whether doctors are covered under consumer protection Act or not. In a landmark case in 1995, the Supreme Court decision in Indian Medical Association vs VP Shantha, medical profession has been brought under the Section 2(1) (o) of Consumer Protection Act, 1986 and also, it has included the following categories of doctors/hospitals under this Section:

- All medical/dental practitioners doing independent medical/dental practice unless rendering only free service.
- Private hospitals charging all patients.
- All hospitals having free as well as paying patients and all the paying and free category patients receiving treatment in such hospitals.
- Medical/dental practitioners and hospitals paid by an insurance firm for the treatment of a client or an employment for that of an employee.

The medical profession has also been included within the ambit of a 'service' as defined in the Consumer Protection Act; 1986. This defined the relationship between patients and medical professionals as contractual and not a master-servant relationship as argued by the medical professionals. Patients who had sustained injuries in the course of treatment can now sue doctors in consumer protection courts for compensation.

As per the Consumer Protection Rules, 1987, the maximum time limit for a claim to be filed under CPA is 2 years from the date of occurrence of the cause of action. There are no court fees to be paid to file a complaint in a Consumer Forum/Commission. Further, a complainant/opposite party can present his case on his own without the help of a lawyer. The courts have responsibility to punish the doctors who are guilty and at the same time to protect the honest doctors from undue harassment at the hands of patients and their relatives.

Legal statutes concerning protection and promotion of rights of persons with disability

8. *Protection of Human Rights Act (PHRA), 1993:* This is an Act for providing the constitution of a National Human Rights Commission (NHRC), State Human Rights Commission in States and Human Rights Courts for enhanced protection of human rights and for matters connected therewith or incidental thereto. This was introduced in 1993, and was amended in 2006. NHRC has been influential in bringing many mental health reforms in past two decades.[26]

9. *Persons with Disabilities Act (PDA), 1995:* Persons with Disabilities Act (PDA), 1995 was enacted to eliminate discriminations and to avert abuse and exploitations of persons with disability. It provides barrier free environment and spelled out responsibilities for the government for planning strategies for a comprehensive development programs and special provision for amalgamation of disabled into the social mainstream. Under this Act,

both mental retardation and mental illness are categorized in conditions of disability. Thus, the mentally ill are also enabled to benefits which are available to disabled as provided under the Act. This Act is reviewed in the light of the UNCRPD-2006.[27]

10. *National Trust for the Welfare of Persons with Autism, Cerebral Palsy, Mental Retardation and Multiple Disabilities Act, 1999:* This Act seeks to provide for the constitution of a body at the National level for the Welfare of Persons with Autism, Cerebral Palsy, Mental Retardation and Multiple Disabilities and for matters connected, to enable and empower persons with disability to live as independently and as fully as possible within and as close to the community to which they belong and to facilitate the realization of equal opportunities, protection of rights and full participation of persons with disability.[28]

11. *Right to Information Act (RTI Act), 2005:* In 2005, the Parliament enacted—Right to Information Act (2005).[29] The legislation confers on all citizens the right of access to the information and, correspondingly, makes the dissemination of such information an obligation on all public authorities (any government or non-government agency owned, controlled, regulated or substantially financed by government), promoting transparency and accountability. Interestingly, the Act in section 8, restricts to disclose any information provided under fiduciary relationship like that of doctor-patient relationship. But the appellate authority, central information commission (CIC) in some specific instances have instructed hospitals to provide medical records under RTI including sensitive psychiatry case records over riding code of medical ethics regulation, 2002 of confidentiality. Also, Prabhat Kumar vs Directorate of Health Services, 2014 case, CIC extended its coverage over to private hospitals stating since private hospitals are under regulations of public authority like IMC Act, CPA Act, Directorate of Health Services and Clinical Establishments (Registration & Regulation) Act 2011.[30] It stated that all hospitals whether private or government are under jurisdiction of RTI and all hospitals have duty to provide information in compliance with IMC Act, CPA and RTI Act.

12. *United Nations Convention for Rights of Persons with Disabilities (UNCRPD), 2006:* UNCRPD was adopted in December 2006; India ratified it in May, 2008. The countries that have signed and ratified it have an obligation to harmonize their laws and policies in tune with it. This convention has been a paradigm shift with regards to disabilities changing from a social welfare domain to a human right matter. This new paradigm is founded on conjecture of legal capacity, equality and dignity. Article 3 enlists the general principles of equality, non-discrimination, accessibility, respect for inherent dignity and individual autonomy. According to Article 12 of the convention, person with disability will enjoy legal capacity on an equal basis for all aspects of life. Article 4 makes it obligatory responsibility of state to provide "reasonable accommodation", i.e. make appropriate modifications in existing system so that persons with disability can enjoy the entitlements without discrimination. Article 15 calls for freedom from inhuman or degrading treatment and article 16 calls for freedom from exploitation, violence and abuse. It explicitly prohibits any kind of forced treatment or restriction on one's liberty on grounds of disability without consent of person. It lays down right to health, right to access treatment and related information, lays down standards of living for persons with disability and mandates putting up adequate safeguard mechanisms in place as oversight monitoring agencies.[31-34]

Legal statutes concerning interface of civil law and mental health

13. *Indian contract laws:* According to Indian Contract Act, 1872, any person of sound mind can make a contract. Section 12 of the Act stipulates that a person is said to be of sound mind for the purpose of making a contract, if, at the time when he makes it, he is capable of understanding it and of forming a rational judgment as to its effect upon his interest. A person, who is usually of unsound mind, but occasionally of sound mind, may make a contract when he is of sound mind. A person, who is usually of sound mind, but occasionally of unsound mind, may not make a contract when he is of unsound mind. It means a person with mental illness who is currently free of the psychotic symptoms can make a contract, whereas a person who is currently intoxicated or delirious cannot make a contract.[33]

14. *Marriage and divorce:* Under Hindu Marriage Act, 1955, conditions in respect of mental disorders, which must be fulfilled before the marriage is solemnized under the Act,[35] are as follows:
- Neither party is incapable of giving a valid consent as a consequence of unsoundness of mind.
- Even if capable of giving consent, must not suffer from mental disorders of such a kind or to such an extent as to be unfit for marriage and the procreation of children.
- Must not suffer from recurrent attacks of insanity.

The expression "mental disorder" means mental illness, arrested or incomplete development of mind. The expression "psychopathic disorder" means a persistent disorder or disability of the mind (whether or not including subnormality of intelligence) which results in abnormally aggressive or seriously irresponsible conduct on the part of the other party, and whether or not it requires or is susceptible to medical treatment.

Marriages in contravention to the provision in respect of mental disorders come under voidable category. Voidable marriages (Sec. 12) are those which may be annulled by a decree of nullity on the given grounds but may continue to be legal till the time it is annulled by a competent court. According to the Section 13 of the Act, divorce or judicial separation can be obtained if the person has been incurably of unsound mind, or has been suffering continuously or intermittently from mental disorder of such a kind and to such an extent that the petitioner cannot reasonably be expected to live with the respondent. The expression "incurably" of unsound mind cannot be so widely interpreted as to cover feeble minded persons or persons of dull intellect who understand the nature and consequences of the act and are therefore able to control them and their affairs, and their reaction in the normal way [A.I.R. 1969 Guj-48 and 78 CLT (1994) 561]. When there was sufficient evidence for the court to conclude that the slight mental disorder of the wife was not of such a kind and to such an extent that the husband could not reasonably be expected to live with her, divorce could not be granted (A.I.R., 1982 CAL 138). Each case of schizophrenia has to be considered on its own merits.[16] Under Special Marriage Act, 1954, the grounds for marriage, divorce and judicial separation are practically the same as those in the Hindu Marriage Act, 1955. The Special Marriage Act, 1954 is meant for any person in India and Indian nationals abroad, irrespective of the faith that the individual may profess. A marriage solemnized in any other form can be registered under this Act.[35]

Under the prevalent Muslim Law, marriage is a type of contract. Therefore, a Muslim who is of sound mind and has attained puberty is qualified to marry. However, if the guardian of a person of unsound mind considers such a marriage to be in his interest and in the interest of society and is willing to take up all the monetary obligations of the marriage, then such a marriage can be performed. *Talaq* (divorce) under Muslim Law has to be for a reasonable cause and must be preceded by attempts for reconciliation by two arbiters. In practice, a Muslim has the right to divorce his wife merely by pronouncing the word Talaq thrice, however, this practice is under criticism and a bill against it is pending in the parliament. According to Muslim Marriage Act, 1939, a woman married under Muslim Law is entitled to obtain a decree of divorce if her husband has been insane for a period of 2 years.

Under Christian Law, marriage is voidable, if either party was a lunatic or idiot. Christians can obtain divorce under Indian Divorce Act. 1869 (as amended in 2001) on grounds of unsoundness of mind provided: (i) it must be incurable (ii) it must be present for at least 2 years immediately preceding the petition. Divorce is not admissible on ground of mental illness under the Parsi Marriage and Divorce Act, 1936. However, divorce can be obtained if the defendant at the time of marriage was of unsound mind, provided the plaintiff was ignorant of the fact and the defendant has been of unsound mind for a period of 2 years upwards and immediately preceding the application.

15. *Testamentary capacity:* Testamentary capacity is the legal status of being capable of executing a Will, a legal declaration of the intention of a testator with respect to his property, which he desires to be carried into effect after his death. Indian Succession Act, 1925 Testamentary capacity requires a person's full sense and mental sanity to have confirmed and signed the Will after understanding what his assets comprised and what he is doing by making a Will. He understands in full mental capacity to whom he is naming the assets to and how are they related to him and what repercussions it may have later.[17]

16. *Transplantation of Human Organs Act, 2014:* The primary legislation related to organ donation and transplantation in India, Transplantation of Human Organs Act, was passed in 1994[36] and is aimed at regulation of removal, storage and transplantation of human organs for therapeutic purposes and for prevention of commercial dealings in human organs. Amendments were made in 2009 and 2011, which were gazette notified in 2014. The Act mandates that organ donation can be done for therapeutic purposes only. It mandates brain death certification from a medical board and psychiatry clearance is required for mental state of living donors.

17. *Protection of Women from Domestic Violence Act (PWDVA) 2005:* The Protection of Women from Domestic Violence Act 2005 is an Act to protect women from domestic violence. It was brought into force from 26 October 2006. The Act provides for the first time in Indian law a definition of "domestic violence", with this definition being broad and including not only physical violence, but also other forms of violence such as emotional/verbal, sexual, and economic abuse. It is a civil law meant primarily for protection orders and not meant to penalize criminally. The Act does not extend to Jammu and Kashmir, which has its own Act, enacted in 2010, the Jammu and Kashmir Protection of Women from Domestic Violence Act, 2010.[37]

Legal statutes concerning interface of criminal law and mental health

18. *Protection of children from sexual offences Act (POCSO Act) 2012:* This Act provides for a variety of offenses under which an accused can be punished. It defines a child as a person under age of 18 years. It encompasses the biological age of the child and silent on the mental age considerations.[38]

- It recognizes range of activities as sexual offences including all forms of penetration other than peno-vaginal penetration, acts of immodesty against children, sexual harassment, using children for pornographic purposes and even online sexual abuse.
- This is a gender-neutral Act including boys also as potential victims besides girls as against to previous laws.
- It mandates all individuals including health professionals to report any such incidence that comes to their notice to legal agencies with punishment of six months for failure reporting.

   The Act has been criticized for three provisions, first mandatory reporting of all cases by health professionals may attach stigma for health care seeking and many of the families may resort to seeking illegal medically harmful quackery practices of medical termination of unwanted conception. Secondly, it criminalizes a consensual sexual intercourse which is between two people under the age of 18. Thirdly, it talks of physical age and is silent on sexual assault of a female with mental age less than 18 years. In a recent case filed in SC, where a woman of biological age 38 years but mental age 6 years was raped. The victim's advocate argues that "failure to consider the mental age will be an attack on the very purpose of act." SC has reserved the case for judgment and is determined to interpret whether the 2012 act encompasses the mental age or whether only biological age is inclusive in the definition.[27]

19. *Laws concerning criminal liability:* The Indian Penal Code (IPC, 1860) says that "Nothing is an offence, which is done by a person who, at the time of doing it, by reason of unsoundness of mind, is incapable of knowing the nature of the act, or that he is doing what is either wrong or contrary to law," (Sec 84).[22] Law presumes every person of age of discretion to be sane and defense on ground of insanity needs to be proved. If defense is proven on ground of insanity, such persons are acquitted to be detained in safe custody either to a Psychiatric Hospital or to be released to a relative on surety bond under Sec. 335 (i) of the CrPC, 1973. It is seen that there have been occasions of lesser sentence due to mental illness.

Legal statutes concerning mental health professional training

20. *Rehabilitation Council of India Act (RCIA), 1992:* In 1992, the RCI Act was enacted and the Rehabilitation Council of India became a Statutory Body in 1993. The Act was amended in 2000 to make it more broad-based. The mandate given to RCI is to regulate and monitor services given to persons with disability, to standardize syllabi and to maintain a Central Rehabilitation Register of all qualified professionals and personnel working in the field of Rehabilitation and Special Education. The Act also prescribes punitive action against unqualified persons delivering services to persons with disability.[39]

MENTAL HEALTHCARE REFORMS IN INDIA

Although the National Mental Health Program is in place since 1982 and was restrategized in 1996. Mental Health Policy of India was introduced in October 2014, policy and programming in mental health so far have been more reactive than proactive. Tragedies like Erwadi and various public interest litigations (PILs) that have been filed before the honorable Supreme Court have been major driving forces of change. Some of the PILs have not only focused on institutional treatments but also focused on economic, social, and cultural rights of persons with mental illness. A series of reports from the National Human Rights Commission[33] highlights the gross deficiencies that existed in institutional care of persons with mental illness. These reports also demonstrated the positive changes that could be brought about with persistent monitoring, collaboration, and proactive intervention.[40] The positive changes noticed are:

1. Improvement in structural facilities and living conditions
2. Improved budgets
3. Voluntary admissions became more frequent than court admissions
4. Greater community participation, and the need for rehabilitation of persons with mental illness received greater focus.

However, these reports have also highlighted the negative aspects in terms of inadequate human resources and poor psychosocial interventions, among others. Meantime, the need to deliver the least restrictive care for persons with mental illness and by extension to develop adequate community care facilities for persons with mental illness has been the driving philosophy of the National Mental Health Policy. However, a recent report compiling state and union territory reports of the status of mental health care reveals extremely low coverage of primary mental health care in the country. The recently published Mental Health Survey Report[22] carried out in 12 states of the country estimates the prevalence of mental disorders at 10.6%, and the mental health care gap that has been calculated in these states as varying between 70.4% and 86.3%. In reality, given the huge inequity of mental health care resources across different states, and local ecologies that may aggravate mental distress, the mental healthcare treatment gap may be much higher. Mental health care, like other health care, requires human resources, facilities, and protected budgets. However, one stark truth is that there needs to be a concerted drive to improve human resources in mental health care, and that will be the biggest challenge in the decades ahead. While there is a need to train all health providers in issues related to mental health, it is also important to develop specialists in different aspects of mental health care. In addition, strengthening undergraduate psychiatry training as well as postgraduate training in psychiatry is of primary importance.

REFERENCES

1. Bar Council of India. Available from: http://www.barcouncilofindia.org. [Last accessed 2012 Jun 21].
2. Jiloha RC. Native Indian: In search of identity. Blumoon Books Publishers New Delhi, 1994.
3. Glenn HP. Legal Traditions of the World: Oxford University Press; 2000;255-76.
4. Nambi S. Forensic psychiatry revisited. Indian J Psychiatry. 2010;52.
5. Rappeport JR. Ethics and forensic psychiatry. In: Bloch S, Chodaff P (Eds). Psychiatric Ethics. Oxford: Oxford University Press; 1981.

6. Agrawal AK. Mental health and law. Indian J Psychiatry. 1992;34:65-6.
7. Singh MP. In: Shukla's VN Constitution of India. (9th ed). Lucknow: Eastern Book Company; 1994;165.
8. Somasundaram O, Kumar MS. Changing patterns of admission in a state mental hospital. Indian J Psychiatry. 1984;26:317-21.
9. Sharma S, Varma LP. History of mental hospitals in Indian sub-continent. Indian J Psychiatry. 1984;26:295-300.
10. Banerjee G. The Law and Mental Health: an Indian Perspective, 2001. Available from: http://www.psyplexus.com/excl/lmhi.html. [Last accessed 2017 Jun 21].
11. Somasundaram O. The Indian Lunacy Act, 1912: the historic background. Indian J Psychiatry. 1987;29:3-14.
12. Narayan CL, Narayan M, Shikha D. The ongoing process of amendments in MHA-87 and PWD Act-95 and their implications on mental health care. Indian J Psychiatry. 2011;53:343-50.
13. Math SB, Nagaraja D. Mental health legislations: an Indian perspective. In: Nagaraja D, Murthy P, (Eds). Mental Health and Human[Downloaded free fromhttp://www.indianjpsychiatry.org on Wednesday, December 27, 2017, IP: 14.139.58.50]
14. United Nations. Universal Declaration of Human Rights; 1948. Available from: http://www.un.org/en/universal-declaration-human-rights/. [Last accessed on 2016 Dec 01].
15. Trivedi JK. The Mental Health Act 1987. In: Agarwal AK, Trivedi JK, Sinha PK and Katiyar M (Eds). Ethies in Psychiatry. Lucknow: LPH; 1989 .pp. 158-60.
16. Banerjee G. The Law and Mental Health: An Indian Perspective, 2001. Available from: http://www.psyplexus.com/excl/lmhi.html.
17. Somasundaram O, Kumar MS. Changing patterns of admission in a state mental hospital. Indian J Psychiatry. 1984;26:317-21.
18. Sharma S, Varma LP. History of mental hospitals in Indian sub-continent. Indian J Psychiatry. 1984;26:295-300.
19. The Narcotic Drugs and Psychotropic Substances Act (NDPSA), 1985. Government of India Publication, New Delhi.
20. Mental Health Act, 1987. Government of India Publication, New Delhi.
21. Mental Healthcare Act, 2017. Government of India Publication, New Delhi.
22. Murthy P, Sekar K. A decade after the NHRC quality assurance initiative: Current status of government psychiatric hospitals in India. In: Nagaraja D, Murthy P, (Eds). Mental Health and Human Rights. Bangalore, New Delhi; 2008 .pp.113-28.
23. Murthy P, Malathesh BC, Kumar CN, et al. Mental health and the law: an overview and need to develop and strengthen the discipline of forensic psychiatry in India. Indian J Psychiatry. 2016;58:181-6.
24. The Cigarettes and Other Tobacco Products (Prohibition of Advertisement and Regulation of Trade and Commerce, Production, Supply and Distribution) COTP Act, 2003. Government of India Publication, New Delhi.
25. The Consumers Protection Act, 1986. Ministry of Law, Government of India Publication, New Delhi.
26. Protection of Human Rights Act (PHRA), 1993. Government of India Publication, New Delhi.
27. Persons with Disabilities (Full Participation and Equal Opportunities) Act, 1995. Government of India Publication, New Delhi.
28. National Trust for the Welfare of Persons with Autism, Cerebral Palsy, Mental Retardation and Multiple Disabilities Act, 1999. Government of India Publication, New Delhi.
29. Right to Information Act (RTI Act). Ministry of Law, Government of India Publication, New Delhi. 2005.

30. Directorate of Health Services and Clinical Establishments (Registration & Regulation) Act, Government of India Publication, New Delhi, 2011.
31. The Rights of Persons with Disabilities Act, 2016. Government of India Publication, New Delhi.
32. Murthy P, Isaac MK. Five-year plans and National Human Rights Commission. Quality Assurance in Mental Health. New Delhi: National Human Rights Commission; 1999.
33. Nagaraja D, Murthy P, (Eds). Mental Health and Human Rights. Bangalore, New Delhi: National Institute of Mental Health and Neuro Sciences, India and National Human Rights Commission; 2008.
34. Murthy P, Kumar S, Desai N, Teja BK. National Human Rights Commission. Report of the Technical Committee on Mental Health; 2016. Available from: http://www.nhrc.nic.in/Documents/Mental_Health_report_vol_I_10_06_2016.pdf. [Last accessed on 2016 Dec 01].
35. Rao TS, Nambi S, Chandrashekhar H. In: Gautam S, Avasthi A, (Eds). Marriage, Mental Health and the Indian Legislation. In Clinical Practice Guidelines on Forensic Psychiatry: Indian Psychiatric Society; 2009 .pp. 113-28.
36. The Transplantation of Human Organs Act. Ministry of Law Government of India Publication, New Delhi, 1994.
37. Protection of Women from Domestic Violence Act (PWDVA), 2005. Government of India Publication, New Delhi.
38. Protection of Children from Sexual Offences Act (POCSOA), 2012. Government of India Publication, New Delhi.
39. Rehabilitation Council of India Act (RCIA), 1992. Government of India Publication, New Delhi.
40. Gururaj G, Varghese M, Benegal V, et al. National Mental Health Survey of India, 2015-16. National Institute of Mental Health and Neuro Sciences, NIMHANS Publication No. 128;2016.

SECTION II
Medicolegal Responsibilities in Doctor-patient Relationship

CHAPTER

Medical Jurisprudence and Medical Negligence

> **LEARNING OBJECTIVES**
> - Forensic psychiatry vs medical jurisprudence
> - Role of medical councils
> - Rights, duties, and responsibilities of a doctor
> - Doctor patient relationship
> - Privileged communication
> - Medical malpractice
> - Psychiatric negligence

Jurisprudence is a term derived from Latin words, *juris*, which means law, and *prudential*, which means knowledge or skill. Medical jurisprudence is the application of knowledge of law in relation to practice of medicine.[1] It includes:
- Doctor-patient relationship
- Doctor-doctor relationship
- Doctor-State relationship

Medical jurisprudence covers a wide range of areas which need to be understood for conceptualization of medical jurisprudence.

Forensic science refers to a group of scientific disciplines which are concerned with the application of their particular scientific area of expertise to law enforcement, criminal, civil, legal and judicial matters.[2] Forensic science is a multidisciplinary subject dealing with examination of objects, substances (including blood/drug samples), chemicals paints/explosives/toxins), tissue traces (hair/skin) or impressions (fingerprints/tyre marks) left at the scene of crime.

Forensic Psychiatry (Legal medicine or State medicine) refers to the application of principle and knowledge of mental health sciences to legal purposes and legal proceedings so as to aid in the administration of justice.

Medical etiquette are the principles and conventional customs of courtesy observed between members of same profession for example, not charging fellow doctors and their family members for professional services offered. *Medical ethics* is concerned with moral standards and conscience for the members of the medical profession in their dealings with each other, their patients and the State. It is a set of self-imposed regulations and discipline assumed voluntarily by medical professionals.

INDIAN MEDICAL DEGREES ACT, 1916

This Act was passed to regulate the grant of titles implying qualification in Western Medical Science.[2]

THE INDIAN MEDICAL COUNCIL (IMC) ACT, 1956

The Medical Council of India was established in 1934 under the Indian Medical Council Act, 1933. In 1956, this Act was repealed and a new one was enacted. Further amendments were carried out in 1964, 1993 and 2001. The government superseded the MCI by issuing an ordinance in May 2010 and constituted a board of governors (BoG), comprising of not more than 7 members with one of them as chairperson till the new council was to be elected (time frame given was of 2 years). The government was liable to get the ordinance converted into a bill within 6 weeks from the date of the commencement of Parliament. Since then, the health ministry sought extension of the tenure of BoG governing MCI four times till 2013. With the government unable to get the Indian Medical Council (Amendment) Bill passed in Parliament, the old IMC Act that provided autonomy to the regulatory body was restored.

MEDICAL COUNCIL OF INDIA (MCI)[3]

The Medical Council of India is a statutory body responsible for establishing and maintaining uniform standards of medical education, and recognition of medical qualifications. The Medical council of India has specific functions to be carried out in relation to the medical profession.

Functions of MCI

- Maintenance of Indian Medical Register
  - It contains the names, addresses and qualifications of the medical practitioners who are registered with any State Medical Council (SMC).
  - Removal of the name from the register of the concerned SMC will lead to its removal from Indian Medical Register.
- **Regulation** of standard of undergraduate and postgraduate medical education
  - The Council maintains the standards of undergraduate medical education. The council prescribes courses and criteria which a medical institute should fulfill for a particular course of study.
  - The Council sends inspectors to see that the college is adequately spaced, staffed and equipped as per MCI stipulations. The inspector may also visit the institution during the examinations to assess the standard of education.
  - On the basis of the reports of the inspectors, the MCI recommends the recognition or non-recognition of the medical qualification to the Central Government.
  - Such an inspection is held for every medical qualification when it is introduced and every 5 years thereafter.

- The council prescribes the standards of postgraduate medical education for the guidance of the universities.
- **Permission** for establishment of new medical college, new course of study and increase in seats: Permission of the central government is obtained after the recommendations of the council which may either approve or disapprove the scheme.
- **Recognition** of medical qualification granted by universities in India: Any university which grants a medical qualification not included in the 1st Schedule may apply to the Central Government, to have such qualification recognized, and the government, after consulting the council, may amend the 1st Schedule.
- **De-recognition** of medical qualification: It can make representation to the central government to withdraw recognition of a medical qualification of any college, if on receipt of report from inspectors it feels that the standards of resources, training/teaching are not satisfactory.
- **Recognition of foreign medical qualifications** under the scheme of reciprocity: The council may enter into negotiations with the authority in any country outside India under a scheme of reciprocity for the recognition of medical qualifications. A separate examination may be conducted by the MCI to assess the standard of knowledge possessed by such individuals, before recognizing their degree.
- **Appellate powers:** It advises the central health ministry when an appeal is made by a medical practitioner against the decision of the State Medical Council (SMC) on disciplinary matters. Its decision is binding on the appealing party as well as the SMC.
- **Disciplinary control:** The council prescribes minimum standards of professional conduct, etiquette and a code of ethics for medical practitioners. It issues a warning notice periodically which is a list of offences constituting infamous conduct (professional misconduct). It can take actions against erring doctors and issue warning in relation to unethical practices which are regarded as disgraceful in a professional respect.
- **Certificates**: The council is empowered to issue certificates of good conduct and character to medical students/doctors going abroad for higher studies/service.
- **CME programs**: It sponsors and organizes continuing medical education (CME) programs for medical practitioners.
- **Faculty development program:** MCI has undertaken the task of training the medical college faculty up to the level of Associate Professors in MCI Basic Workshop in Medical Education Technologies. Faculty should undergo this training either before joining service or during probation period and once every 5 years thereafter. MCI has asked the health ministry to make it mandatory for all doctors to re-register with the SMCs and MCI every 5 years. This will help in tracking the number of doctors still alive and practicing in the country and registered with MCI.

There is no provision in the existing IMC Act for re-registration or revalidation of doctors. Medical Councils of certain states like Punjab, Delhi, Odisha, Rajasthan and Maharashtra have provision for re-registration of doctors under their respective statutes. Doctors who have already got permanent registration/registration of additional qualification with any SMC are not required/eligible for re-registration with the MCI.

- **Disciplinary control**: The Council is entrusted with disciplinary control over the registered medical practitioner.

   SMC can issue warning, suspension or penal erasure of the name of medical practitioner found indulging in unethical practice, and advises them to conduct themselves according to the ethical norms prescribed by the Council. It can act against doctors for professional negligence too.

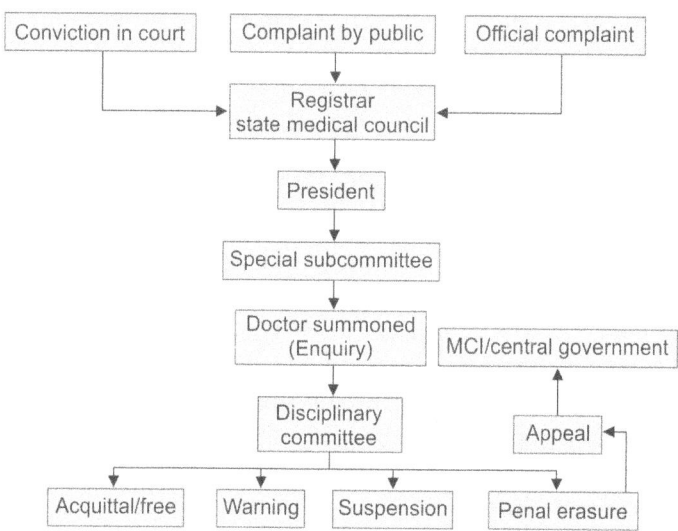

   The SMC takes cognizance of any misconduct (professional) in case:
   – The medical practitioner has been convicted by court for any criminal offence
   – A complaint has been lodged against him by some person or body.
   – Upon receipt of any complaint, the SMC would hold an enquiry and give opportunity to the registered medical practitioner to be heard.
   – If the doctor is found to be guilty of committing professional misconduct, the Council may punish as deemed necessary or may direct the removal of the name of the delinquent practitioner from the register, altogether or for a specified period. Decision on complaint against delinquent physician is taken within a time limit of 6 months.
   – An inquiry against a doctor should be initiated by SMC with which he/she is registered. The role of the MCI is only as an appellate authority to the Central Health Ministry to decide on an appeal against the decision of the SMC on disciplinary matters.
- **Removal of name of medical practitioner:** SMC is empowered to erase from the register the name of any registered medical practitioner with whom it is unable to establish communication.
- **Restoration of name of medical practitioner:** It can direct restoration of any name of registered medical practitioner so removed.

DUTIES OF A DOCTOR

Under the Indian Medical Council Act, 1956, the MCI, with the approval of the Central Government, made the following regulations which are called the Indian Medical Council (Professional Conduct, Etiquette and Ethics) Regulations, 2002 (amended in 2009).[1,4]

Code of Medical Ethics: At the time of registration, all the doctors are self-warned about certain unethical practices (infamous conduct) and the disciplinary action by the SMC (also called as warning notice). The applicant should certify that he/she has read and agreed to abide by the same, and submit a declaration duly signed.

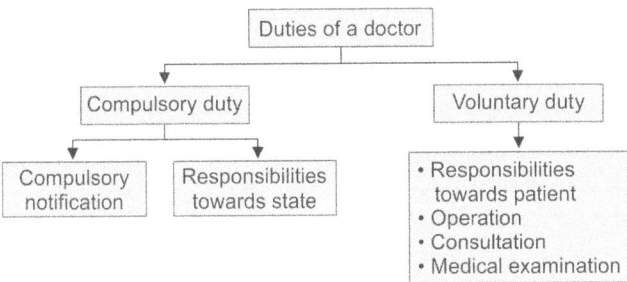

Duties of a Doctor in General

- *Character of physician:* A physician should uphold the dignity and honor of his profession and render service to humanity; reward or financial gain is a subordinate consideration.
- Maintaining good medical practice:
  - The physician should try to improve medical knowledge and skills, and should practice methods having scientific basis. He should participate in professional meetings, i.e. CME programs for at least 30 hours every 5 years.
  - *Membership in medical society:* He should affiliate with associations and societies for the advancement of his profession.
- Maintenance of medical records:
  - Physician should maintain the medical records of his indoor patients for a period of 3 years. In a case where medical records and consent obtained from a patient were not produced, negligence was established.
  - On request for medical records, either by the patients or legal authorities, the same should be issued within the period of 72 hours. This applies to a doctor in his private capacity, in case of indoor patients whom he/she might have treated/ operated in hospital/nursing home.
  - He should maintain a register of medical certificates issued. He should record the signature and/or thumb mark, address and at least one identification mark of the patient and keep a copy of the certificate.

- Display of registration numbers:
  - Physician should display the registration number accorded to him by the SMC in his clinic and in all his prescriptions, certificates, money receipts given to his patients. A doctor was held guilty for printing incorrect information about his qualification on the prescription paper.
  - Physicians should display as suffix to their names only recognized medical degrees or such certificates/diplomas and memberships/honors which confer professional knowledge.
- *Use of generic names of drugs:* Physician should prescribe drugs with generic names, and ensure that there is a rational prescription and use of drugs.
- *Highest quality assurance in patient care:* He should not employ in connection with his professional practice any attendant who is not registered or permit such persons to attend, treat or perform operations upon patients wherever professional discretion or skill is required.
- *Exposure of unethical conduct:* Physician should expose, without fear or favor, incompetent or corrupt, dishonest or unethical conduct on the part of members of the profession.
- Payment of professional services:
  - Physician should clearly display his fees in his chamber and/or hospitals he is visiting.
  - He should announce his fees before rendering service and not after the operation or treatment is underway.
- *Evasion of legal restrictions:* Physician should observe the laws of the country in regulating the practice of medicine and should not assist others to evade such laws.

Duties of a Doctor towards the State

- Poisoning cases:
  - He should assist the police in determining whether the poisoning is accidental, suicidal or homicidal.
  - In case of death, death certificate should mention about the poisoning with recommendation for postmortem examination.
- Notification: Doctor is bound to give information of communicable diseases (notifiable diseases), births, deaths and outbreak of an epidemic to public health authorities. Failing which he is not only liable for criminal penalties, but also negligence suits brought by affected persons.

  A notifiable disease is any disease that is required by law to be reported to government authorities, e.g. cholera, plague, leprosy, diphtheria, typhoid fever, tetanus, measles, tuberculosis, chickenpox, acute poliomyelitis, encephalitis, influenza, dengue fever, hemorrhagic fevers, hepatitis, HIV, etc.

Duties of a Doctor towards Patients

- Exercise reasonable degree of skill and knowledge:
  - It begins the moment the physician-patient relationship is established (i.e. when the physician agrees to treat the patient).

- He owes this duty even when the patient is treated free of charge.
- It neither guarantees cure nor an assured improvement.
- A practitioner (e.g. MBBS) is not liable because some other doctors of greater skill and knowledge (e.g. MD/MS) would have prescribed a better treatment or operated better in the same circumstances.

- Attendance and examination:
  - When a doctor agrees to attend a patient, he is under an obligation to attend to the case, as long it requires attention.
  - He can withdraw after giving reasonable notice or when he is asked by the patient to withdraw.
  - If the doctor is called by police to attend a case of road side accident, he may give first aid and advice, but no doctor-patient relationship is established.
- Furnish proper and suitable medicines:
  - He should give a legible prescription. He should write in capital letters—mistakes arising out of illegibly written names of medicines as opposed to other kinds of indecipherable documents—can be very dangerous.
  - Doctor is held responsible for any temporary or permanent damage in health, caused to the patient due to wrong prescription.
- Instructions: Doctor should give full instructions to his patients or their attendants regarding use of medicines (quantities and timings), injections (whether to be given intramuscularly or intravenously) and diet.
- Prognosis: The patient or his relatives should have such knowledge of the patient's condition as will serve the best interests of the patient and the family.
- Control and warn:
  - Doctor should warn patients of the side-effects involved in the use of prescribed drug, otherwise it might amount to negligence.
  - If the doctor fails to inform the known dangerous effects of a drug/device, he becomes liable not only for the harm suffered by the patient but also for injuries his patient may cause to third parties.
- Third parties: If a patient suffers from an infectious disease, the doctor should warn not only the patient, but also third parties who are close to the patient.
- Children and disabled persons being incapable of taking care of themselves, the doctor should arrange for their proper care, e.g. supervised application of hot water bottles.
- Consent: A person must be told of all the relevant facts in non-medical terms and in a language he/she understands and then obtain consent.
- Interventions:
  - Doctor should explain the nature and extent of intervention, and take consent of patient.
  - He should take proper care to avoid mistakes, such as operating on the wrong patient or on wrong limb, or leave any instrument or swab inside a body cavity.
  - He should not delegate his duty to operate a patient to another doctor.

- He should not experiment without valid reason or valid consent from the patient. He should avail the assistance of qualified and experienced anesthetists.
- Death on operation table should be followed by postmortem examination.
- Investigations:
  - All cases of accident, unless they are minor, should be X-rayed.
  - For proper diagnosis and to know the progress, the doctor should advise investigations, like biopsy, X-rays, CT scan, etc.
  - Wrong interpretation of X-ray is liable to be held as negligent.
- Emergency cases:
  - He has moral, ethical and humanitarian duty to help the patient in saving his life.
  - In medicolegal injury cases, a doctor is obliged to give medical aid and to save life of the patient.
- Professional secrecy/medical confidentiality, The doctor is obliged to maintain the secrets that he comes to know concerning the patient in the course of a professional relationship, except when he is required by the law to divulge the secrets or when the patient has consented for its disclosure.
  - It is a fundamental tenet that whatever a doctor sees or hears in the life of his patient must be treated as totally confidential. Disclosure would be failure of trust and confidence.
  - The patient can sue the doctor for damages or face disciplinary action by the SMC, if the disclosure is voluntary and has resulted in harm to the patient and is not in the interest of public. Following principles should be followed:
    - Physician should not answer any query by third parties, even when enquired by close relatives, either with regard to the nature of illness or any subsequent effect of such illness on the patient, without his/her consent.
    - If the patient is major (≥ 18 years), physician should not disclose any facts about the illness without his consent to parents or relatives even though they may be paying the doctor's fees. In case of minor or persons with mental illness, guardians or parents should be informed of the nature of illness.
    - A doctor should not disclose the illness of his patient without his consent, even when requested by a public or statutory body, except in case of notifiable diseases. If the patient is minor or persons with mental illness, consent of the guardian should be taken.
    - Even in case of husband and wife, the facts relating to the nature of illness of one must not be disclosed to the other, without the consent of the concerned person. Particular caution is required over the disclosure of sexual matters, such as pregnancy, abortion or venereal disease, as disclosure might cause conflict between them.
    - In divorce and nullity cases, no information should be given without the consent of the concerned person.
    - When a domestic servant is examined at the request of the master, the physician should not disclose any facts about the illness to the master without the consent of

servant, even though the master is paying the fees. Similarly, the medical officer of firm or factory should not disclose without the patient's consent.
- Medical officers in government service are also bound by code of professional secrecy, even when the patient is treated free.
- A person in police custody as an undertrial prisoner has the right not to permit the doctor who has examined him, to disclose the nature of his illness to any person. If convicted, he has no such right and physician can disclose the findings to the authorities.
- Any information regarding a dead person may be given only after obtaining the consent from a relative.
- In examination of a dead body, certain facts may be found, the disclosure of which may affect the reputation of the deceased or cause mental torture to his relatives, and as such, the autopsy surgeon should maintain secrecy.
- The medical examination for life insurance policy is a voluntary act by the examinee, and consent to the disclosure of findings may be taken as implied.

Duties of a Doctor in Consultation

- Consultation for patient's benefit is of foremost importance. Unnecessary consultations should be avoided.
- Statement to patient after consultation should take place in the presence of the consulting physician, except if otherwise agreed. Differences of opinion should not be divulged unnecessarily.
- Treatment after consultation: The attending physician should make subsequent variations in the treatment, if any unexpected change occurs. The attending physician may prescribe medicine at any time for the patient, whereas the consultant may prescribe only in case of emergency or as an expert when called for.
- Patients referred to specialists: When a patient is referred to a specialist by the attending physician, a case summary of the patient should be given to the specialist, who should communicate his opinion in writing to the attending physician.

Consultation is advised with a specialist in the following conditions:
- In case of emergency
- If the patient requests consultation
- If quality of care or management can be considerably enhanced
- In cases where diagnosis remains obscure
- In case of homicidal poisoning
- In connection with organ transplantation
- When treatment or operation involves risk of life
- When operation affecting vitality, intellectual or generative functions is to be performed
- When an operation involves mutilation or destruction of an unborn child
- When an operation is to be performed on a patient who has received injuries in a criminal assault

- To take decision about termination of pregnancy case, after 12 weeks and upto 20 weeks of pregnancy

A referring physician is relieved of further responsibility when he completely transfers the patient to another physician.

The referring physician may be held liable under the doctrine of negligent choice, if it can be proved that the consultant was incompetent or had a reputation as an errant physician.

Responsibility of Doctors towards Each Other

  i. **Conduct in consultation:** No insincerity, rivalry or envy should be indulged in. All due respect should be observed towards the physician in-charge of the case, and no statement or remark be made, which would impair the confidence the patient has reposed in him.
  ii. **Consultant not to take charge of the case:** Consultant should normally not take charge of the case, especially on the solicitation of the patient or friends.
  iii. **Appointment of substitute:** A physician should accept to attend another physician's patients during his temporary absence from his practice, only when he has the capacity to discharge the additional responsibility along with his other duties.
  Privileged Communication
  It is a statement, made bonafide upon any subject matter by a doctor to the concerned authority having corresponding interest, due to his legal, social or moral duty to protect the interests of the community or of the state.
  - It is an exchange of information between two individuals in a confidential relationship, and an exception to professional secrecy.
  - To be privileged, it must be made to the person who has a duty towards it. If made to more than one person or to a person who has not got a direct interest in it, the plea of privilege fails.
  - Doctor should first persuade the patient to obtain his consent before notifying the proper authority. However, disclosure can be done without consent (if consent is not forthcoming).
  - Doctor has a statutory duty to notify births, deaths, still births, infectious diseases, therapeutic abortions, drug addictions, epidemic and food poisoning to public health authorities.

Following are the situations requiring privileged communication:
  i. **Suspected crime:**
  If the physician learns of a crime, such as assault, terrorist activity, traffic offence or homicidal poisoning by treating the victim or assailant, he is bound to report it to the nearest Magistrate or police officer.
  - But sometimes, the issue of confidentiality clashes with the need to protect some individual or the public from possible further danger (e.g. a below-age of consent girl came to a doctor with STD). The doctor is usually required to obtain a list of the patient's sexual contacts to inform them that they need treatment. However, the patient may be reluctant to divulge the names of her older sexual partners, for

fear that they will be charged with statutory rape. The same issue may arise where a doctor suspects a child or an elderly person, disabled or incompetent person is being abused, but here the overriding consideration is the safety of these individuals. It has been made mandatory to report to the police any case of sexual abuse in children (≤18 years) as per the Protection of Children from Sexual Offences Act, 2012.
- At times, assault may occur within a family, e.g. between spouses or close relatives, the victim may not wish to bring criminal charges, and so the doctor must not assume that consent for disclosure has been given.
- The doctor knowing or having reason to believe that an offence has been committed by a patient when he is treating, intentionally omits to inform the police, can be punished with imprisonment upto 6 months and with/without fine (Sec. 202 IPC).

ii. **Patient's own interest:** Doctor may disclose patient's condition to his relatives so that he may be properly treated, e.g. to warn parents/guardians of patient's melancholia or suicidal tendencies.

iii. **Self-interest:** In case of civil and criminal suits by the patient against the physician, evidence about patient's condition may be given.

iv. **Negligence suits:** When doctor is employed by opposite party to examine a patient who has filed a suit for negligence, the information thus acquired is not a professional secret (no physician-patient relationship) and the doctor may testify to such information.

v. **Court ordered examination:** If a court orders an examination for the purposes of reporting back to the court about the physical or mental condition of the person, then he/she should be told that examination findings is not confidential. The report becomes part of the court record.

vi. **Court of law:** Doctor cannot claim professional secrecy concerning the facts about illness of his patient in court of law. He has to answer the questions about patient's confidential matters to avoid risk penalties for contempt of court. A doctor can disclose and discuss the medical facts of a case with other doctors and paramedical staff, such as nurses, radiologist and physiotherapist to provide better service to the patient.

To protect life of others. This gave rise to concept of duty to warn as detailed below.

Duty to Warn Famous Tarasoff Case

The California Supreme Court decision in Tarasoff v. Regents of the University of California (1974; 1976) set a standard for practitioners to reveal confidential information in their duty to warn others of the potential dangers from a client. Briefly, the Tarasoff case involved a murder victim, Tatiana Tarasoff, who was killed by an alleged acquaintance, Prosenjit Poddar. Poddar who was a client of Dr. Lawrence Moore, a psychotherapist employed by the University of California. Prosenjit Poddar had stated during a therapy session that he intended to kill Tarasoff because she had rejected him as a lover. He was assessed as a danger and was held briefly and released. Shortly after his temporary confinement, he did indeed kill Tarasoff during an attack with a pellet gun and knife. The victim's parents sued the therapist, campus police, and everyone who had contact with the case at the University of California (Board of Regents) for wrongful death. They asserted that if the therapist knew that Poddar was indeed a danger and there was intent related to his threat to his victim, that they had a duty to warn her. In the majority decision, the court found that the "protective privilege ends where the public peril begins" [17 Cal.3d 425, 441 (1976)]. The decision had a significant impact on the legal requirements for a clinician and certainly affected a client's confidentiality. If, during the course of therapy, a clinician assesses a client as a danger to someone, he or she has a duty and is legally compelled to warn the intended victim.

Actually, a *privilege* is a legal rule that protects communications within certain relationships from compelled disclosure in a court proceeding. While some use the terms 'privileged' and 'confidential' interchangeably, they all protect communications made in confidence in the context of the professional relationship. Like other confidentiality statutes, the privilege statutes grant control over the release of the information to the individual and also define circumstances under which the information may be released without the consent of the individual. In medical context, this term is being used to indicate that the information is shared with one particular individual having corresponding interest.

The term '*medical malpractice*' covers all failures in the conduct of doctors, where it impinges upon their professional skills, ability and relationships.

It divided into two broad types:
i. **Professional misconduct**—where the personal, professional behavior falls below that which is expected of a doctor.
ii. **Medical negligence**—where the standard of medical care given to a patient is considered to be inadequate.

A medical practitioner should not commit any of the following acts which may be construed as unethical:

- **Advertising:** *He should not:*
    - Solicit patients directly or indirectly, by a physician or a group of physicians or by institutions.
    - Make use his name for any advertising through any mode (such as in the form of strips on the cable television), so as to invite attention to his professional position.
    - Give any recommendation, endorsement or statement with respect of any drug, surgical or therapeutic appliance with his name, signature or photograph (**no association with manufacturing firms**) nor shall he boast of cases, operations or cures or permit the publication of report there of through any mode.
    - Print self-photograph or any such material of publicity in the letterhead or on sign board of the consulting room. A medical practitioner is, however, permitted to make a formal announcement in press regarding the following:
        - On starting or resumption or change of type of practice.
        - On changing address.
        - On temporary absence from duty.
        - Public declaration of charges.
        - Acquiring new equipment or starting a new procedure or operation (as per Punjab Medical Council).

The advertisement in the press should be in black and white, and < 15 × 10 cm in size. It should not carry photograph of the doctor/building/equipment/procedure (as per Punjab Medical Council).
- **Patent and copyrights:** He may patent surgical instruments, appliances, procedures and medicine. However, it is unethical, if the benefits of such patents are not made available in situations where the interest of large population is involved.
- He should not **run an open shop for dispensing of drugs and appliances** prescribed by other physicians.
- **Rebates and commission (dichotomy/fee splitting/'cut practice'):** He should not give or receive any gift or commission in consideration of referring, recommending or procuring of patient for medical, surgical or other treatment, or for getting specimen or material for diagnostic purposes.
- **Secret remedies:** He should not prescribe or dispense secret remedial agents of which he does not know the composition.
- **Human rights:** He should not aid or abet torture or be a party to either infliction of psychological or physical trauma.
- **Euthanasia:** He should not practice euthanasia.
- **Pharmaceutical and allied health sector industry:** A medical practitioner should not receive any gift, cash or monetary grants, travel facility or accept any hospitality, like hotel accommodation from any pharmaceutical industry for vacation or for attending conferences, seminars, workshops or CME program as a delegate.

Recently, the MCI has fixed the quantum of punishment: doctor taking bribe (gifts, cash or travel facility) worth '1000–5000 will receive a warning; taking' 5000–10000: suspension from the SMC for 3 months, taking '10000–50,000: suspension of 6 months, and bribes ≥ 50,000: suspension for 1 year.

PROFESSIONAL MISCONDUCT

Any conduct of the doctor which might reasonably be regarded as disgraceful or dishonorable as judged by professional men of good repute and competence. It involves abuse of professional position.

The following acts of commission or omission on the part of a physician constitutes professional misconduct:
- Any **unethical practice** as outlined above.
- If he **does not maintain the medical records** of his indoor patients for a period of 3 years and refuses to provide the same within 72 hours when the patient requests for it.
- If he **does not display the registration number** accorded to him by the SMC in his clinic, prescriptions and certificates issued by him.
- Physician posted in **rural area is found absent on more than two occasions** during inspection by the Head of the District Health Authority or the Chairman, Zila Parishad.
- Physician posted in a **medical college** as teaching faculty or otherwise is **found absent on more than two occasions**; the same is construed as misconduct, if it is certified by the Principal/Medical Superintendent.

- Providing **falsified and misleading information** to the MCI via Form A. The form is filled by the doctor when he/she joins a medical college.

Further, he should not
- **Commit adultery or misbehave** with a patient.
- Be **drunk and disorderly** so as to interfere with proper practice of medicine.
- Be **convicted by court of law** for offences involving moral turpitude/criminal acts.
- Do **sex determination tests** with the intent to terminate the life of a female fetus.
- **Issue false, misleading or improper certificates** for subsequent use in the courts or for administrative purposes.
- **Violate the provisions of Drugs and Cosmetics Act.** He should not: sell Schedule 'H' and 'L' drugs and poisons to the public, except to his patient. Prescribe steroids/psychotropic drugs when there is no medical indication.
- **Supply or sell addiction forming drugs** to a patient other than medical grounds.
- **Give cover,** i.e. assist someone who has no medical qualification to attend, treat or perform an operation, in cases requiring professional discretion or skill.
- **Perform an illegal abortion/operation** for which there is no medical, surgical or psychological indication.
- **Issue certificates of efficiency in modern medicine** to unqualified or non-medical person.
- **Disclose professional secrets.**
- **Refuse on religious grounds** sterilization, birth control, circumcision and medical termination of pregnancy when it is indicated.
- **Publish photographs/case reports** of his patients **without their consent** in any medical or other journal or social media in a manner by which their identity could be made out.
- **Use touts or agents** to entice patients.
- **Claim to be specialist** when he has no special qualification in that branch.
- **Undertake in-vitro fertilization or artificial insemination** without the informed consent of the female patient and her spouse as well as the donor.
- Do clinical **drug trials** or other **research** involving patients or volunteers not abiding by the guidelines of ICMR.
- **Advertise**
    - Contribute to the lay press articles and give interviews regarding diseases and treatments which may have the effect of advertising himself. He can write to the lay press under his own name on matters of public health, hygiene or deliver public lectures, give talks on the radio/ FM/TV/internet for the same purpose.
    - Use an unusually large signboard and write on it anything other than his name, qualifications, title, name of his speciality and registration number.
    - Affix a signboard on a chemist's shop or in places where he does not reside or work.
    - Give his name, address and speciality in the yellow pages of the telephone directory in bold letters.

The instances of offences and professional misconduct which are given above *do not constitute a complete list of the infamous acts* which calls for disciplinary action. Circumstances may arise from time to time in relation to which there may occur questions of professional misconduct which do not come within any of these categories.

Important offences as 6 As:
1. Association with unqualified persons
2. Adultery
3. Advertising
4. Addiction
5. Abortion (criminal)
6. Alcohol.

The name of the doctor is removed from the SMC register in following conditions:
- After the death of registered medical practitioner.
- When entries of the medical practitioner are erroneous or fraudulent.
- In case of professional misconduct which is known as *penal erasure*. When the name is permanently removed, it is termed as **professional death sentence**.
- When the registered medical practitioner is not traceable at the address recorded with the council.

RIGHTS AND PRIVILEGES OF REGISTERED MEDICAL PRACTITIONERS

- Right to choose his patient—he may refuse any patient without reason, but he should not refuse emergency treatment required by the patient.
- Right to use title and description of the qualification to his name.
- Right to practice medicine.
- Right to dispense medicine to his patient.
- Right to possess and supply dangerous drugs to his patients.
- Right to give evidence in the court of law, as an expert witness.
- Right to issue medical certificates and medicolegal reports.
- Right to recovery of fees—if the patient does not pay the justified fees, help of court can be taken.
- Right for appointment in public and local hospitals.

PRIVILEGES AND RIGHTS OF PATIENTS

- **Access** to healthcare facilities and emergency services regardless of age, sex, religion, social or economic status.
- **Choice:** To choose his own doctor freely.
- **Continuity:** To receive continuous care for his illness from doctor/institution.

- **Comfort:** To be treated in comfort during illness and follow-up
- **Complaint:** Right to complain and redressal of grievances.
- **Confidentiality:** All information about his illness should be kept confidential.
- **Dignity:** To be treated with care, compassion, respect without any discrimination.
- **Information:** Should receive full information about his diagnosis, investigations, treatment plans, alternative therapy, procedures, diagnosis, complications and side-effects.[5]
- **Privacy:** To be treated in privacy.
- **Refusal:** Can refuse any specific or all measures.
- **Records:** Can have access to his records and demand summary or other details.

DUTIES OF A PATIENT

- He should furnish the doctor with complete information about the facts and circumstances of his illness.
- He should strictly follow the instructions of the doctor as regards diet, medicine and lifestyle.
- He should pay a reasonable fee to the doctor.

DOCTOR–PATIENT RELATIONSHIP

It is of two types:
- **Therapeutic relationship:** A doctor is free to accept or refuse to treat a patient, subject to constraint of his work, except in emergencies.[6] He may refuse to treat the patient in following circumstances:
  - Beyond his practicing hours.
  - Not belonging to his specialty.
  - Doctor or any other family member is ill.
  - Doctor having important social function in family.
  - Illness beyond the competence and qualification of the doctor or beyond the facilities available in his setup.
  - Doctor is having alcohol.
  - Patient is malingering.
  - Patient has been defaulting in payment.
  - Patient or his relatives are abusive/uncooperative
  - Patient refuses to give consent.
  - Patient demanding specific drugs, like amphetamine, steroids, etc.
  - Patient rejecting low-cost remedies in favor of high cost alternatives.
  - At night, on grounds of security, if patient is not brought to him.
  - An unaccompanied minor or female patient.
  - When doctor remains engaged with an emergency or more serious case.
  - Any new patient, if he is not the only doctor available.

- **Formal relationship:** It pertains to the situation where the third party has referred the person/patient for impartial medical examination; for example,
  - Pre-employment.
  - Insurance policy.
  - Yearly medical checkups
  - Cases of rape or victims of crimes, medicolegal cases
  - In certain psychiatric illnesses referred by court/police
  - Doctor has to comply with the directive of the party demanding such examination.

MEDICAL NEGLIGENCE

The failure to exercise reasonable care and skill of an ordinary prudent medical practitioner in the circumstances; a breach of duty to act with care appropriate to the situation, which resulted in bodily injury (harm/loss) or death of the patient.

Negligence consists of two acts:
Not doing something that a reasonable man, under the circumstances would do **(act of omission)**; or
Doing something which a reasonable prudent man under the circumstances would not do **(act of commission)**.

According to Black's Law Dictionary, medical negligence requires that the plaintiff establish the following **(4 Ds)**:

i. Existence of the physician's *duty* of care to the plaintiff, based on the existence of the physician patient relationship.
ii. Applicable standard of care and its violation *(dereliction of duty)*, i.e. a breach in the duty caused by the defendant's negligent act or omission.
iii. *Damage* (a compensable injury), i.e. pain and suffering, disability and disfigurement, past and future medical bills, lost wages, wrongful death, etc.
iv. Causal connection between the violation of care and the harm complained of *(direct causation)*, i.e. a direct link between the defendant's negligent act or omission and an injury suffered by the plaintiff. In a lawsuit for malpractice or negligence (civil), the 'patient' is known as the *plaintiff* and the 'physician' becomes the *defendant*. Malpractice requires the demonstration of negligence or substandard practice that caused of harm. To successfully sue a physician for malpractice, the plaintiff must prove damage has been caused by the doctor's conduct.

'Damage' should be distinguished from 'damages'. *Damage* (injury or harm) to the patient may be physical, mental or financial. *Damages* are assessed by the court based on parameters, like loss of earning, medical and surgical costs, or reduction of quality of life. Potential damages (financial compensation) in negligence suits fall into three categories:
   (i) **Economic** or the monetary costs of an injury (e.g. medical bills or loss of income)
   (ii) **Noneconomic** (e.g. pain and suffering, loss of ability to have sex)
   (iii) **Punitive** or damages to punish a defendant for willful and wanton conduct.

Types of Medical Negligence

There are two types of medical negligence:
i. Civil
ii. Criminal.

Civil Negligence

Question of civil negligence arises:
- When a patient, or in case of death, any relative brings suit in a civil court for realization of compensation from his doctor, if he has suffered injury due to negligence.
- When doctor brings a civil suit for the realization of his fees from patient or his relatives, who refuse to pay the same, alleging professional negligence.

  Civil negligence involves:
  - Such act on the part of the treating physician which causes some suffering, harm or damage to the patient
  - Damage is such, which can be compensated by paying money
  - Does not come under the purview of CrPC and IPC
  - Does not demand legal punishment.

Criminal Negligence

- Criminal negligence is more serious than civil negligence.
- Practically limited to cases in which the patient has died.
- Mostly associated with drunkenness or impaired efficiency due to the use of drugs by doctors.
- Doctor shows gross incompetency and inattention in the selection and application of remedies, undue interference by him or criminal indifference to the patient's safety.
- **Sec. 304-A IPC** deals with criminal negligence; "whoever causes the death of any person by doing any rash or negligent act not amounting to culpable homicide is punished with imprisonment up to 2 years and with/without fine".[7]
- The concept of negligence differs in civil and criminal law. What may be negligence in civil law may not necessarily be negligence in criminal law. For an act to amount to criminal negligence, the degree of negligence should be much higher, i.e. gross or of a very high degree. Negligence which is neither gross nor of a higher degree may provide a ground for action in civil law but cannot form the basis for prosecution.
- The Supreme Court has held that to prosecute a doctor for criminal negligence, it must be shown that the accused did something or failed to do something which in the given facts and circumstances no doctor in his ordinary senses and prudence would have done or failed to do. The expression 'rash or negligent act' as occurring in Sec. 304-A IPC has to be read as 'grossly'.

Examples of Medical Negligence

A physician may be liable to both civil and criminal negligence by a single act, e.g. if he performs an unauthorized operation on a patient, he may be sued in civil court for damages and prosecuted in criminal court for assault.

The police sometime register the cases of professional negligence deaths under Sec. 304 IPC which is non-bailable offence, whereas if it is registered under Sec. 304-A IPC, the offence is bailable. The basic difference is that in Sec. 304, the act is intentional, while in 304-A, the act is never done with the intention to cause death.

Medical Negligence and Culpability of Doctor

Burden of Proof

The accused (doctor) is innocent until proven guilty, and the prosecution must prove the case against him/her. The plaintiff (patient) bears the burden of proof and must convince the judge by a preponderance of the evidence that its case is more plausible.

- In civil cases, a preponderance of the evidence is at least 51%. It means that judges in a medical negligence case must be persuaded that the evidence presented by the plaintiff is more plausible as the proximate cause of the injury than any counter argument offered by the defendant.
- In criminal cases, the prosecutions must prove their case 'beyond reasonable doubt' akin to a 98 or 99% certainty.

A doctor can be held liable for negligence only if one can prove that she/he is guilty of a failure that no doctor with ordinary skills would be guilty of if acting with reasonable care.[8] An error of judgment constitutes negligence only if a reasonably competent professional with the standard skills that the defendant professes to have, and acting with ordinary care, would not have made the same error.[9]

In Calcutta Medical Research Institute vs Bimalesh Chatterjee, it was held that the onus of proving negligence and the resultant deficiency in service was clearly on the complainant.[10] In Kanhaiya Kumar Singh vs Park Medicare and Research Centre, it was held that negligence has to be established and cannot be presumed.[11]

Even after adopting all medical procedures as prescribed, a qualified doctor may commit an error. The National Consumer Disputes Redressal Commission and the Supreme Court have held, in several decisions, that a doctor is not liable for negligence or medical deficiency if some wrong is caused in her/his treatment or in her/his diagnosis if she/he has acted in accordance with the practice accepted as proper by a reasonable body of medical professionals skilled in that particular art, though the result may be wrong. In various kinds of medical and surgical treatment, the likelihood of an accident leading to death cannot be ruled out. It is implied that a patient willingly takes such a risk as part of the doctor-patient relationship and the attendant mutual trust.

Recent Supreme Court rulings

Before the case of Jacob Mathew vs State of Punjab, the Supreme Court of India delivered two different opinions on doctors' liability. In Mohanan vs Prabha G Nair and another,[12] it ruled that a doctor's negligence could be ascertained only by scanning the material and expert evidence that might be presented during a trial. In Suresh Gupta's case in August 2004, the standard of negligence that had to be proved to fix a doctor's or surgeon's criminal liability was set at "gross negligence" or "recklessness."

In Suresh Gupta's case, the Supreme Court distinguished between an error of judgment and culpable negligence. It held that criminal prosecution of doctors without adequate medical opinion pointing to their guilt would do great disservice to the community. A doctor cannot be tried for culpable or criminal negligence in all cases of medical mishaps or misfortunes.

A doctor may be liable in a civil case for negligence but mere carelessness or want of due attention and skill cannot be described as so reckless or grossly negligent as to make her/him criminally liable. The courts held that this distinction was necessary so that the hazards of medical professionals being exposed to civil liability may not unreasonably extend to criminal liability and expose them to the risk of imprisonment for alleged criminal negligence.

Hence, the complaint against the doctor must show negligence or rashness of such a degree as to indicate a mental state that can be described as totally apathetic towards the patient. Such gross negligence alone is punishable.

On September 9, 2004, Justices Arijit Pasayat and CK Thakker referred the question of medical negligence to a larger Bench of the Supreme Court. They observed that words such as "gross", "reckless", "competence", and "indifference" did not occur anywhere in the definition of "negligence" under Section 304A of the Indian Penal Code and hence they could not agree with the judgement delivered in the case of Dr Suresh Gupta.

The issue was decided in the Supreme Court in the case of Jacob Mathew vs State of Punjab.[13] The court directed the central government to frame guidelines to save doctors from unnecessary harassment and undue pressure in performing their duties. It ruled that until the government framed such guidelines, the following guidelines would prevail:

A private complaint of rashness or negligence against a doctor may not be entertained without prima facie evidence in the form of a credible opinion of another competent doctor supporting the charge. In addition, the investigating officer should give an independent opinion, preferably of a government doctor. Finally, a doctor may be arrested only if the investigating officer believes that she/he would not be available for prosecution unless arrested.

Preventing Medical Litigation

Some ways/methods to minimize litigation are sited below:
- *Awareness of potential areas of litigation and medicolegal problems:* Doctor should be aware of the risks involved in certain procedures and should have clear knowledge of the changes in legislation which might influence his practice.
- *Good 'doctor-patient' relationship:* Sympathy, good rapport and taking keen interest in the patient's apprehensions and complaints are hallmarks in gaining the patient's confidence. A suspicious patient who has no faith in the physician is a potential litigant.

- *Appropriate training and maintenance of authorized protocol:* Up-to-date and adequate training of medical and nursing staff is needed. It is dangerous to venture beyond one's capability and qualifications. Maintaining a time-tested, well accepted protocol is necessary. It is wise to seek a second opinion.
- *Maintaining standard medical service:* Limited work load and adequate infrastructure are needed to maintain good quality service. Minimum standard for nursing homes or hospitals, whether public or private, must be maintained.
- *Proper counseling and informed consent:* Counseling and informed consent is mandatory before each medical/investigative/operative procedure.
- *Proper investigation:* Any noninvasive/invasive procedures should be done, provided the risks and benefits are duly informed, and written consent has been taken.
- *Adequate supervision and timely referral:* Adequate supervision by a well-organized graded system is recommended. Early detection of complications by resident doctors and timely notification of the consultant, especially in emergency cases, may prevent mishaps.
- *Therapeutic intervention:* Therapeutic procedures should always be performed in places where there is sufficient equipment and qualified staff. Junior doctors should be trained well and supervised in surgical care of the patient.
- *Meticulous record keeping:* Often proper record keeping can prove the doctor innocent in the court. However, fabrication of records after any mishap is dangerous.
- *Morbidity and mortality audits:* Discussions, analysis and constructive criticism of errors and omissions help in improving and maintaining standard of patient care.
- *Medical indemnity insurance:* The doctor must cover himself with indemnity insurance.
- *Medical defense procedure:* Efficient defense lawyer is important to defend one against a malpractice and negligence suit. The lawyer must be aware of the expected standard of patient care.

In case of alleged negligence, following may be helpful for defense:
- No duty owed to patient, i.e. no doctor-patient relationship was established.
- Duty discharged according to prevailing standards.
- *Informed consent for the act:* The patient was duly informed of the consequences.
- Patient was guilty of contributory negligence.
- Therapeutic misadventure.
- Medical maloccurrence.
- Error of judgment. The court has held that the error of judgment is not negligence. If, e.g. one of the risks inherent in an operation takes place or some complication ensues which lessens the benefit that was hoped for, he makes an error of judgment. Moreover, doctor is not responsible if patient does not respond to the treatment.
- Mistake of fact is a situation where a person not intending to do unlawful act, does so because of wrong conclusion or understanding of fact. The guilty mind was never there while doing the act. It can be a factor in reducing civil liability but not criminal liability.
- Res judicata means 'the things have been decided'. According to this principle, once the case is completed between two parties, it cannot be tried again between the same parties. Suppose a patient sues a hospital for any malpractice and the things are decided, he cannot subsequently sue the doctor again separately for the same negligence.

- *Limitation:* The case against the doctor should be filed within 2 years from the date of alleged negligence.
- No fee was charged for the treatment cannot be a defense.

Psychiatry Malpractice Lawsuits and their Causes

Psychiatric treatment is often a difficult process for both doctor and patient. Because of this, strict guidelines have been set out to help doctors make the right diagnoses and prescribe the proper treatments, while providing the best standard of care for patients, and protecting the patient and other individuals from harm. Medical malpractice in the psychiatric fields is as common as other medical fields and often involves more than just the traditional doctor or patient.

Common Forms of Psychiatric Negligence

- *Failure to conduct a proper suicide risk assessment:* The standard of care requires physicians to conduct a proper risk of suicide assessment on every potentially suicidal patient. If a doctor fails to properly assess the patient considering all the relevant factors such as patient history, age, gender, sexual orientation, employment and living standards, then he is at risk for potential litigation.
- *Improper diagnosis or treatment:* While some people believe that many psychiatric diagnoses are ill-defined, this is simply not the case. Any mental health professional should be able to come to a definitive diagnosis assuming the proper patient assessment has occurred. However, if an improper diagnosis is made or if a doctor prescribes the incorrect treatment, a patient or their family has a strong case for malpractice against the doctor or mental health professional.
- *Failure to warn:* Extending further from the traditional doctor and patient relationship, courts have ruled that if a patient makes threats during sessions against another person, the clinician has a duty to warn this person of the potential threat if they believe it is credible. This can often be a difficult determination for the clinician as he/she must balance doctor/patient confidentiality versus their responsibility for the safety of others. If a patient acts on these threats, the victim's families have a reasonable malpractice case to pursue.
- *Boundary violations:* It has been established that there must exist a boundary between the healthcare professional and their patients. If the professional violates these boundaries or attempts to use his/her position as a means to, for example, illicit sexual encounters with their patients, he/she are guilty of malpractice and may be even other felony crimes.

Courts are increasingly recognizing the standard of care required for mental healthcare professionals and, in some areas, their responsibilities can extend far beyond just their patients. It is important for every mental healthcare professional to provide the highest standard of care possible at all times and to maintain the safety of not only their patients but any individuals that have been threatened by the patient. Failure to provide this type of care is grounds for malpractice and mental healthcare professionals are often held liable for these mistakes.

REFERENCES

1. Medical jurisprudence. In: Rao NG (Ed). Textbook of Forensic Medicine and Toxicology, 2nd edn. Jaypee Brothers Medical Publishers (P) Ltd; 2010.
2. Medical Council of India, Appendix I, 1593, in Gazette of India, (Chaitra 16, 1924, Part – III, Section 4), April 26, 2002.
3. Indian Medical Council (Professional conduct, Etiquette and Ethics, Regulations) by MCI, Arman–E-Galib Marg, Kotla Road, New Delhi, 2002.
4. Dikshit PC, HWV Cox (Eds). Medical Jurisprudence and Toxicology, 7th edition. Lexis Nexis Butterworths, 2002.
5. Committee of Bioethics 1993-94: Informed consent, parental permission and assent in paediatric practice. Paediatrics. 1995;2:314-17.
6. Laughron W, Bakken GM. The psychotherapist's responsibility toward third parties under current california law. Western State University Law Review. 1984;12(1):1-33.
7. Kaushal KA. Medical Negligence and Legal Remedies with Special Reference to COPRA, 2nd edition. Universal Law Publication, 2016.
8. Observations of Lord President Clyde in Hunter vs Hanley (1955) SLT 213. In: Nathan HL. Medical Negligence. London: Butterworths; 1957.
9. Whitehouse vs. Jordan (1981) 1 All ER 267 the House of Lords.
10. Calcutta Medical Research Institute vs Bimalesh Chatterjee I (1999) CPJ 13 (NC).
11. Kanhaiya Kumar Singh vs Park Medicare & Research Centre III (1999) CPJ 9 (NC).
12. Mohanan vs Prabha G Nair and another (2004) CPJ 21(SC), of 2004 Feb 4.
13. Criminal Appeal Nos 144-145 of 2004.

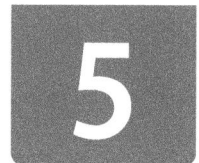

CHAPTER 5

Consent and Capacity Assessment

> **LEARNING OBJECTIVES**
> - Definition, types, legal relevance
> - Doctrine of informed consent
> - Age for consent
> - Capacity assessment
> - Invalid consent
> - When one need not obtain consent
> - Consent in mental healthcare
> - Consent in organ transplantation
> - Consent in research work
> - Caution for consent

Over the years, doctor-patient relationship has turned from traditional paternalistic mode to one incorporating elements of shared decision making, giving autonomy and freedom of expression to both parties. With this, the time has also seen a surge in malpractice suits and lack of consent or inadequate consent or blanket consent has been a point of contention in many of them. Thus, awareness about principles and legality surrounding consent is of paramount importance. Much more important in mental health, where at times nature of illness may have bearing on capacity to give consent, raising several ethical and legal issues.

Definition: Consent (Co= Mutual, Common; Assent= Agreement) means voluntary agreement, compliance or permission.[1]

According to the Section 13 of the Indian Contract Act, two or more persons are said to consent when they agree upon the same thing in the same sense (meeting of the minds).'[2]

■ LEGAL RELEVANCE OF OBTAINING CONSENT

1. To examine, treat or operate upon a patient without consent is assault (battery) in law, even if it is beneficial to the patient and done in good faith.[3]
2. If a doctor fails to give the required information to the patient before taking consent to a particular intervention/treatment, he/she may be charged for negligence.
3. Not taking consent is considered as deficiency in medical services under the section 2(1) of the Consumer Protection Act, 1986.[4]

TYPES OF CONSENT

Consent is broadly of two types; implied and expressed.[5]

1. *Implied consent*: When the patient presents himself at the doctor's clinic or outpatient, it is held to imply that he is agreeable to be examined. Complex procedures other than inspection, palpation, percussion and auscultation do not come under it. For other examinations, like withdrawal of blood for diagnostic purposes, expressed permission should be obtained.
2. *Expressed consent*: Specifically stated by the patient in distinct and explicit language. It can be:
    i. *Oral/verbal consent* is obtained for relatively minor examinations or therapeutic procedures, preferably in presence of disinterested party, like patient's attendant or nurse.
    ii. *Written consent* is to be obtained for:
        - All major diagnostic procedures
        - Psychotherapy

Specific therapeutic interventions such as ECT, rTMS, Clozapine or Disulfiram treatment

- **Oral consent** is legally valid when taken for some specific procedures like injecting medication, drawing blood for pathological examination, gynecological examinations etc. Oral consent can be proved in court if it was taken in the presence of witnesses or if the doctor records in the case record of the patient that oral consent was taken.
- For major procedures and surgery, **written consent** should be taken but if for some reason only oral consent is possible then the doctor should enter it into the case record of the patient.
- The value of **signed written consent** is important for those cases that go to court as a written consent will be of great value for the doctor when he defends himself. According to the Indian Medical Council (Professional Conduct and Ethics) Regulations 2002, before performing an operation written consent should be obtained.
- **Signed by both parties:** Those doctors who take consent to be legal contracts between two parties feel that both the doctor and patient should sign the consent form as this is the basic requirement of a contract, otherwise it becomes null and void. Two witnesses who are uninterested third parties should preferably also sign it.

IMPORTANT ELEMENTS OF CONSENT[5]

i. Voluntariness
ii. Doctrine of informed consent
iii. Capacity to consent (age and mental capacity)

For a consent to be valid all three elements should be present:

i. *Voluntariness:* Consent is said to be free when it is not caused by coercion, undue influence, fraud, misrepresentation, or mistake

ii. *Doctrine of informed consent:* Consent should be on the basis of adequate information concerning the nature of the treatment procedure. Consent should be informed and based on intelligent understanding. The doctor must disclose information regarding:
   - His/her condition or nature of illness
   - Purpose or necessity for further testing
   - Natural course of condition and possible complications
   - Nature of procedure or treatment proposed
   - Risks and benefits of treatment or procedure
   - Risks and benefits of alternative treatment or procedure
   - Prognosis in the absence of intervention
   - Duration and approximate cost of treatment
   - Expected outcome and follow-up.

   Dos and Don'ts
   - The information provided to patients should be simple, clear, in a language patient understands and should include any possible major complications to assist the patient in deciding whether to undergo or decline a procedure (informed refusal).
   - Remote or theoretical risks involved which may frighten or confuse the patient and result in refusal to take treatment may be omitted.
   - There are no clear specifications laid down regarding the quantum of information to be given for informed consent. Therefore, it implies reasonable information which a doctor gauges fit, considering best practices.
   - The standard to which physicians are held in negligence suits is that of a 'reasonable physician' dealing with a 'reasonable patient.'

iii. *Capacity to consent* (age and mental capacity):
   a. **Age for capacity to consent**

   Indian law is not very clear regarding capacity to consent for treatment in general, though Mental Health Care Act (MHCA) 2017 lays it for mental health related decisions. According to **Section 90 IPC,** a child less than **twelve years** of age or insane person cannot give valid consent. By implication from Section 90 IPC, one can say that in general a boy or girl can consent to medical or surgical treatment if he or she is above twelve years of age provided the treatment is intended for his or her benefit and is undertaken in good faith.[6,7]

   Section 88 and Section 90 of the IPC suggest that the age for giving valid consent for any medical procedure is **twelve years.** Hence, a doctor taking consent for medical or surgical treatment from a person aged twelve years or more can be legally said to have taken a valid consent and cannot be held criminally liable on this account.[6,7]

   However, **Sections 87 IPC** mentions eighteen years as the age for giving consent for acts not intended and not known to be likely to cause death or grievous hurt. These acts are not necessarily for the benefit of the person.[6,7]

   Another school of thought however feels that valid consent can only be given at or above **eighteen years** of age. They feel that consent is a contract between two parties

and as the **Indian Contract Act** states that to enter into a contract both parties must be at least eighteen years of age, this should be the age for giving valid consent in medicine. However, it should be noted that the Indian Contract Act is for conditions like marriages, financial agreements etc. and is not specific for the medical profession.[2]
- Guidelines by Ministry of Health and Family Welfare for sexual assault victims examination mention, consent for examination and treatment to be obtained from victim above 12 years of age.[8]
- MHCA 2017 mentions minor as less than 18 years and declares their legal guardian to be their nominated representatives and ones responsible for decision making of mental health care and treatment.[9]

b. **Mental capacity**
Definition: Mental capacity refers to a person's ability to understand, retain, and weigh up information relevant to a decision to arrive at a choice, and then to communicate that choice (Health Concept).[10]
Competence: It refers to the legal consequences of not having the mental capacity (Legal concept).

Capacity includes four key components:
i. *Understanding:* The person needs to recall conversations about issue concerned, to make the link between causal relationships, and to process probabilities for outcomes. Problems with memory, attention span, and intelligence can affect one's understanding.
ii. *Appreciation:* The person should be able to identify the task to be done, likely effect of it on self and others concerned and consequences of it. A lack of appreciation usually stems from a denial or cognitive deficits (lack of a capability to understand) or emotion, or a delusion that the patient is not affected by this situation the same way and will have a different outcome.
iii. *Rationalization or reasoning:* The person needs to be able to weigh the risks and benefits of the decision opted keeping with their goals and best interests, as defined by their personal set of values. This often is affected in psychosis, depression, delirium, and dementia
iv. *Communication:* The person needs to be able to express a choice, and this decision needs to be stable enough to be implemented. Changing one's decision in itself would not bring a patient's capacity into question, so long as the patient was able to explain the rationale behind the switch. Frequent irrational changes back and forth however in the decision-making, could bring capacity into question.[10]

Presumption of capacity: Every person is assumed to be capable and competent to make decisions unless proven otherwise. The presence of a major mental disorder does not in and of itself imply incapacity in decision-making functions.[11]

Capacity is task specific: Despite presence of a mental disorder that may affect capacity, a person may still have the capacity to carry out some decision-making functions. Capacity and competence are task specific, for example.[12]

i. *Capacity to make a treatment decision:* The person must have the ability to: (a) understand the nature of the condition for which the treatment is proposed; (b) understand the nature of the proposed treatment; and (c) appreciate the consequences of giving or withholding consent to treatment **(Table 1)**.

ii *Capacity to select a nominated representative:* The person must have the ability to: (a) understand the nature of the appointment and the duties of the nominated representative as a substitute decision-maker; (b) understand the relationship with the proposed nominated representative; and (c) appreciate the consequences of appointing the nominated representative.

iii. *Capacity to make a financial decision:* The person must have the ability to: (a) understand the nature of the financial decision and the choices available; (b) understand the relationship to the parties to, and/or potential beneficiaries of, the transaction; and (c) appreciate the consequences of making the financial decision.

Table 1: Capacity assessment for treatment-related decision and MHCA **(Flowchart 1)**.

Construct	Assessment	MHCA sections on Capacity
Understanding the relevant information	Ask individual to paraphrase the information explained regarding mental illness and treatment options	**4.(1a) understand the information** that is relevant to take a decision on the treatment or admission or personal assistance
Appreciate the situation and its consequences	Ask individual to describe about medical condition and proposed treatment and likely consequence of taking and not taking treatment	**4.(1b) appreciate** any reasonably **foreseeable** consequence of a decision or lack of decision on the treatment or admission or personal assistance
Reason about treatment options	Ask individual patient to compare treatment options and consequences and to offer reasons for selection of option	
Communicate a choice	Clearly indicate preferred treatment option	**4.(1C) communicate the decision** under sub-clause (*a*) by means of speech, expression, gesture or any other means
The process of reaching on this decision, i.e. the reasoning used to form opinion is more important than the outcome, i.e. the final decision) IF THE DECISION MAKING PROCESS AND REASONING IS INTACT AND EVEN IF IT IS NOT IN ACCORDANCE WITH MEDICAL ADVISE, IT HAS TO BE RESPECTED For example, a person who refuses to have a blood transfusion because it is against their religious beliefs would not be thought to lack capacity. They still understand the reality of their situation and the consequences of their actions. But someone with anorexia who is severely malnourished and rejects treatment because they refuse to accept there is anything wrong with them would be considered incapable. This is because they are regarded as not fully understanding the reality of their situation or their consequences.		Section 4 (3) Where a person makes a decision regarding his mental healthcare or treatment which is perceived by others as inappropriate or wrong, that by itself, shall not mean that the person does not have the capacity to make mental healthcare or treatment decision, so long as the person has the capacity to make mental healthcare or treatment decision under subsection (*1*).

Capacity assessment should be time limited: Capacity changes over time. A finding of lack of capacity should be time-limited (i.e. it will have to be reviewed from time to time), because a person may regain some or complete functionality over time, either with or without treatment of the mental disorder.

CHAPTER 5: Consent and Capacity Assessment

Flowchart 1: Assessing capacity for treatment-related decision.

Provide adequate & relevant information: Inform about illness/condition, treatment/Care proposed, alternative options of other treatment modality and consequence of no treatment/Care. Inform patient also not just caregiver.

WAY OF PROVIDING INFORMATION: Information should be given in language and manner so that patient and caregiver can understand easily. Aim should be to convey about benefits of treatment without coercing, keeping patient's best interest and preferences in mind. Involving patient in **COLLABORATIVE DECISION MAKING** establishes good therapeutic alliance and reduces perceived coercion, promotes autonomy).

If patient has not understood, think **can it be done differently or by a different mental health professional** in a better way, try it.

↓

Assess capacity by assessing understanding, appreciation of consequences and communication

↓

1. Assess **UNDERSTANDING** (It assesses assimilation of FACTUAL knowledge): Ask individual to paraphrase the information explained regarding mental illness/condition and treatment/care options

↓

2. Does individual **APPRECIATE** consequences (It assesses a REASONING and ANALYSIS): Ask individual to describe about medical condition and proposed treatment and likely consequence of taking and not taking treatment

↓

3. COMMUNICATING choice (It assesses judgment): Ask individual what **DECISION** individual arrived at and **WHAT ARE THE REASONS FOR CHOSING A PARTICULAR OPTION** (more important is the reasoning i.e. the process of reaching on this decision than the outcome i.e. the final decision)

↓

OUTCOME OF ASSEESSMENT: For decision on the treatment or admission or personal assistance, **PATIENT HAS** : (a) **Understood the information** provided, or (b) **Appreciated** any reasonably **foreseeable consequence of a decision or lack of decision** or (c) Been able to **communicate the decision by any means**

If answer to any of a/b/c is NO	If answer to ALL a and b and c is YES
Capacity is impaired	Capacity is intact

Therefore, because capacity may fluctuate from time to time, and is not an "all or nothing" concept, it needs to be considered in the context of the specific decision or function to be accomplished.

Determination of incapacity may be made by a health professional, but a judicial body would determine incompetence.

Capacity is the test for competence, and people should not be judged as lacking competence only because they are incapable of making specific kinds of decisions at a specific time.[12]

INVALID CONSENT

Following are the situations in which the consent becomes invalid:[13]
1. If it is not an informed consent.
2. Given for committing a crime or an illegal act, such as criminal abortion.
3. Obtained by misrepresentation of facts or fraud.
4. Given by one who had no legal capacity to give it, for example, a minor or person with mental illness and impaired decision-making capacity.

Exceptions to Obtaining Consent

1. In **medical emergencies** consent need not be obtained if circumstances are such that it is impossible for that person to give consent (Section 92 IPC).[7]
2. Locoparentis: In an emergency involving children when their parents or guardians are not available, consent is taken from the person in charge of the child, e.g. school teacher.[7]
3. **Provision of emergency treatment in mental healthcare Act 2017**[9]
   According to the Chapter XII Section 94 of the Act, following provisions are described:
   Allowed treatment: Any medical treatment, including treatment for mental illness, may be provided by any registered medical practitioner to a person with mental illness either at a health establishment or in community, subject to the informed consent of the nominated representative, if available, and where it is immediately necessary to prevent—
   i. death or irreversible harm to the health of the person; or
   ii. the person inflicting serious harm to himself or to others; or
   iii. the person causing serious damage to property belonging to himself or to others where such behavior is believed to flow directly from the person's mental illness.
   Prohibited treatment: It does not allow medical officer or psychiatrist to give treatment which is not directly related to the emergency situations described above or use electroconvulsive therapy.
   Time frame for emergency treatment: Emergency treatment in this section shall be limited to seventy-two hours or till the person with mental illness has been assessed at a mental health establishment, whichever is earlier except in national disasters (7 days).
4. **Court ordered evaluations** for competency to stand trial, consent is not required. In such a case a psychiatrist should inform the subject and explain that the evaluation is legally required and if the subject refuses to participate in the evaluation this fact will be included in any report or testimony.[13] **An arrested person** can be examined without consent if requested to do so by a police officer not below the rank of a Sub-Inspector (Section 53 IPC) if examination may provide evidence to the commission of the offence. (This includes examination of blood, bloodstains, semen, swabs in cases of sexual offences, sputum and sweat, hair samples and fingernail clippings using modern and scientific techniques including DNA profiling.[13]
5. A **prisoner can be treated without consent** in the interest of society.[13]

With regard to any person charged with criminal acts who has not been arrested, *ethical considerations preclude forensic evaluation prior to access to, or availability of legal counsel.* The **only exception is an examination for the purpose of rendering emergency medical care and treatment.**[13]

Consent for Removal of Organ for Transplantation
- *From a living person*: Section 3 of "The Transplantation of Human organs Act, 1994" defines authorizes the removal of any of his/her organs for therapeutic purposes. Therefore, it is illegal to remove of organs from the body of a person of less than 18 years even with his/her consent. If the person is above 18 years, conscious and of sound mental health his/her own consent is required for removal of organs from his/her body.[14]
- *From a dead body*: (1) No organ can be removed, it in request is to be carried out on the dead body. (2) To remove organs from the body, there must exist an oral or written consent of the deceased that have been obtained at any time in the presence of two or more witness, during his last illness. Even if the consent was given by the deceased during life, permission must be obtained from the person in possession of the body.[14]

Consent for. For video and audio recording: Doctor should inform the patient before recording (except in situations in which consent may be understood from patient's cooperation with a procedure, e.g. radiographic investigation) and obtain his consent. But doctor may record without consent in exceptional circumstances, such as when it is believed that child has been victim of abuse. If a recording has been made in the course of investigation or treatment of a patient but the doctor now wishes to use it for another purpose, e.g. Publication in textbook, journals, etc., the patient's consent must be obtained.[13]

Consent for research: before obtaining consent from the potential subject the doctor must inform about:
- Purpose of the study.
- How the research relates to the subject's underlying condition and the impact on his wellbeing.[13]

■ CAUTIONS TO EXERCISE WHILE TAKING CONSENT
i. Nothing is said to be done in good faith which is done without due care and attention (Sec. 52 IPC).[7]
ii. In civil cases, examination should not be done without the consent of the person.[13]
iii. In criminal cases, the victim cannot be examined without his/her consent. The court cannot force a person to get medically examined.[13]
   - In rape cases, victim should not be examined without her written consent.
   - In medico-legal cases of pregnancy, delivery and abortion, the woman should not be examined without her consent.
iv. Under Sec. 54 CrPC, an arrested person may be examined by a doctor at his request to detect evidence in his favor, a copy of the report is to be furnished by the doctor to the arrested person.[7]

v. Consent of one's spouse is not necessary for the treatment of other. Husband or wife has no right to refuse consent to any intervention, which is required to safeguard the health of the partner.[13]
vi. For contraceptive sterilization and artificial insemination, consent of both husband and wife should be obtained.[13]
vii. Consent is procedure specific: Consent given for a diagnostic procedure cannot be considered as consent for therapeutic treatment. Consent given for a specific treatment/procedure is not valid for conducting some other treatment/procedure.
viii. Consent for examining or observing a patient for educational purpose must be taken separately and not to be subsumed in blanket consent for treatment.[13]
ix. **Blanket consent is not valid:** Consent should be procedure specific. An all-encompassing consent to the effect 'I authorize so and so to carry out any test/procedure/surgery in the course of my treatment' is not valid.
x. **Fresh consent should be taken for a repeat procedure** or a prior consent mentioning number of sessions needed to be taken in anticipation, e.g. in ECT.
xi. **Patient has the right to refuse treatment**: Competent patients have the legal and moral right to refuse treatment, even in life-threatening emergency situations. In such cases informed refusal must be obtained and documented, over the patient's witnessed signature.
xii. **Consent should be properly documented.**
xiii. **Unilaterally executed consents are void**: Consent signed only by the patient and not by the doctor is not valid.[15]
xiv. **Witnessed consents are legally more dependable:** The role of a witness is even more important in instances when the patient is illiterate, and one needs to take his/her thumb impression.
xv. **Patient is free to withdraw his consent anytime:** When consent is withdrawn during the performance of a procedure, the procedure should be stopped. The doctor may address to patient's concerns and may continue the treatment only if the patient agrees. If stopping a procedure at that point puts patient's or other's life in danger, the doctor may continue with the procedure till such a risk no longer exists.
xvi. **Consent for illegal procedures is invalid:** There can be no valid consent for direct ECT which is prohibited procedure as per MHCA.
xvii. **Consent is no defense in cases of professional negligence.**

REFERENCES

1. Palmer RN. A Physician's Guide to Clinical Forensic Medicine. Humana Press, New Jersey 2000;17-23.
2. Singh A. Textbook on Law of Contract and Specific Relief (2016 ed.). Eastern Book Company. p. 488. ISBN 9789351453482.
3. Consent & capacity Assessment, 2008, 2SCC 1 Para 32.
4. Kumar V. An Analysis of Consumer Protection Laws in India. iPleaders. Available at: https://blog.ipleaders.in/analysis-consumer-protection-laws-india/ Retrieved 10 December 2017.

5. Yadwad BS, Gouda H. Consent—Its Medico Legal Aspects J Assoc Physicians India. 2005;53:891-4.
6. Mukesh Yadav. Age of Consent in Medical Profession: A Food for Thought. JIAFM, 2007; 29 (2) ISSN: 0971-0973 80 -5
7. Ram Narain Lal, Beni Prasad. The Indian Penal Code 1860 (Act No XLV) As Amended up to date. Law Publishers. Allahabad 1980.
8. Guidelines and protocols of Medico-legal care for survivors/victims of sexual violence. Ministry of Health and Family Welfare. Government of India. November 2014.
9. The Mental Healthcare Act 2017. Ministry of Law and Justice, Government of India Publication, New Delhi.
10. Appelbaum PS. Assessing Competence to Consent to Treatment. The New Engl and Journal of Medicine. 2007;357:1834-40.
11. Kim SYH. When does decisional impairment become decisional incompetence? Ethical and methodological issues in capacity research in schizophrenia. Schizophr Bull. 2006;32:92-7.
12. Competence, capacity and guardianship chapter in book: WHO resource book on mental health human rights and legislation. World Health Organization. 2005;39-40.
13. Pillay VV. Textbook of Forensic Medicine and Toxicology. 14th Edition-2004. 27-29.
14. Transplantation of Human Organs Acts Amendment 2011. Gazette of Government of India. Ministry of Health and Family Welfare, notified on 27 March 2014. Available at: https://mohfw.gov.in/sites/default/files/THOA-Rules-2014%20%281%29.pdf. Last accessed on 07.02.18.
15. Kumar A. Mullick P, Prakash S. et al. Consent and the Indian medical practitioner. Indian J Medical Anesthesia, 2015;59(11): 695-700.

CHAPTER

Psychiatry Case Records and Right to Access Records

> **LEARNING OBJECTIVES**
> - Medical records: Definition, general principles
> - Confidentiality and psychiatry case records
> - Fiduciary relationship
> - Legislative statutes of relevance to medical records
> - Right to Information Act 2005 and medical records
> - Some relevant case laws in healthcare setting in RTI
> - Mental Health Care Act (MHCA) 2017 and medical records

Medical records refer to documents containing a written account of any patient's medical history, physical findings, results of diagnostic tests, medications, therapeutic procedures and day-wise progress notes recorded by a medical practitioner.[1]

GENERAL PRINCIPLES CONCERNING IMPORTANCE OF MEDICAL RECORDS

- It is a documentary evidence of patient's ailment, management done and response to same.
- As far as ownership of record is considered, medical records are property of the hospital and personal data included in them is the property of patient.
- Whether record keeping be manual or electronic, it is responsibility of the doctor and hospital to maintain its safety and ensure confidentiality.
- Consent of patient is mandatory for using any data for research purpose, however, for evaluating quality of health care provided and statistical purpose, hospitals have right to use the data without jeopardizing patient's confidentiality or divulging any individual's identity in public domain.
- *Records concerning medicolegal cases (MLC):* Original X-ray/CT/MRI films of such cases should be kept safely in hospital. They are not to be released to patient, however, copies of report of same can be given. It should also not be given to police. However, photocopy of record can be given on request of investigating officer (IO).
- An unsigned medical record has no legal validity.
- The patient or their nominated representatives have right to ask for copies of medical records. Failure to provide same amounts to deficiency in hospital service and institutional negligence.[2]

- *Medical records as evidence in court:* As per amendment of section 3 of the Indian Evidence Act, 1872 done in 1961, medical records are acceptable as documentary evidence.
- Any medical record written after discharge or death retrospectively has no legal value.
- Tempering with records is an offence.
- Changing the records is not permitted, in case of any correction, the written part can be struck out by a horizontal line with signature and then can be rewritten mentioning the date and time of re-writing.

Legal context of relevance: Medical records with or without health professional expert can be summoned in a court of law in the following cases:

1. Medical negligence cases under Consumer Protection Act or in criminal courts
2. Motor accident claims tribunal-related accident cases
3. Corroborating nature of injury or weapon used in criminal cases
4. Road traffic accident cases under the Motor Accident Claims Tribunal (MACT) Act for deciding on the amount of compensation
5. In insurance claims to determine cause of death and illness duration
6. For determining compensation as per Workmen's Compensation Act according to the nature of injury
7. Right of patient to access information under Right to Information Act, 2005
8. Right of patient to access information under Mental Health Care Act, 2017.

Court can issue orders to only verify or present medical records alone in court. In that case, hospital's medical record officer can also present it to the court. In some cases, doctors are summoned to appear in the Court of Law along with medical documents and give evidence based on the same.

PRIVACY, CONFIDENTIALITY AND PSYCHIATRY CASE RECORDS

General Confidentiality Principles for Healthcare Settings

Privacy and confidentiality are important cornerstone of a doctor-patient relationship. A client must feel enough comfort to report to the doctor about physical complaints, mental agony, and sensitive personal information of relevance for enabling physician to undertake a holistic evaluation. A patient shares such information deposing great trust in doctor and presuming, it will be used for health purpose only and confidentiality shall be ensured. Health-related information or any personal information shared during that process can have significant repercussions if divulged in public domain. Certain medical and psychiatric illnesses have significant social stigma attached to them and can lead to loss of job opportunity, relationship discord and social alienation. In a healthcare context, patient confidentiality and the protection of privacy is the foundation of the doctor-patient relationship. Thus, it is imperative for healthcare professionals to maintain confidentiality as a duty towards patient.

Element of Fiduciary Relationship in a Patient-doctor Relationship

Fiduciary: This has been derived from latin word "fiducia" meaning "trust". The Advanced Law Lexicon defines "fiduciary" as a person who holds a position of trust with another party (individual or group of persons) and is obliged to act for benefit of that party within scope of that relationship.[3]

Fiduciary Relationship

The Advanced Law Lexicon defines "fiduciary" as a relationship wherein one party places trust on the fiduciary who has duty to act in benefit of former."[3]

"Fiduciary relationship usually arise in one of the four situations:[3]

1. When one person places trust in the faithful integrity of another, who as a result gains superiority or influence over the first,
2. When one person assumes control and responsibility over another,
3. When one person has a duty to act or give advice to another on mattes falling within the scope of the relationship, or
4. When there is a specific relationship that has traditionally be recognized as involving fiduciary duties, as with a doctor and patient.[3]"

Fiduciary Duty

It is the highest standard of duty as a fiduciary should fulfill following rules:

1. *No conflict rule:* A fiduciary must not place himself in a position where his own interests conflict with that of his customer or the beneficiary. There must be real sensible possibility of conflict.
2. *No profit rule:* A fiduciary must not profit from his position at the expense of his customer, the beneficiary.
3. *Undivided loyalty rule:* A fiduciary owes undivided loyalty to the beneficiary, not to place himself in a position where his duty towards one person conflicts with a duty that he owes to another customer. A consequence of this duty is that a fiduciary must make available to a customer all the information that is relevant to the customer's affairs
4. *Duty of confidentiality:* Fiduciary must only use information obtained in confidence and must not use it for his own advantage, or for the benefit of another person."[3]

In a Judgment, Supreme Court of India v. SC Agarawal & Anr. WP (C) No. 227/2009, dated 20.09.2009 (Del), it is discussed that the following kinds of relationships may broadly be categorized as fiduciary:[4]

1. Lawyer/client
2. Doctor/patient
3. Trustee/Beneficiary (Section 88, Indian Trust Act,1882)
4. Legal guardians/wards (Section 20, Guardians and Wards Act,1890)
5. Parent/child
6. Liquidator/company
7. Receivers, trustees in bankruptcy and assignees in insolvency/creditors.

FIDUCIARY RELATIONSHIP AS APPLIED IN HEALTHCARE SETTING

- Doctors by virtue of their knowledge and skill are in a position to influence and have a duty to advise the patient.
- Patient vests interest in judgment and skill of doctor.
- Doctors have a duty to act in best interest of patient.
- *Hippocratic Oath:* Trust is the most important construct on which doctor-patient relationship is based and it is very well reflected in Hippocratic Oath, where it is said that doctors must act for benefit of the patient and should strictly refrain from any wrongdoing or exploitation of patient.
- As per the ethical principles of doctor-patient relationship, doctors are expected to demonstrate:
    - Duty to confidentiality towards information received in therapeutic relationship
    - To show undivided loyalty by keeping duty towards patient more important than anything, e.g. a doctor treating patients during epidemic of a contagious disease keeping patients interest as priority than his own interests (risk of contracting disease)
    - No conflicting duty and no profit rule by avoiding entering into any other relationship with patient, e.g. personal or business related which if done will be constituted as "boundary crossing or violation."

Thus, doctors share fiduciary relationship with their patient and are legally bound to maintain privacy and confidentiality unless some larger public interest is being served as decide by competent authority.

PRINCIPLES OF CONFIDENTIALITY SPECIFIC FOR MENTAL HEALTH SETTINGS

Besides above general principles, psychiatry case records unlike many other medical records are also different in following dimensions:[5]

1. *Personal and sensitive information:* Unlike physical illnesses case records, psychiatry case records have information which is sensitive and personal in nature containing some historical facts, recollections, fears, fantasies, sexual history, etc.
2. *Compartmentalized confidentiality:* History collected is from many other informants besides patient and is provided on the grounds of maintaining compartmentalized confidentiality for only purpose of facilitating holistic treatment. Many a times, information is divulged by several informants on pretext of maintaining compartmentalized confidentiality by therapist to facilitate treatment, but avoid any untoward ramifications of disclosure of such sensitive information on one's personal, interpersonal or professional life.
3. *Objective, subjective and deductive impressions:* Besides objective facts, health records also contain certain subjective and deductive impressions made by therapist.
   Thus, psychiatry case records cannot be equated loosely with any other record and case by case discretion has to be exercised.
- **Legislative statutes of relevance to medical records—confidentiality and disclosure (Table 1):** There are no definite guidelines in India regarding how long to retain

medical records. The hospitals follow their own pattern retaining the records for varied periods of time.

  i. *"Consumer Protection Act, 1986:* Hon'ble Supreme Court in a matter ("Indian Medical Association vs VP Shantha & Ors on 13 November, 1995") stated that as consumer of service patients have right to know about the details of services provided and hence both public and private medical services are under ambit of Consumer Protection Act.[4] Under the provisions of the Limitation Act, 1963, and Section 24A of the Consumer Protection Act, 1986, a complaint has to be filed within 2 years, thus, it is prudent to maintain records for 2 years for outpatient records and 3 years for inpatient and surgical cases. However there are provisions of the Consumer Protection Act allowing for condoning the delay in appropriate cases. Thus, in some cases, records may even be needed after 3 years. It is important to note that in pediatric cases a medical negligence case can even be filed by the child after acquiring the age of majority."
  ii. *Code of Medical Ethics Regulations, 2002:* All registered medical practitioners are bound by medical ethics code of Indian Medical Council, which states as follows in regard of medical record keeping and confidentiality:[6]
      - *Record maintenance:* Section 1.3 states that medical records of indoor patients must be maintained for three years and should be produced on request of patient or authorized attendant or legal authorities within 72 hours.[5]

Table 1: Legislative statutes of relevance to medical records—confidentiality and disclosure.

Consumer Protection Act, 1986	• Both private as well as public medical services are covered under Consumer Protection Act • Patients as a consumers of services have right to know details about the services provided to them • Maintain records for 2 years for OPD and 3 years for inpatient and surgical cases
Code of Medical Ethics Regulations, 2002	• All registered medical practitioners in India, both private as well as government service are bound to code of medical ethics of Indian Medical Council • Indoor medical records to be maintained for 3 years and to be produced on request of patient or authorized attendant or legal authorities within 72 hours • Ensure confidentiality • Maintain record of medical certificate issued
Directorate General of Health Services (DGHS), Ministry of Health and Family Welfare	• Responsibility of hospital to keep medical records is: • *Digitalized format:* Up to 10 years or as per availability • *Hard copy:* Three years for outpatient and inpatient and in MLC cases, for 10 years or till case is dismissed
Right to Information Act, 2005	• The legislation confers on all citizens the right of access to the information and, correspondingly, makes the dissemination of such information an obligation on all public authorities, promoting transparency and accountability • Section 8 information forbidden from disclosure: Information obtained in Fiduciary relationship
Mental Health Care Act (MHCA), 2017	• Chapter V Section 25 patients will have right to access their 'basic medical records (BMR).' For OPD/IPD/Camps, BMR has been defined differently in Chapter II Section 6 of "The Mental Healthcare (Rights of Persons with Mental Illness) Rules, 2018"

- *Confidentiality:* Section 2.2 states that physician must respect the information about patient including his life and character and should not be disclosed unless required by law. However, physicians may disclose the information, if he consider potential harm to a healthy person weigh over privacy of patient and should act as he wish his own family member be treated in similar manner.
- *Disclosure:* Section 7.14 states that disclosure of patient's information shall be professional misconduct except if disclosed to (i) the court of law under orders of the presiding Judge, (ii) safeguard serious and identifiable risk to a specific person or community, and (iii) public health authorities in case of communicable/notifiable diseases.
- *Medical certificates record maintenance:* Section 1.3.3 states that "Maintain a register of certificates with the full details of medical certificates issued with at least one identification mark of the patient and his signature".
- *Computerization of records:* Section 1.3.4 states that "Efforts should be made to computerize medical records for quick retrieval."

iii. *Directorate General of Health Services (DGHS), Ministry of Health and Family Welfare guidelines for patient record retention:* Responsibility of hospital to keep medical records is: up to 10 years or as per availability in **digitalized format.** In **hard copy,** it is 3 years for outpatient and inpatient and in MLC cases, for 10 years or till case is dismissed.[1]

iv. *Medicolegal records:* The records that are the subject of medicolegal cases should be maintained until the final disposal of the case even though only a complaint or notice is received.

v. *Pre-Natal Diagnostic Test Act, 1994 (PNDT):* The provisions of specific Acts like the Pre-Conception Pre-Natal Diagnostic Test Act, 1994 (PCPNDT), Environmental Protection Act, etc. necessitate proper maintenance of records that have to be retained for periods as specified in the Act. Section 29 of the PNDT Act, 1994 requires that all the documents be maintained for a period of 2 years or until the disposal of the proceedings. The PNDT Rules, 1996 requires that when the records are maintained on a computer, a printed copy of the record should be preserved after authentication by the person responsible for such record.[1]

vi. *Right to Information Act, 2005:*[7] In 2005, the Parliament enacted Right to Information (RTI) Act (2005). The legislation confers on all citizens the right of access to the information and, correspondingly, makes the dissemination of such information an obligation on all public authorities, promoting *transparency and accountability.*[7]
- *Coverage:* It covers whole India except Jammu and Kashmir (Jammu and Kashmir passed its own *Freedom of Information Act* in 2004).
- *Jurisdiction:* Covers **offices of Public Authorities** established, owned or substantially financed by the Central Government, the State Governments and the Administration of the Union Territories (will include, *Panchayats,* municipalities and other local bodies) including non-governmental agencies also receiving government funding.

- *Implementation and supervision:* Every public authority to have public information office (PIO) appointed in each concerned department for answering RTI queries. Supervisory role lies with Central Information Commission (CIC) and State Information Commission (SIC) in each state.
- **What is Information (Section 2)?**
  Any records, documents, memos, emails, opinions, advices, press releases, circulars, orders, logbooks, contracts, reports, papers, samples, models, data material held in any electronic form.
- **What is Record (Section 2)? Record means: Section 2**
  a. Any document, manuscript and file;
  b. Any microfilm, microfiche and facsimile copy of a document;
  c. Any reproduction of image or images embodied in such microfilm (whether enlarged or not); and
  d. Any other material produced by a computer or any other device.
- **What is Right to Information (Section 2)?**
  – Right to inspect works, documents, records
  – Right to take notes, extracts or certified copies
  – Right to take samples
  – Right to obtain information in electronic form
  – Right to information whose disclosure is in the public interest

  Information which cannot be denied to Parliament or State Legislature shall not be denied to any person.
- **What is exempted from disclosure under Right to Information (Section 8)?**
  – Information that would prejudicially affect the sovereignty, integrity, security, scientific or economic interest and relation with a foreign state
  – Information which would lead to commission of an offence
  – **Information whose release is forbidden by a court or tribunal or disclosure which might constitute contempt of court**
  – Information whose release may lead to breach of privileges of Parliament or State Legislatures.
  – Commercial and trade secrets, intellectual property, etc. that would harm competitive position of third party.
  – Information available to a person in his fiduciary relationship (information shared between client and lawyer or landlord and tenant or patient and doctor) unless larger public interest [Section 8(1)e]
  – Information received in confidence from a foreign government
  – If information disclosure endangers life and physical safety of any person
  – If it is about a source of information or assistance given in confidence of law enforcement or security purposes
  – **If it is likely to impede investigation and prosecution processes** [Section 8(1)h]
  – Cabinet papers including deliberations of Ministers, Secretaries and other officers (but decisions and related reasons contained in them will be made public after the decision has been taken and the matter is complete or over)

- Personal information the disclosure of which has no relationship to any public activity or interest, or which would cause unwarranted invasion of the privacy of the individual unless the larger public interest justifies disclosure (Section 8(1)j)

  All exemptions subject to public interest override. If public interest outweighs harm to the public authority information must be disclosed. The power to decide whether public interest is with the Public Information Officer and the Appellate Authorities.

- **Partial disclosure under Right to Information (Section 10)?**
  Partial access to information contained in records covered by exemption clause is allowed.
- **Who is third party? (Sections 2, 11)**
  Any person other than the requestor of information. This category includes another Public Authority also.[7]

Debatable issues

- What is a *public authority?*
  The definition of 'public authorities' under **RTI Act** has been a contentious issue. In past few years even many private entities (such as schools, colleges and sports associations) have been declared public authorities under RTI Act.
  "Public authority" is defined in Section 2(h) of the RTI Act. It states: "public authority" means any authority or body or institution of self-government established or constituted:[7]
  a. By or under the Constitution;
  b. By any other law made by Parliament;
  c. By any other law made by state legislature;
  d. By notification issued or order made by the appropriate government, and includes any:
     i. Body owned, controlled or substantially financed;
     ii. Non-government organization substantially financed, directly or indirectly by funds provided by the appropriate government;

The Act thus defines public authorities in two parts:[8]

1. *The first part of the definition* [clauses 2(h)-(a) to (d)] clearly delineate bodies created by the Constitution of India (Union and State Executives, Election Commission, etc.), by laws made by Parliament and state legislatures (Central and state universities, regulators such as RBI, SEBI, TRAI, etc.), and by government orders or notifications (Planning Commission) as public authorities.

   Area of controversy: That has emerged in relation to the first part of the definition—i.e. bodies created by law—was regarding whether entities registered under various laws become public authorities merely by reason of their incorporation or registration. The Delhi High Court has decided this issue, and unambiguously stated that the mere establishment of a body under a statute will not automatically render it a public authority for the purposes of the RTI Act.[7] Therefore, companies incorporated under the Companies Act, 1956, societies and trusts registered under laws providing for their creation and registration do not become public authorities merely by virtue of Section 2(h)(d) of the RTI Act.

2. *The second part of the definition* broadens the scope of the definition of a public authority to include anybody owned, controlled or substantially financed, and any non-governmental body substantially financed by the appropriate government. *This second part of the definition has been the subject of much controversy largely because it leaves the question of what constitutes (a) ownership, (b) control or/and (c) substantial financing open to interpretation.*[8]

Some relevant case laws passed by CIC/SIC under RTA 2005 concerning hospitals:

Since "public interest" has no clear definition and has been subject to interpretation by competent authorities [Central Information Commission (CIC) and State Information Commission (SIC)] on merit of individual cases, so, for a better understanding, some of the case laws have been highlighted below as per systematic analysis done by Jain et al in 2017:[9]

- Case laws regarding exempting authorities form information disclosure
  - In an RTI case "Arjesh Kumar Madhok vs. Centre for Fingerprinting & Diagnostics, 2007", CIC exempted authority from providing child's medical test information to father stating that tests were done on mother's request which fulfills fiduciary relationship and there is no public interest apparent for CIC to invade into an individual's privacy.[10]
  - In RTI case "Shravan Kumar vs IHBAS, 2009," citing similar grounds, CIC exempted hospital from disclosing wife's medical information to husband.[11]
- Case laws regarding information disclosure instruction to authorities
  - In an RTI case "Surupsingh Hrya Naik vs State of Maharashtra, 2007," SIC mandated hospital to disclose information in public interest regarding a patient who was an influential politician and had spent most of his imprisonment period in a luxurious hospital facility for some suspected medical conditions.[12]
  - In an RTI case "Rashmi Dixit Matiman vs IHBAS, 2011" where patient herself was denied information by psychiatry hospital authority stating that while obtaining information from family and relatives, doctors are bound to maintain compartmentalized confidentiality and they on the same grounds also had fiduciary relationship with family members and relatives. CIC instructed hospital to provide information to the patient. Case is further subjudice in a higher court of law.[13]
  - In an RTI case "Jyoti Jeena vs IHBAS, 2015" wife asked for husband's medical records stating she was subject to physical torture due to husband's mental illness. Hospital refused to provide information to any third party under section 8(1)(e). However, CIC concluded that wife has right to know the information to facilitate exercising her right to seek divorce under Hindu Marriage Act and she should be prevented from further cruelty perpetrated by husband because of mental illness and considered in favor of disclosure of information by hospital in larger public interest, decision was further challenged in higher court of law and stay was taken on previous orders. The case raises an important debate that will giving information to spouse regarding a person's mental illness irrespective of index patient's consent not violate the rights of persons with mental illness. The case provokes several ethical and legal debates for entire mental health fraternity and legal parlance.[14]

- "CIC also extended its coverage over to private hospitals stating since private hospitals are under regulations of public authority like IMC Act, CPA Act, Directorate of Health Services and Clinical Establishments (Registration & Regulation) Act 2011, thereby all hospitals whether private or government are under jurisdiction of RTI and all hospitals have duty to provide information in compliance with IMC Act, CPA Act and RTI Act ("Prabhat Kumar vs Directorate of Health Services, 2014")". [9,15]

vii. *Mental Health Act (MHA) 1987:* MHA states that the board of visitors can inspect admission documents, medical certificates and document their findings for record but are not entitled to inspect personal records which in the opinion of the medical officer are confidential in nature. However, it neither defines nature of what to be considered as "personal record" nor established any data retention, security or access standards for records.[16]

viii. **Mental Health Care Act (MHCA) 2017**
- **Right to information** of Chapter II, Section 22 of MHCA states that: A person with mental illness and his nominated representative shall have the rights to the following information, namely:
  a. Criteria of admission and provisions of Act under which admitted
  b. Of his right to make an application to the concerned Board for a review of the admission
  c. Nature of person's mental illness and the proposed treatment plan which includes information about treatment proposed and the known side effects of the proposed treatment
  d. Receive the information in a language and form that such person can understand.
     In case complete information cannot be given to the person with mental illness at the time of the admission or the start of treatment, it shall be given to nominated representative of patient at that time and to the index patient when he/she is in a position to receive it.
- **Right to confidentiality** of Chapter II, Section 23 of MHCA states that: A person with mental illness shall have the right to confidentiality in respect of his mental health, mental health care, treatment and physical health care. The right to confidentiality of person with mental illness shall also apply to all information stored in electronic or digital format in real or virtual space. All health professionals shall have a duty to keep all such information confidential except when release of information is needed to:
  a. Enable nominated representative from fulfilling his duties under this Act
  b. Provide care and treatment by other health/mental health professionals
  c. To protect any other person from harm or violence
  d. To protect against the harm identified shall be released
  e. Is necessary to prevent threat to life
  f. Upon an order by concerned Board or the Central Authority or High Court or Supreme Court or any other statutory authority competent to do so and
  g. Protect larger public interests of public safety and security.

- Chapter II, Section 24 is regarding **Restriction on release of information in respect of mental illness.** It states that no photograph or any other information relating to a person with mental illness undergoing treatment at a mental health establishment shall be released to the media without the consent of the person with mental illness.
- Chapter II, Section 25 is regarding **Right to access medical records.** It states that all persons with mental illness shall have the right to access their basic medical records as prescribed in Chapter II Section 6 of "The Mental Healthcare (Rights of Persons with Mental Illness) Rules, 2018". But rule is silent about period till when record is to be retained. Also the rules mention, A person with mental illness may apply for a copy of his **basic inpatient medical record** by making a **request in writing in Form-A,** and **within fifteen days** from the date of receipt of the request, MHE to provide same in Form B, but what is status of OPD records is not clear.
- The **mental health professional in charge of such records may withhold specific information** in the medical records if disclosure would result in:
  a. Serious mental harm to the person with mental illness; or
  b. Likelihood of harm to other persons.

When any information in the medical records is withheld from the person, the mental health professional shall inform the person with mental illness of his right to apply to the concerned Board for an order to release such information.[17]

Full information disclosure to patients and relatives cannot be a simple exercise to be uniformly followed in all cases. It raises a bigger issue of having a formal assessment of capacity of client to receive the information and the likely impact of receiving the information on one's mental health in the best interest of patient. Also, distinction in disclosure has to be maintained in request received from patient vis-a-vis as any other family member other than index client to prevent abuse of such information against index client except when warranted by court of law. Keeping in mind the sensitive nature of psychiatry information, the laws should not deter patients and family members from sharing the complete information or therapist from documentation. So, a fine balance needs to be strike between duty of therapists toward patients and public interests. Determining when to disclose overriding patient's right of confidentiality over a larger public interest is going to be difficult task for public information officers and appellate authorities cognitively as well as ethically.

REFERENCES

1. Biswas G. Medical jurisprudence and ethics. Review of Forensic Medicine and Toxicology, 3rd edn. Jaypee Brothers Medical Publishers; 2015.
2. Thomas J. Medical records and issues in negligence. Indian J Urol. 2009;25(3):384-88.
3. Available at: www.dhirassociates.com/images/Fiduciary-Relationship-RBI-NEW.pdf. Last accessed on 07.02.18.
4. Available at: https://indiankanoon.org/doc/84476ZASdrc632/ Last accessed on 07.02.18.
5. Available at: https://indiankanoon.org/doc/723973/ Last accessed on 07.02.18.
6. Available at: https://www.mciindia.org/.../rulesnregulations/codeofMedicalEthicsRegulations2002 Last accessed on 07.02.18.

7. Nayak V, Rodrigues C. The Right to Information Act, 2005: Summary. Commonwealth Human Rights Initiative, New Delhi. Available at: www.humanrightsinitiative.org/programs/ai/rti/india/.../rti_act_2005_summary.pdf. Last accessed on 07.02.18.
8. Available at: www.accountabilityindia.in/sites/.../rti_brief_no._5-_who_is_a_public_authority_0.pd. Last accessed on 07.02.18.
9. Jain S, Jain H, Srivastava AS, et al. Indian legislation "Right o Information Act": An ethical dilemma for medical professionals. Asian J Psych 2007;25:161-2.
10. Arjesh Kumar Madhok vs. Centre for Fingerprinting & Diagnostics, 2007. [WWW Document], n.d. URL http://cic.gov.in/CIC-Orders/Decision_26102007_06.pdf Last accessed on 07.02.18.
11. Shravan Kumar vs IHBAS, 2009. [WWW Document], n.d. URL https://indiankanoon.org/doc/1396043/ Last accessed on 07.02.18.
12. Surupsingh Hrya Naik vs State of Maharashtra, 2007. [WWW Document], n.d. URL https://indiankanoon.org/doc/570038/ Last accessed on 07.02.18.
13. Rashmi Dixit Matiman vs IHBAS, 2011. [WWW Document], n.d. URL https://indiankanoon.org/doc/111032562/ Last accessed on 07.02.18.
14. Jyoti Jeena vs IHBAS, 2015. [WWW Document], n.d. URL https://indiankanoon.org/doc/51016925/ (Accessed 28 August 2016). Narayanan V, Bista B, Koshy C, et al., 2010. Last accessed on 07.02.18.
15. Prabhat Kumar vs Directorate of Health Services, 2014. [WWW Document], n.d. URL http://jksic.nic.in/E%20-library/Prabat%20Kumar%20-%20Fortis.pdf Last accessed on 07.02.18.
16. Mental Health Act 1987, Government of India Publication, New Delhi.
17. Mental Healthcare Act 2017, Government of India Publication, New Delhi.

SECTION III

General Principles of Forensic Psychiatry Evaluation

CHAPTER 7

Approach to a Forensic Psychiatry Interview and Case Taking

> **LEARNING OBJECTIVES**
> - Basic principles of forensic psychiatry assessment
> - Indications of forensic interview
> - Conducting assessment

Sound case assessment is the foundation stone of a good case analysis in forensic psychiatry. Quality of a forensic psychiatry report depends on how well the foundation has been laid. Current chapter will discuss basic principles of forensic psychiatry assessment.

CONTEXT OF FORENSIC PSYCHIATRY INTERVIEW[1]

Psychiatry assessment varies in its form and detail as per the context for which assessment is sought for and its implications needed thereof. A psychiatry assessment in its approach and purpose will differ for the same patient of psychosis being evaluated in hospital setting for treatment purpose than to a court ordered evaluation of same patient for fitness to stand trial in a jail setting. In forensic psychiatry evaluation, following things will prominently differ from usual therapeutic assessments:

Difference of purpose: Duty of forensic psychiatrist is towards state's welfare and to assist law enforcement agencies in reaching to a fair decision than towards individual therapeutic benefit.

Difference of relationship: Relationship between patient and doctor is an evaluator-evaluee relationship in forensic psychiatry setting than usual therapeutic one and it differs in principles of confidentiality, ethics, and interview technique used.

Indian perspective: Unlike west, no separate specialization in forensic psychiatry is available In India, neither for teaching and training nor for service delivery. General psychiatrists only end up taking forensic psychiatry assessments simultaneously carrying out the conflicting dual roles of therapist and forensic assessor. Thus, it is prudent for all psychiatrist to have basic knowledge of forensic psychiatry assessment.

INDICATIONS OF FORENSIC INTERVIEW IN INDIA

During these different stages, role of psychiatrist can be in following areas.

Competence Assessment for Various Civil Responsibilities
- Fitness for making will
- Fitness for marriage and divorce
- Fitness for child custody
- Fitness for entering into a contract
- Fitness for duty.

Competence Assessment and Management Issues in Criminal Cases
Pre-trial Stage
- Assessment of Fitness for interrogation
- No person with mental illness should be detained unlawfully in prisons on name of "preventive detention"
- Screening for mental illnesses in accused and offering appropriate treatment
- Assessment of Fitness for standing trial (if invoked during enquiry stage).

Trial Stage
- Assessment of Fitness for standing trial (if noticed or invoked during trial stage)
- Insanity defense Assessment
- Appearing as expert witness
- Screening for mental illnesses in accused and offering appropriate treatment in prison setting for under trials.

Post-trial Stage
- Screening for mental illnesses and offering appropriate treatment in prison settings for convicts
- Assessment of Fitness for execution.

Conducting Assessments
Accepting Instructions
Before undertaking any assessment, following are important considerations:
- *Written referral letter/Order for assessment:* Instead of accepting verbal instruction from patient or families, it is always better to get written letter from the agency interested in seeking report (Court or employer or others as case may be)
- *Clarify terms of assessment:* Go through the order received and be clear about the focus of assessment needed and your role as expert. If order is not clear, write back to clarify
- Determine if any potential conflict of interest from your side in the index case as assessor
- Identify limitations of assessment or if it is beyond your clinical domain. In such cases, it is prudent to inform the ordering agency beforehand

CHAPTER 7: Approach to a Forensic Psychiatry Interview and Case Taking

- Estimate the time and resources needed and is your center equipped for same.
  Most important task is to understand the right psycholegal question to be answered as per the need of agency ordering or requesting evaluation.

Setting the Stage for Assessment

- Mention **identification mark** of the evaluee
- Take photograph of the evaluee
- **Informed written consent** regarding following:
  - No doctor-patient relationship
  - Who ordered assessment?
  - Who all will have access to records?
  - Does client has right to refuse assessment or not and legal implications thereof
  - Inform about the **limitations of confidentiality**
  - Verbal interview
  - Need of psychological testing
  - Interview with collateral sources
  - Mandatory reporting of any information suggesting harm to others or crime against state, e.g. child abuse
- *Collateral information:* Information has to be collected from various sources including:
  - All previous medical records including psychiatric records.
  - Interview of different sources familiar to patient.
  - Useful records in civil and criminal cases[2]
    - *Personal records:*
      - Past and present mental health treatments
      - Medical history and treatments
      - Educational history
      - Occupational history
      - Substance abuse treatment
      - Histories of arrest, detention or incarceration
      - Psychological testing results
    - *Criminal assessments:*
      - Police investigation reports
      - Jail psychiatrist behavior report
      - Police interrogation tapes and interview transcripts
    - *Civil assessments:*
      - Job description (nature of patient's job)
      - Employers' report of behavior at work place
      - Educational history

Conducting Forensic Interview[2]
Safety Considerations
There are no unique safety concerns for forensic psychiatry evaluation in specific, but certain evaluations specific for criminal cases may take place at the setting psychiatrist has little control over. Thus, it is important to not compromise one's own safety and be cautious of following:
- Ensure safety of evaluator and evaluee
- Never perform evaluation is isolated settings
- Ensure maximum privacy
- Consider and negotiate need of presence of third parties cautiously
- Be well aware of entry and exit strategies.

Interview Style[2]
- Open-ended questions
- Neutral attitude
- Be cautious of countertransference
- Multiple interviews at different cross sections, if necessary
- *Forensic empathy:* Kenneth Appelbaum describes "forensic empathy" as the quest for "awareness of the perspectives and experiences of interviewees," to allow their voices and concerns to be aired in the assessment process".[2,3] Shuman further differentiates two fine nuances about empathy, as per him, it can be receptive and reflective empathy. 'Receptive empathy' as the "perception and understanding of the experiences of another person." Reflective empathy, however, is problematic, in that it involves communicating an "interpretation or understanding to the defendant in a manner that implies a therapeutic alliance".[2,4] "Such an implication may undermine objectivity and respect for persons, as it may work against the warnings about limits of confidentiality and the lack of a therapeutic relationship that are critical to ethical forensic practice. Recent work has concluded that empathy may help promote rapport, and therefore experts may use a moderate degree of empathy. Thus, the use of clinical skill is essential to the assessment process, but the expert must be vigilant about the manner in which such skills are deployed in the forensic assessment. The evaluator must also be vigilant for signs in himself of inappropriate emotional reaction to the evaluee or the circumstances of the case".[2]

Recording During Interview
- Take notes carefully
- Consider recording the interview in audio- or video-format
- Notify evaluee of the recording.

Important Components of Assessment
- History of present psychiatric illness
- Past medical or psychiatry history

- Substance use
- Legal history of relevance
- History concerning the question in focus of assessment
- Mental status examination
- Psychological testing appropriate to question of assessment
- Need of other tests as appropriate (EEG, MRI, etc.)
- Physical examination
- Examination by all other medical professionals or other mental health professionals as needed.

Specific situations like aggressive patients, uncooperative patients, children or persons with intellectual disability require special skill to be individualized in specific cases. Assessment of clients with malingering, evaluee from different cultural background, ethical questions surrounding assessment and reporting back to the concerned agency are discussed in subsequent chapters **(Table 1)**.

Table 1: Approach to a forensic psychiatry case.

1. Accepting instructions	• Written referral letter/Order for assessment • Clarify terms of assessment: Role of Expert and What is the 'psycholegal question' asked • Ensure no potential conflict of interest of any of the assessor • Identify and inform concerned agency limitations of assessment if any
2. Informed written consent regarding	• No doctor-patient relationship • Who ordered assessment? • Who all will have access to records? • Does client has right to refuse assessment or not and legal implications thereof • Inform about the limitations of confidentiality
3. Sources of information	Relevant documents are provided before actual examination which include: • Case summary • Prosecution witness statements • Police interviews with the defendant • Medical records
4. Assessment (i) The environment	• Ensuring that staff know where you are, roughly how long will interview go • Make sure that there is unimpeded route from chair to exit • Quiet room • Assessor should introduce himself to the defendant • Inform about the purpose of the assessment • Inform about the approximate time needed for the interview • Areas to be covered in the interview • Explaining the absence of confidentiality is necessary
(ii) The interview	• Adopt techniques designed to determine whether there is feigning or exaggeration of symptoms • Attention to be paid to non-verbal cues • Interviewer should be sensitive to emotional problems • Cover psychiatric history and mental state examination, • Open questions should precede closed ones • Mindful of potential diagnoses

Contd...

Contd...

(iii)	Detailed evaluation	• Detailed history includes; history of present illness, past psychiatric history, history of substance abuse, general medical history, developmental, psychosocial and socio-cultural history, occupational history and legal history • Physical examination and investigations • Neurological and Mental state Examination
(iv)	Assessment of personality	• Minnesota Multi-phasic Personality Inventory (2nd Edition).[MMPI-2] • Personality Assessment Inventory [PAI]
(v)	Tools to assess malingering	• Miller Forensic Assessment of Symptoms • Structured Inventory of Malingering Symptoms
(vi)	Psychological testing	• Cognitive tests, Projective Tests, Objective tests • Specific tests to evaluate competency
(vii)	Other tests	• Narco-analysis, Voice Stress analysis, Polygraphy, Galvanic Skin response, Thermal Image, Brain finger printing, Brain Imaging

CONCLUSION

Forensic psychiatrists play a sensitive role. They need to step out of the usual role of confidential doctor-patient relationship in many ways, providing valuable confidential information about evaluee to judicial officers, e.g. lawyers/courts thereby carrying out duty towards state welfare, maintaining a neutral attitude In the truthful pursuit of finding an objective answer to psycholegal question forensic psychiatrist must do a fine balancing act between the interests of referring authority as well as evaluee.

REFERENCES

1. Eastman N, Adshead G, Fox S, et al. Forensic Psychiatry. Oxford Specialists Handbooks. London: Oxford University Press, 2017.
2. AAPL Practice Guideline for the Forensic Assessment. Available at: jaapl.org/content/43/2_Supplement/S3. Last accessed on 07.02.18.
3. Appelbaum PS. The parable of the forensic psychiatrist: ethics and the problem of doing harm. Int J Law Psychiatry. 1990;13:249-59.
4. Griffith EE. Ethics Behav Brodsky SL, Wilson JK: Empathy. 1993;66(3):289-302.

CHAPTER

Special Investigative Techniques in Forensic Psychiatry

> **LEARNING OBJECTIVES**
> - Deception detection tests (DDT)
> - Polygraph testing
> - Brain mapping and brain fingerprinting
> - Narco-analysis
> - Provisions in Indian Law for DDTs
> - National Human Rights guidelines for use of DDT

To improve the evidence gathering procedure without use of 'physical torture' and having more reliability of a scientific technique, deception detection tests (DDT) are being utilized now a days by investigative agencies. These tests include polygraph, narco-analysis and brain-mapping and are becoming popular as they can pave the way to the information concealed by guilty. In India, currently they are not accepted as a proof against guilty at any stage of trial but they facilitate the investigative prong. Its use is still surrounded by many clinical ethical and legal dilemmas. Some of these techniques have been reviewed with relevance to their utility, merits and demerits.[1]

POLYGRAPH TESTING

A polygraph *(lie detector)* is a device which makes a continuous record of several physiological variables, such as *blood pressure, heart rate, respiration* and *electrodermal reaction,* while a series of questions are being asked, in an attempt to detect lies. The above measurements are believed to be indicators of anxiety due to sympathetic stimulation that accompanies the telling of lies. However, if the evaluee is anxious from other reasons, it may lead to a false positive test. A polygraph test is also known as a *psychophysiological detection of deception* (PDD) examination. The term 'polygraph' was used first time in 1908 by James MacKenzie in his invention, the 'ink polygraph' which was used for medical reasons. Marston nevertheless remained its primary advocate for judicial use.[2]

Procedure[2]

The polygraph uses two major techniques: the Relevant/Irrelevant Technique (RIT) and the Control Question Technique (CQT).

A typical polygraph test starts with a pre-test interview to gain some preliminary information, which will later be used for 'Control Questions' or C (control questions that most people will lie about may be such as: 'have you ever stolen money?' or 'have you ever committed such crime before?' etc.). The tester will explain how the polygraph is supposed to work, with an emphasis on the nature of the test as a lie detector, and an emphasis that answers must be truthful. The subject is then asked to deliberately lie, which the tester claims to have detected on the test. This is followed by 'the actual test' wherein some of the questions asked are 'Irrelevant' or IR ('Is your name Rob/Tom?'), others are 'probable-lie'; and the remainder are the 'Relevant Questions' or R in which the tester is really interested in.

Accuracy

Examiners maintain that the accuracy is 90% and the errors tend to be false negative rather than false positive, i.e. a person who actually lied is reported as 'truthful'.

Admissibility of Polygraphs in the Court[1]

1. *US courts*: While lie detector tests are commonly used in police investigations, no one can be forced to take the test in court. The US Supreme Court leaves it to individual jurisdictions as to whether polygraph results could be admitted as evidence in court cases.
2. *Europe:* Polygraphs are not considered reliable evidence and are not generally used by police forces.
3. *Canada:* The test may be used for screening candidates for government jobs. The Supreme Court does not accept it as evidence in court.
4. *Australia:* The High Court has not yet considered the admissibility of polygraph evidence.

Brain Fingerprinting (Brain Mapping)

BRAIN MAPPING AND BRAIN FINGERPRINTING

Brain mapping is a group of neuroscience techniques based on the mapping of quantities or properties (biological) onto spatial representations of the brain. While various brain imaging techniques (e.g. CT, MRI, PET, SPECT) measure properties such as cerebral blood flow, metabolism or structural integrity, EEG (quantitative EEG) measures electrical activity of the brain which is usually known as brain mapping.[1,2]

Brain fingerprinting, invented by *Lawrence Farwell*, is a computer-based test that is designed to provide evidence of information regarding crimes. This test detects the presence or absence of information, and not guilt or innocence per se. This investigative technique is based on the recognition of familiar stimuli by measuring electrical brain wave responses to words, phrases, pictures, acronyms, etc. that are presented on a screen. The basis for the test is that the suspect's reactions to the details of an event or activity will be displayed through changes in his brain waves if the suspect had prior knowledge of the event or activity. Lawrence Farwell used P300 wave for detecting these changes and called this technique as MERMER, i.e. 'memory and encoding related multifaceted electroencephalographic response.'[1,2]

Procedure

An elastic cap (headband) with 19 electronic sensors is placed on the shaven scalp of the subject and connected to the recording device that measures the EEG. The subject is shown stimuli consisting of sounds, words, phrases or pictures on a computer screen.

It detects response to the stimuli related to the crime or other investigated situation. The theory is that the suspect's reaction to the details of an event or activity will reflect, if the suspect had prior knowledge of the event or activity. As the test is based on EEG signals, it does not require the subject to issue verbal responses to questions or stimuli.[1,2]

Principle

Farwell's brain fingerprinting originally used the *P300 brain response* (emitted from an individual's brain approximately 300 milliseconds after it is confronted with a stimulus of special significance) to detect the brain's recognition of the known information. Later, he used the Memory and Encoding Related Multifaceted Electroencephalographic Response (MERMER), which includes the P300 and additional features and is reported to ensure better of accuracy than the P300 alone.[1,2]

Uses

i. *Criminal cases*: To check if the interviewee is revealing the truths about the facts of the case.
ii. *Medical diagnosis*: For assessment of brain function in diseases that affect cognition such as dementias.
iii. *Advertisement*: Evaluates the effectiveness of advertising by measuring brain responses.
iv. *National security*: Screening employees, especially in military and foreign intelligence and counterterrorism.
v. Insurance fraud.[1,2]

Drawbacks

The test may not be useful in a case in which:
- Two suspects were present at a crime—one as a witness and the other a perpetrator.
- Investigators do not have sufficient information about a crime so as to test a suspect for crime-relevant information stored in the brain.[1,2]

Brain Fingerprinting vs Polygraph

Brain fingerprinting is not influenced by the subjects' emotional responses, relying only on the information stored in the brain. In this aspect, it differs significantly from the polygraph, which measures emotion-based physiological signals.[1,2]

Legal Aspects[2]

The United States: An Iowa Court in the US accepted brain fingerprinting as scientific evidence in the reversal of the murder conviction of Terry Harrington.

India: Data from Brain Electrical Oscillation Signature (BEOS) profiling has been admitted as evidence in the court in a murder trial in India.

There has been not even a single case, in which the court has convicted a subject based *only* on the results of the brain fingerprinting. In fact, in the cases, wherein results of such tests were positive, but were not supported by other oral or documentary evidences, the subjects in those cases have been acquitted of the charges against them.

Brain Signature Profiling (BSP) or BEOS is another EEG procedure which was developed in 2003 by *CR Mukundan* which is similar to brain fingerprinting. In the case mentioned above, the woman was convicted of murdering her former fiancé based on BEOS profile. But subsequently, the Mumbai High Court suspended her sentence and released her on bail due to a lack of sufficient evidence.[3]

NARCO-ANALYSIS

Greek word 'narke' means 'anesthesia' or 'torpor' numbness/ apathy/dormancy, etc. The term 'analysis' has been used in Pierre Janet's sense of a process that, by means of partial dissolution of consciousness, undoes the complex syntheses of waking mental life and accesses mental content that is more automatic.

Definition: It is a scientific procedure used to obtain information from an individual in a natural sleep-like state.

Principle: The narco-analysis procedure depends on the effect of biomolecules on the bioactivity of the individual.
- A person is able to lie by using his imagination. During the test, the subject's imagination is suspended by placing them in a semi-conscious state. In this state, it becomes difficult for him to lie, and his answers would be restricted to facts he is already aware of. The level of awareness is suspended to an extent that the subject is not able to speak spontaneously, but is able to answer specific, short, succinct queries.
- In such sleep-like state, efforts are made to obtain 'probative truth' about the crime.

Procedure: The individual is put to trance-like state and loses all his inhibitions by administering *sodium amytal or thiopentone sodium*, (known as 'truth drug' or 'truth serum') 2.5–5% solution, slow IV.

Other Methods
- 0.5 mg scopolamine hydrobromide (commonly used) subcutaneously, followed by 0.25 mg every 20 minutes (average 3–6 injections), till proper stage of questioning is reached.[3]
- 100 mg sodium seconal, 15 mg morphine and 0.5 mg of scopolamine hydrobromide may be given IV.

The dose is dependent on the examinee's features such as sex, age, health and physical condition. A wrong dose can result in a person going into a coma or even death.

Team required: A team comprising of an anesthetist, psychiatrist, clinical/forensic psychologist, audio-videographer and supporting nursing staff does the test. The forensic psychologist will prepare the final report about the findings, and these are used as evidence along with the audiovisual recordings of the session.

The procedure has been criticized at various platforms, voicing the technique as 'betrayal through medicine/pharmacological torture.[1,2]

Legal Aspects Specific to India for DDTs

Indian Supreme Court in 2010 declared that narco-analysis, polygraph tests and brain-mapping cannot be done without the consent of the individual. If the person consents for such methods, then any information obtained can be used for further probe. Results of such tests will not be admissible as evidence, even if done with consent.[4]

Use of such methods are illegal and against following principles of constitution:[5]
- 'Right against self-incrimination' enumerated in Article 20(3) of the Constitution, which states that no person accused of an offence shall be compelled to be a witness against himself/herself, and
- Article 21 (Right to life and personal liberty) has been expanded to include a 'right against cruel, inhuman or degrading treatment'.

NATIONAL HUMAN RIGHTS GUIDELINES FOR USE OF DDT

Indian Supreme Court in 2010 has left the scope only for the voluntary administration of Polygraph, Narco-analysis and Brain Electrical Activation Profile (BEAP) test techniques in the context of criminal justice, provided that certain safeguards are in place. Even when the subject has consented to any of these procedures, the test results cannot be used as standalone evidence because these do not involve conscious control of the responses obtained under these testing conditions. However, any information or material that is subsequently obtained with the help of voluntarily administered test results can be admitted, in accordance with Section 27 of the Evidence Act, 1872. The National Human Rights Commission (NHRC) had published *'Guidelines for the Administration of Polygraph Test (Lie Detector Test) on an Accused'* in 2000. These guidelines should be strictly adhered to and have been given below:[6]

1. A polygraph test can only be administered after obtaining consent from the accused. An option should be given to the accused whether he/she wishes to avail such tests.
2. If the accused volunteers for a Lie Detector Test, he should be given access to a lawyer and the physical, emotional and legal implications of such a test should be explained to him by the police and his lawyer.
3. The consent should be recorded before a Judicial Magistrate.
4. During the hearing before the Magistrate, the person alleged to have agreed should be duly represented by a lawyer.

5. At the hearing, the person in question should also be told explicitly that the statement that is made shall not be a 'confessional' statement to the Magistrate but will have the status of a statement made to the police.
6. The Magistrate shall consider all factors relating to the detention including the length of detention and the nature of the interrogation.
7. The actual recording of the Lie Detector Test shall be done by an independent agency (such as a hospital) and conducted in the presence of a lawyer.
8. A full medical and factual narration of the manner of the information received must be taken on record.

REFERENCES

1. Biswas G. Review of Forensic Medicine and Toxicology. Jaypee Brothers Medical Publishers (P) Ltd, 3rd ed, 2015.
2. Vij K. Textbook of Forensic Medicine and Toxicology: Principles and Practice. Jaypee Brothers Medical Publishers (P) Ltd, 5th ed.
3. Singh DK. Constitutionality and evidentiary value of narco-analysis, polygraph and BEAP tests. Int J Law. 2017;3(4):84-9.
4. Smt. Selvi and Ors vs. State of Karnataka. Smt. Selvi and Ors vs State of Karnataka Judgment on 5th May 2010. Available from:http://supremecourtofi ndia.nic.in.
5. Math SB. Supreme Court judgment on polygraph, narco-analysis and brain-mapping: a boon or a bane. Indian J Med Res. 2011;134(1):4-7.
6. National Human Rights Commission Guidelines. Available from: http://nhrc.nic.in/Documents/sec-3.pdf.

CHAPTER

Ethical Issues in Forensic Psychiatry

> **LEARNING OBJECTIVES**
> - Ethics: concept and application in psychiatry
> - Forensic psychiatry ethics
> - Limitation of confidentiality
> - Consent for forensic psychiatry
> - Dual agency
> - Research involving prisons
> - Interrogation and participation of mental health professionals

Word "ethics" is derived from *Ethikos*: Which means rules of conduct that govern natural disposition in human beings. Dorland's dictionary describes medical ethics as "the values and guidelines that should govern decisions in medicine". Accordingly, one has to observe the ethics in different situations.[1]

Most visible activities in clinical practice of medicine involve:[1]
- *Professional ethics*: The appropriate manner of behavior expected from an individual in a professional role.
- *Medical ethics*: Standards of professional conduct expected from medical professionals, usually resulting from the degree of trust involved in their interactions with individuals.
- *Ethical conflicts*: Discord between how one wants to behave and the ethical behavior expected in that context.
- *Ethical dilemmas*: Conflict between different ethical perspective or values.

For any profession, there are certain ethical requirements which can be counted as follows:
- Accountability
- Optimization of quality and quantity
- Ethical choices made have consequences, both for the individual and for the others
- Conflicts need to be avoided and if occur should be resolved
- Ethical dilemmas should be solved.

The Hippocratic Oath has paternalism in doctor-patient relationship.

ETHICS AND PSYCHIATRY

Line of demarcation between normal and abnormal is hazy in psychiatry, and the validity of diagnosis and treatment can be questioned in psychiatric practice. Psychiatric treatment can be used for vested interests. Close relationship between the therapist and the patient can lead to intense transference which could be maliciously utilized by the either party. Poor insight may affect patient's decision making which can raise certain ethical and forensic issues. The confidence reposed in therapist by a psychiatric patient can be exploited. In forensic psychiatry when the patient knows that his mental health report may be used against him in the court of law, doctor-patient relationship and confidentiality may be seriously affected. Following are the basic principles required to be observed by a practicing psychiatrist:[2]

1. Respect for autonomy
2. Beneficence
3. Nonmaleficence
4. Justice

Respect of Autonomy

Patient's personal autonomy needs to be respected. He should be given sufficient time to explain his problems and then should be given appropriate professional information so that he understands the benefits, the risks, and potential costs of all options. Patient's individual rights should be given due respect. He has the right to choose someone else to decide best course of action on his behalf. Professional information can be used by the physician to persuade the patient to make a choice, however, the patient cannot be coerced to make him accept the decision. Relevant information should not be withheld from the patient.

Beneficence

It is the professional responsibility of the physician to promote the well-being of his patients as well as the society at large. The physician must, at times, heed to the patients' interests even at their own expense. Physician's action should have limits in a beneficent manner for the patient and should not manipulate by controlling information, should provide complete and factual information.

Nonmaleficence

Primum non nocere means first do no harm; that is what is expected from a physician. He should be careful in decision making and in his actions. He should be adequately trained in what is being done by him. He should be open to seeking second opinion from his professional colleagues. He should avoid creating risk by his action or inaction. In decision making, the helpful effects should overweigh the harmful ones.

Justice

Aristotle wrote, "Justice involves treating equals equally and those not equal differently." Justice derives from genuine concern for the wellbeing of people, and includes reward, punishment and equitable distribution of social benefits. This principle is also important for research purposes.

LEGAL AND MORAL RESPONSIBILITY

Criminal responsibility of an individual is often assigned on the basis of an assessment of his volition, i.e. on how he chooses to act. Choice can include the choice to do nothing (which may lead to crime of omission); therefore, being reckless or negligent can represent choices as much as can an intention to commit an offence.

In moral philosophy, the knowledge of wrongness of the action is required for it to be mentally blameworthy. The law rarely has such a requirement; in fact, it is a general principle that, 'ignorance of the law is no excuse.' Moreover, the law ignores the question of whether the individual even had the capacity to take into account the wrongness of the action, and with the exception of children holds individuals responsible even if they lacked a capacity for moral reasoning unless they have other deficits of mental function that render them unfit to plead. This reflects the different and overlapping social function of law and morality.[3]

PERSONAL BELIEFS AND PROFESSIONAL OPINION

The different views of professionals about the nature of volition and free will may have an impact on their professional stance and behavior. Those who take a strict deterministic view may not see the mentally ill as having any control over their volition and by extension their offending behavior; those who take a more experiential view, or those who have strong religious views, may be more inclined to want them held at least partially responsible even when the illness is severe and involves a loss of touch with reality. These views also have significant influence on how risk is assessed and managed. Practitioners should be aware of their own views and how they may influence their professional judgment or the objective of their opinion.

ETHICS AND FORENSIC PSYCHIATRY

Forensic psychiatry deals with application of technical skills of psychiatry in civil and criminal cases, correctional settings and legislative domains. As discussed above in the clinical psychiatry patient's interests are of central importance and ethical principles of beneficence and nonmaleficence take precedence. On the other hand, in the forensic psychiatry duty towards welfare of public or society at large state is at the center, hence, principles of social welfare and justice become more important. These contradictions challenge the value system underlying the practice of forensic psychiatry. This brings to question whether forensic psychiatry contradicts the core ethical values medicine.[4]

The two disciplines of forensic psychiatry and clinical psychiatry are based on such divergent principles that they can be compared to opponents in a game of tennis, continuously shuttling ethical dilemmas across a moral field.

The ethical dilemma is basically at two fronts, first is while carrying out the role of forensic expert for evaluation, when, purpose is only court ordered assessment and no therapeutic relationship exists, thus, irrespective of the consequences of that report for the patient, one has to strive for honesty and objectivity to give a scientific opinion for fair trial to proceed. For example, a client awaiting capital punishment is referred for mental state assessment, so that he can be executed if found healthy; and a report mentioning no mental illness can hasten the process of execution, but, forensic psychiatrist has to maintain objectivity and should opine honestly. Secondly, is about the role of a psychiatrist in correctional setting. It is a unique triangular relationship, besides the therapeutic relationship with client; psychiatrist also owes a responsibility towards director of the prison as employer. Forensic psychiatrists often work with the mentally ill offending patients and their role in the criminal justice may increase the severity of the sentence for the patient.[5] Forensic psychiatrists operate outside the expected medical role, and different ethical principles guide actions in both roles.[6] Aforementioned rinciples of beneficence and nonmaleficence cease to hold the same importance in the forensic setting. The principles of truth and objectivity are of a greater significance in forensic practice.[8] Any information obtained during forensic assessment can be used against an individual by the prosecution. Confidentiality is not an obligation in the practice of forensic psychiatry. The two main guiding principles of objectivity and respect may not be enough in the practice of forensic psychiatry. Professional integrity and ethical principles of medical practice may influence decision-making in forensic psychiatry.

The forensic psychiatrist frequently attempts to find a balance between the traditional ethical principles in medicine and the expected ethical standards in forensic medicine. The American Academy of Psychiatry and the Law (AAPL) in 2005 has issued highest standards of practice as ethical guidelines for forensic psychiatry. Forensic psychiatry follows:[6]

i. Respect for person
ii. Honesty
iii. Justice
iv. Social responsibility

However, in therapeutic relationship of correctional settings, the traditional ethical principles are practiced. The following issues need to be addressed specifically in forensic psychiatry:

Confidentiality

Forensic assessments must respect individual's right of privacy and the maintenance of confidentiality. Within legal boundaries, confidentiality must be maintained to the greatest extent possible, and the examinee must be aware of the concept of medical confidentiality. Forensic evaluation is one of the circumstances where privileged communication, or breach of confidentiality is valid, but there are rules that guide such a breach. Any disclosure of information should be informed to the client and this information should involve:[3,7]

a. The details of the party which has requested the evaluation, and the intended recipients of the report.
b. Other parties who will gain access to the report
c. Information about privileged communication and limits of confidentiality.
d. Information about the nontherapeutic nature of assessment.
e. The primary forensic query to be addressed in the evaluation.
f. The nature of information to be assessed and the methods of eliciting this information.
g. The type of legal proceedings in which this assessment will be used.
h. Information about issues which warrant mandatory reporting.
i. Rights of the examinees during the forensic assessment.

Consent

Informed consent is one of the core values of the ethical practice of medicine and psychiatry. However, in particular situations such as court-ordered evaluations for competency assessment or involuntary commitment, neither assent nor informed consent is required. In these situations, the examinee must be made aware of the fact that refusal to cooperate will be documented in any report or testimony. An impression of inability to cooperate must be included in the report. Consent in correctional settings is different from forensic evaluations alone, where rules and regulations of jurisdiction will apply.[3,7]

Honesty and Striving for Objectivity

As previously discussed, forensic psychiatrists work on the guiding principles of honesty and objectivity. All professional psychiatric assessments must be based on objective assessment of the data made available. Although they may be retained by one party to a civil or criminal matter, psychiatrists should adhere to these principles when conducting evaluations, applying clinical data to legal criteria, and expressing opinions. Forensic psychiatrists must be able to distinguish between verified and unverified information, and between information that merely poses as an objective truth whereas in reality is merely inferential. Psychiatrists should not distort their opinion in the service of the retaining party.[3]

Qualifications

Expertise in the practice of forensic psychiatry should be claimed only when the practicing psychiatrist has knowledge, skills, training, and experience. The forensic psychiatrist should know both principles of clinical psychiatry as well as the legal system of a country.[3]

Producing a Forensic Report without a Clinical Interview

The clinical interview is an integral part of the forensic evaluation, and is the most preferred situation for an accurate assessment. However, in some instances an interview is not possible because either the evaluee declines to participate, or circumstances do not allow an interview to take place. It sometimes becomes imperative to conduct an assessment without the interview to prevent unnecessary delays in the legal process due to noncompliance of the evaluee. Ethical guidelines for both psychologists and psychiatrists acknowledge the occasions where an interview is not feasible but there is sufficient collateral information to formulate an opinion with a reasonable degree of clinical certainty. Mental health practitioners must state clearly in their work product (whether oral or written) the limitations of formulating such a report.[7]

Dual Agency

Dual agency refers to a situation in which the clinician must simultaneously serve a clinical therapeutic role in a legal case, and a forensic role with different purposes of legal evaluation. Dual agency may occur when:

1. A company hires a psychiatrist who owes a treatment duty to his patient—an employee of the same company—and a simultaneous obligation to the company to return the patient to work immediately
2. A military psychiatrist owes a treatment duty to his enlisted patient and a simultaneous duty to the military to maintain security
3. A jail psychiatrist owes a treatment duty to his inmate patient (who is awaiting his trial) and a simultaneous duty to the state to get a confession from the inmate
4. A state-employed psychiatrist owes a duty to the best interest of his death row patient and a simultaneous job assignment to get the execution done.[4] A treating psychiatrist asked for forensic evaluation, which is common in Indian setting. Clearly, the two roles of *the psychiatrist in these examples conflict with each other.*

ETHICAL ISSUES IN FORENSIC PSYCHIATRY RESEARCH

1. While conducting research in psychiatric patients one has to take into account the 'lack of judgment, and decision-making capacity to participate in research. The most common ethical dilemma in forensic psychiatry is between the two principles of (a) beneficence or promotion of welfare and (b) respect for justice. The forensic psychiatrist often has to make a choice between well-being of the patient and well-being of the society as a whole. In India, the psychiatrists practicing forensic psychiatry have the dual role of both carrying out forensic assessments as well as providing medical treatment. In settings with well established forensic services one way of overcoming this dilemma has been to have forensic psychiatrists carrying out mental assessments of mentally ill offenders on behalf of the legal system, and treatment provision by a different set of treating professionals. The ultimate aim of the forensic psychiatrist should be revelation of truth as part of pursuit of justice without affecting privacy and autonomy of the patient. As per the American Academy of Psychiatry and Law, forensic evaluation should never be conducted for either prosecution or government until the patient has had access to legal counsel.[5,6]
2. Forensic psychiatry is more than just providing expert witness in a trial. It sometimes provides contrasting points of view to the legal system, illuminating ethical issues often disregarded by the law. It comes with a wealth of knowledge and methodological viewpoints that can ensure a more holistic approach to the delivery of justice.[3]
3. Forensic psychiatry is a fascinating specialty, which, if done right, brings forth continuous ethical challenges for its practitioners. It is an opportunity to preserve the ethical heritage of medical practice, regardless of the side one picks.

ETHICS IN RESEARCH INVOLVING PRISONERS

From the dawn of modern civilization, prisoners have been used as research subjects. The exploitation is even more starkly apparent when researchers come from developed countries and study subjects are from developing countries. As an example, Louis Pasteur once wrote to Emperor Dom Pedro II of Brazil, proposing to test his anti-rabies vaccine on prisoners condemned to death, which was declined, but emperor offered to test for more prevalent yellow fever vaccine for greater benefit for society. In the Tuskegee study in the United States, hundreds of detainees were inoculated with malaria in order to discover effective means of preventing and treating the disease that devastated the American troops. Nazi Germany was a hotbed for unethical scientific experiments carried out by physicians in concentration camps. In the post world-war II era, the indignation over the behavior of the defeated nations led to the establishment of the Nuremberg Code governing research on human subjects in general and to determine their applicability to prisoners.

Such atrocities in the name of human experimentation gained the terms "human guinea pig" and "cheaper than chimpanzees" for the coerced participants, as a way to address the demeaning nature of the work. A complete ban on such research has therefore been proposed. Subsequently, the United Nations, in its Body of Principles for the Protection of All Persons Under Any Form of Detention or Imprisonment, established that "no detained or imprisoned person shall, even with his consent, be subjected to any medical or scientific experimentation which may be detrimental to his health."

As a result of the international furore against unethical medical research on human subjects, the number of studies involving prisoners has declined considerably in the last two decades. However, no clear definitions exist regarding the ethical guidelines to conduct research involving prisoners. Considering the fact that relatively minor remunerations such as better standards of living, transfer to another cell block, and better nutrition may "buy" inmates as study participants, mental competence and non-coercive participation do not suffice as adequate criteria to conduct prison-based research. On the other hand, providing explicit advantages to study participants in prisons, such as fiduciary benefits or a reduced sentence are unethical practices at face value.

The ethical problem of *The Free Will* is even more paramount in the context of research in prisons. Simply by virtue of being incarcerated, there is a restriction on the liberty at which prisoners can give an informed consent. Additionally, mentally ill prisoners are even more vulnerable, as the mental illness further impairs their competence.

To achieve equilibrium between the need to conduct research in prison settings and the protection of the rights of prisoners, the following basic principles have been proposed.[8]

- *Incentives to participate should be avoided*: Appropriate medical amenities and adequate nutrition should be a mandatory provision for all prisoners provided by the state, and not incentives to encourage participation in research projects. Reduced sentences or other such explicit benefits undermine the authority of the judicial system and should therefore not be used as incentives. Payments, if made, should be limited to what is normally paid to other prisoners for their labors within the prison.
- *Therapeutic research should be distinguished from non-therapeutic research:* Therapeutic research potentially precludes the potential therapeutic benefit to non-participants, and should be designed in a way to prevent such an event. Non-therapeutic research must only be permitted under special circumstances, where a clear potential benefit can be demonstrated for the concerned population.

- *Pro-active role of ethics in research committees (ERC):* Prisoners are a vulnerable population in general because of their suspensions of autonomy and of the inherent abuse well known in prison systems. To prevent further abuse of the incarcerated through medical research, an Ethics Review Committee (ERC) should carefully evaluate: the scientific validity of proposed projects; the qualifications of the researchers; the estimated risks; the cost-benefit ratio; the rules governing the recruitment of subjects; the guarantee of confidentiality; the safeguards against the release of confidential data; and any potential conflicts of interest among the researchers. In addition, the ERC should ensure monitoring the execution of the project, going beyond the call of duty and simple bureaucratic requirements.

Participation of Mental Health Professionals in Interrogation[9,10]

Guantanamo incidence: In 2002, American soldiers captured a man, and transferred him to the detention center at Guantanamo Bay. The man was labeled a "high-value detainee." Former Secretary of Defense Donald Rumsfeld authorized extraordinary interrogation techniques being designed by mental health professionals for high-value detainees. Special teams were created to work on interrogations called Behavioral Science Consultation Teams (BSCTs) headed by a psychologist. Their job was not simply to monitor interrogations but to employ their knowledge of human psychology to better exploit a prisoner's psychological and cultural vulnerabilities for the purposes of extracting information.

The prisoner in question was interrogated using very aggressive and controversial techniques. These included being deprived of sleep for more than a week at a time, having hypothermia induced by air conditioning, being exposed to barking, growling dogs, to which the prisoner has a phobia, being forced to take many bags of intravenous fluids and then to urinate on himself. Throughout the prisoner's interrogation he was monitored daily by physicians.

A psychologist suggested that the prisoner be placed in a swivel chair so that he could be prevented from focusing his eyes on one spot. The interrogators employed dehumanizing techniques such as leashing the prisoner like a dog and making him bark, and remarking that the prisoner's life was worse that of the rats inhabiting the compound.

Professional Bodies Stand

This followed American Psychological Association's stand in 2002 to condemn any torture but it allowed its members to participate in interrogative techniques with the larger interest of safeguarding public against terrorism and helping military. This was in stark contrast to the position held by American Medical Association and American Psychiatric Association which strongly condemned any form of torture. In 2005, the Board of Trustees of the APA prepared a Position Statement entitled Psychiatric Participation in Interrogation of Detainees. This statement explicitly stated that psychiatrists should not participate in any form of legal interrogation, whether coercive or not, in both the civil as well as military setting. This was approved in 2006 and reaffirmed by assembly in 2014.[11-14]

The concentrated focus on thinking through ethics quandaries encourages forensic practitioners to reflect regularly on the ethics dimensions of their work and provides them with the tools to create ethics-based solutions that are transparent and understandable and best serve their clients. Knowledge of and observance of the ethical principles that govern forensic practice are essential to physicians who give expert opinions regarding individuals involved in civil or criminal trials, as well as to those who treat individuals deprived of their freedom. Adhering to these principles is the only way to ensure that the basic rights of all citizens are respected. However, the practice of carrying out biomedical research in prisons in ethical way is a public health necessity, since only through knowledge of this situation can we intervene in an efficacious manner and provide benefits to this vulnerable population. These principles provide a roadmap for specialists in these evolving fields to recognize dilemmas.

REFERENCES

1. Rao NG. Textbook of Forensic Medicine and Toxicology, Second edition. Jaypee Brothers Medical Publishers (P) Ltd; 2010.
2. Sidhu N, Srinivasraghavan J. Ethics and Medical Practice: Why Psychiatry is Unique. Indian Journal of Psychiatry. 2016;58(Suppl 2):S199-S202. doi:10.4103/0019-5545.196838.
3. Nigel Eastman, Gwen Adshead, Simone Fox, et al. Forensic Psychiatry. Oxford Specialists Handbooks. London: Oxford University Press; 2017.
4. Appelbaum PS. The parable of the forensic psychiatrist: ethics and the problem of doing harm. Int J Law Psychiatry. 1990;13:249-59.
5. Appelbaum PS. A theory of ethics for forensic psychiatry. J Am Acad Psychiatry Law. 1997;25:33-247.
6. American Academy of Psychiatry and the Law Ethics Guidelines for the Practice of Forensic Psychiatry Adopted May, 2005. Available at http://www.aapl.org/ethics.htm. Last accessed on 12 June 2018.
7. Stone JH, Grady JO, Tylor AV (Eds). Ethics in Psychiatry. Faulk's Basic Forensic Psychiatry, 3rd Edition. Blackwell Science Publishers. Maldain MA, USA.1999. pp. 14-9.
8. Taborda, JG, Arboleda-Flórez, J. Forensic psychiatry ethics: expert and clinical practices and research on prisoners. Revista Brasileira de Psiquiatria. 2006;28(Suppl. 2):s86-s92.
9. Halpern AL, Halpern JH, Doherty SB. "Enhanced" interrogation of detainees: do psychologists and psychiatrists participate? Philosophy, ethics, and humanities in medicine : PEHM. 2008;3:21. doi:10.1186/1747-5341-3-21.
10. Behnke S. Ethics and interrogations: comparing and contrasting the American Psychological, American Medical and American Psychiatric Association positions. Monitor on Psychology. 2006;37:1-4.
11. American Psychological Association Reaffirmation of the American Psychological Association Position Against Torture and Other Cruel, Inhuman, or Degrading Treatment or Punishment and Its Application to Individuals Defined in the United States Code as "Enemy Combatants" http://www.apa.org/governance/resolutions/councilres0807.html 2007, Aug 19.
12. American Psychiatric Association: Psychiatric participation in interrogation of detainees http://www.psych.org/Departments/EDU/Library/APAOfficialDocumentsandRelated/PositionStatements/200601.aspx
13. Levin A. Psychologists adopt resolution updating position on torture. Psychiatr News. 2007;42:2.
14. American Psychiatric Association Position Statement on Detainee Interrogation, Paragraph 1. 2006.

CHAPTER 10

Ethnicity, Culture and Forensic Psychiatry

> **LEARNING OBJECTIVES**
> - Concept of culture
> - Impact of culture on distress
> - Cultural explanations
> - Pathways into care
> - Epidemiological problems
> - Management issues
> - Race and ethnicity
> - Ethnicity in forensic psychiatry

"Human behavior is conceived of as an outcome of genetic and biochemical characteristics, past learning experiences, motivational states, psychosocial antecedents and the cultural context in which it unfolds."[1] Ethnicity and culture have an important role in pathways into care. For mentally ill-offenders and forensic patients, ethnicity and culture become even more significant as most of the patients in forensic settings go through secondary care but occasionally through court diversion schemes. Understanding culture and cultural impact on pathways into care can lead to early and appropriate identification of and provision for patients. These varied pathways are determined by explanatory models, severity of symptoms, resources available and ease of access to them, and also perceived effectiveness of treatments. Underprivileged group patients in Indian society often differ in their use of health care services as compared to the privileged ones.[2]

WHAT IS CULTURE?

Culture plays a complex role in the natural history and psycho-social development of human behavior. It is a set of norms, and values or reference points utilized by members of a particular society to construct their unique view of the world, and ascertain their identity. Culture has been variously defined, however, according to Orlandi[2] culture comprises shared values, beliefs, norms, traditions, customs art, history, folklore and the institutions of a group of people. Social *norms,* the shared rules, that specify appropriate and inappropriate behaviors;[3,4] *mores,* that people consider vital to their well-being and to their most cherished values[5] and *sanctions,* the socially imposed rewards and punishments that compel people to comply with norms,[6] constitute important ingredients of a culture. A society which is a cohesive group of people shares all the ingredients of the culture among its members. Keeping pace with the times, this definition has also incorporated elements such as financial philosophies, and the ever-changing realities imposed by technological advances. The range of possible interactions between culture and its components, with clinical phenomena in general and psychiatric evaluation and management in particular, is broad and multifaceted.[7]

Tylor, a British anthropologist, defined culture as the complex whole that includes knowledge, beliefs, arts, morals, laws, customs, and any other capabilities and habits acquired by man as a member of society.[8,9] Powys has over-simplified the definition and called culture as that what is left over after one forgets all that one has learned.[10] In simple words, one can define culture as a shared way of life of a group of people.[11]

No matter what definition one follows, culture is an integral part of human beings. An individual is not born with a culture but into one. Removing culture from a person's life leaves nothing but an empty shell, as seen in individuals who are totally de-cultured. Cultures can be individualistic or collectivistic. Each individual in a family living in an individualistic culture has his ego centered on himself with little worries about others, making the society egocentric. Individuals in such cultures have little to do with other families in the society, and sometimes even with other individuals in the same family. On the other hand, individuals in collectivist cultures focus on kinship and extended family. They are more concerned about "what others might think"; the "others" will include family members and the society they belong to. To understand individual patients from other cultures, a degree of cultural competence helps. Cultural competence is good clinical practice because every individual needs to be assessed and managed in his or her cultural context.

Transcultural psychiatry as a subspecialty tries to explore the meanings that cultures give to various presentations of psychopathology. It is concerned not only with diversity but also with uniformity across different cultures. It looks at one culture from the point of another majority culture.

Indian subcontinent is compared to a deep net where various races and people have drifted in somewhere in the remote past and have got caught. The topographical conditions of the sun-continent enforced these diverse people to stay collected in a multiple society creating what is described as 'unity in diversity' and 'cultural homogeneity' giving an mistaken understanding of India's social reality. In contrast to Unity in Diversity there is ethnic diversity which has led to formation of minority group differing from majority prototype in terms of numerical strength and also in terms of access to the resources of power and prestige. Since the societies are governed by the members, it is understandable that this majority group will have the maximum say. Thus, there is a creation of a dialectical interrelationship between majority groups who dominate limited goods of power and prestige and the minority groups who lack them. Deprivation is a key factor in unfolding of human behavior in our Indian society.

Deprivation is the outcome of the vast socioeconomic disparity from the caste-system which is uniquely fitted in our Indian society to hand on the cultural patterns and certain items of culture. There is compartmentalization in the traditional Hindu society in various caste-groups, dictating superior and lesser-beings amid its fellow members. It is an obvious institution of social-inequality, a system of legalized inequality, a variant of ascriptive system of stratification in which allocation of role and status is governed by its own principles, determining social, economic, political, legal and ritualistic structure of individuals in relation to each other.[11]

Preamble of World Health Organization (WHO) succinctly underscores enjoyment of highest standard of health as fundamental right of every human being. Article 25 of Universal Declarations of Human Rights, says that everyone has the right to a standard of living, adequate for health including food, clothing, housing, medical care and other necessary services. Studies reveal that individuals' poorer health status, including higher morbidity, lower life expectancy and higher infant mortality rate is linked to their race, ethnicity and caste. Studies also reveal that discrimination due to caste, or racial origin affects people's health in three ways: (a) health status, (b) access to health care, and (c) in quality of health services.

Health is a state of complete physical, mental and social well-being and not merely the absence of disease or infirmity. It is a basic and dynamic force in our daily lives influenced by our circumstances, beliefs, culture, social, economic and physical environments. Mental Health is appropriate balance between the individual, social group and the larger environment. These three components combine to promote, psychological and social harmony, a sense of well-being, self-actualization, and environmental mastery. In a society where ethnic diversity, minority status, stratification, social mobility, and deprivation operate in such a complex manner, mental health assumes greater significance.

Mental health is not just absence of mental illness but a positive concept of displaying ability for adaptive social and interpersonal relationships and to reach a harmonious relationship with the society. It is the mental health component of overall health that gives quality and meaning to our lives. When individual is unable to cope with change, it not only affects social role but also disturbs psychosocial homeostasis. As such ethnic minorities are subjected to mental health strains, it becomes more important when social changes operate in diverse and complex manner to influence human behavior in Indian society.[11]

IMPACT OF CULTURE ON DISTRESS

Distress across cultures manifests in several ways. Culture influences the way distress is experienced and expressed in individuals,[12] to the extent that rates of psychological distress vary in different ethnic groups.[13] Higher levels of distress are explained by socially disadvantaged, whereas lower rates are explained by culturally specific protective factors such as social cohesion and availability of resources in terms of material goods and economic power.[14] Cultures may differ in recognizing, labeling, and interpreting deviant behaviors influencing help-seeking behavior and the outcome of psychiatric disorders. It would be interesting to understand how cultures affect distress. In collectivist cultures, every individual may put himself after his family members, and in some cases, significant members of the social group. This gives rise to a certain level of family support in such cultures, which may be protective for mental health.[15] On the other hand, an individual from an individualist culture may put his own interest above that of the family or the society, which leads to weaker bonds between them and hence a different impact of distress on these individuals. However, this concept needs more exploration through research. Ross, et al.[16] studied how psychological distress is affected by social class and ethnic identity. It was found that fatalism was more in persons in lower social classes, and this fatalism increases psychological distress. There is association between psychological distress in childhood, adolescence, and adulthood, which is shown by Stansfeld, et al. in the survey of 2,790 males and females, aged between 11-14 years.[15] Their survey found greater rates of depressive symptoms in non-UK white girls, largely of Turkish, Irish, or Greek origin. They also found low risk of psychological distress in Bangladeshi pupils, which might have been because of their preference for conveying psychological distress in somatic symptoms rather by emotional expression, which is a commoner finding in the non-Western cultures. Somatic symptoms are seen to be common expressions of various psychiatric disorders in many different cultures,[17] which often result into nonrecognition of depression.[18] In this context, Bhugra and Mastrogianni have enumerated the emotional lexicon and cultural phrases that could be seen as somatic metaphors of various mental experiences of patients.[19] For example, a Nigerian individual may use the term "biting sensation all over the body" or "heaviness sensation in the head";[20] an Indian woman may use the term "pulling sensation in the brain" for describing a headache, rather than calling it simply a "pain in the head." There is a possibility that in cultures that somatized depression, individuals may frequently visit a general practitioner (GP) complaining of headaches and body pains, be prescribed analgesics for the same, but may perceive no benefit despite adequate doses. Eventually such a patient is referred to a psychiatrist who may overlook the condition as somatization disorder, when in effect the patient is suffering from major depressive disorder; the patient is somatizing his or her depression because of a lack of sufficient words in the language or an inability to psychologize the symptoms. Manson points out how the term *depression* may altogether be absent in the language of some cultures.[21]

CULTURAL EXPLANATIONS

'Interpretive hypothesis' is used to understand the cultural differences and psychopathology[22] which claims that something can be interpreted as something else or that a given concept is useful for describing or understanding something; in simple words.[23] Applying this hypothesis, cultural psychiatry lends some cultural explanation and understanding of mental health problems in different cultures, the aim being to understand a particular psychopathology better if we see it a particular way or through that culture's explanatory model.[24-26]

Cultures provide explanations and causal attributes for somatic and other symptoms.[26] Explanatory models propose that an individual's efforts to make sense of her symptoms and suffering are culturally shaped.[27] Cultural knowledge about symptoms and illness may be encoded in cognitive schemas in individuals, which may include certain beliefs about bodily processes, mechanisms, and their consequences. The strongly held cultural belief and the model of illness play a vital role in determining individuals' use of medical resources. Explanatory models also influence the way patients complain to mental health practitioners about symptoms and whether they somatize or psychologize them. If the cultural background of the health practitioner is different from that of the patient, it may lead to misinterpretation and (mis) labeling of his symptoms and hence under-treatment of the actual underlying disorder.

PATHWAYS INTO CARE

Pathways into mental health care are influenced by one's health beliefs; beliefs of others (especially in a sociocentric society); cultural accessibility, identification and referral system of the services; and their perceived and real efficacy. Individuals recognize health as the norms laid down by the culture in which they are brought up, and these values stay with them unless they are acculturated or assimilated. Thus, if the choice is depends on culture, the various agencies may not be within mental health care services. In addition, identifying agencies of care can help improve the effectiveness of the health services, one's perceptions toward them, and the culturally sensitive framework of the care.[28] Evidences indicate that black and ethnic minority people with mental illnesses differ in their use of services and their treatment compared to whites.[29] Unfavorable experiences with mental health care services discourage ethnic minorities from gaining access to care and staying in touch with service providers. Discontent with the mental health services leads to a "vicious cycle" of undesirable experiences, coercion, disentanglement, and relapse[30] Parkman, et al. found young black men to be dissatisfied with inpatient services in proportion to the contact they had with these services.[31] This dissatisfaction leads to seek alternative help agencies that are influenced by their explanatory models. In a study, Blacks, compared to Asians and Whites, were found to live alone more before admission and had a more complex pathway into care.[32] They also felt less informed about their illness and were perceived as more violent than other ethnic groups. These negative experiences result in avoidance of the mental health services.

Morgan, et al. identified three priority areas for further research: (1) social networks, (2) cultural contexts and mental health beliefs and (3) healthcare services that are available.[33] Future research in this area would provide an insight into how to identify cases and agencies. It would also highlight the reasons why ethnic groups are more likely to contact a voluntary organization than mental health services.[33] More research could result in health professionals developing a complete competency in working with ethnic groups. If Black patients have a more complex pathway and enter mental health services much later than white patients,[34] it is possible that this group may conceptualize their illness experiences in a dissimilar way than other ethnic groups.

Help-seeking is a process is defined by one's social, educational, and cultural background, among other factors. Mechanic found 10 variables that characterize how one reacts to illness: (i) visibility and recognizability of symptoms, (ii) perceived seriousness of symptoms, (iii) extent to which symptoms disrupt life, (iv) frequency of symptoms, (v) tolerance threshold of individual, (vi) cultural beliefs about illness, (vii) denial of symptoms, (viii) needs that compete with illness response, (ix) normalization of symptoms, and (x) treatment available.[35] These factors influence one's response and could explain why Black patients deny illness because of the stigma attached to psychotic illness in their culture.[36] In one of the earliest studies, Kleinman emphasized the significance of health beliefs to determine how and from whom people look for help. He also suggested a healthcare service (HCS) model consisting of the three treatment areas: popular, folk, and professional.[37] The popular area includes "free" help agencies, for instance, receiving advice from family and friends. The patient intellectualizes his illness during this stage in a social framework. The folk area contains looking for help from cultural agencies, for instance, healers, shamans, etc.[38] How the patient recognizes his illness in a cultural framework governs whether he may access the professional sector. The professional sector embodies health services. These sectors are actually not distinct entities but have a liquefied status where people move between the agencies of these sectors. A model was proposed by Goldberg and Huxley which describes the different planes of engagement for minority patients.[39-41] A patient needs to pass through various planes and filters for obtaining specialist care. The first level begins by the patient recognizing his distress in the community and pursuing guidance from family and friends. Each stage depends on whether symptoms are identified and apt help is provided on that particular level. This model helps in identifying the processes through patients pass in accessing care. Thus the first stage comprises of understanding one's illness with the support of caregivers and friends. Morgan, et al. in a review argued that the understanding of various pathways into care is incomplete as it focuses on only medical framework. They stressed that future research must explore the cultural element and its effect on help-seeking behavior.[30] Five of the 26 studies of criminal justice referrals indicated no significant difference between the African Caribbean patients and the white patients.[42-44] Four of eleven studies of GP involvement displayed no significant differences in the ethnic groups. It was seen that white patients were more likely to be recognized in primary care, and black patients were mostly referred to a specialist service if mental illness in them was identified.[30] It was noted by the researchers that because the research has largely been conducted by psychiatrists using survey methods, rates of police/GP involvement, and correlations of referrals and admissions, the models of factors involving admissions were far too narrow. Furthermore, research differs in its patient samples, which do not control for previous contact with the services. This variable is important in how patients access care, and, if not controlled, it disregards whether a patient's previous contact has been favorable or not, which has already been shown to be a significant factor in both engagement and satisfaction. Also, studies differ in how the ethnicity of patients is recognized or rated. This permits for overlap between various cultures, for instance, African Caribbean and Black Caribbean; thus, cultural differences are difficult to determine.

EPIDEMIOLOGICAL PROBLEMS

Among prisoners who were sentenced, prevalence of mental illness in African Caribbean individuals is 6% compared to 2% in the white population.[45] African Caribbean patients in England have greater incidence of schizophrenia and other psychotic disorders than white patients.[30] It is probable that Blacks are over-represented in population in remand and sentenced prison. According to Coid, et al. first admission rates to a forensic unit in half of England and Wales were 5.6 times greater for black males than white population.[46] Similarly, black patients with physical illnesses contact health services at a later stage than white patients.[47-51]

A review[52] focused on whether ethnic groups differ in (1) pathways into mental health care, (2) ongoing care, (3) use of inpatient services, and (4) admissions; it found that black patients were referred to at least three caregivers before entering the mental health care system.[32] More black patients than white had seen a "helping agency" close to entry to psychiatric care.[53]

Thus, feelings of social isolation, living alone, racism, and lack of support, all could contribute to poor mental health. India's minorities face similar mental health issues.[54,55]

MANAGEMENT ISSUES

A desirable approach in management is the biopsychosocial strategy. A clear understanding of the interplay of different factors is crucial in developing and delivering the right treatment strategies. Clinicians need to be certain that the right dosage and right treatment are available and their effects are discussed with the patients and their caregivers. Kennedy and Olsson demonstrated that health care-seeking activities are related to the perceived etiologies of the illness or the cultural knowledge of the person.[53] If the perception of the etiology is more traditional, there are more chances of the patient's choosing a traditional practitioner over the modern clinician, and the more likely the practitioner is to prescribe traditional treatments. There are a number of theories proposed to describe the possible path taken by a sick individual to seek help from a healthcare provider. Parson's sick role theory[56] expects the sick individual to look for medical aid and to conform with treatment in order to recover. While Parson's theory did explain the typically expected and seen behavior in individuals who are ill, it failed to explain the variability that is commonly seen in illness behavior. The various Suchman's stages for illness and medical care,[57] describe a sick individual's moving through five stages in the process of deciding whether to use health care:

- The individual's experience of his or her symptoms, which includes all the associated emotions and the patient's recognition of this experience as being indicative of an illness.
- Sick role assumption by the patient; during this stage he may explore available treatment options, which may include both the Western biomedical treatments and also the culturally viable and sanctioned traditional systems.
- Medical care contact, which happens if the individual pursues a professional health care system.
- The fourth stage is the notion of a dependent patient role by accepting the professional treatment of health care services. However, in case the individual chooses this option over the traditional system and then finds that the treating professional has differing opinions of the illness and the treatment required, there is a good chance that he may shun the idea of continuing with this model of treatment and move back to traditional models.
- Recovery from the illness. understand that the sick individual may spend an ample amount of time exploring the amateur referral system for validation of the sick role and for recommendations regarding consideration of treatment options available, thus affecting the rate and pace at which the individual enters the next stage. The lay referral system includes all the nonprofessional persons, such as various family members, friends who may aid the sick person infer his problem.

Grubin comments that no clear guidelines can be drawn for forensic psychiatrists considering the nature of psychiatry and the realities of law.[58] Forensic psychiatrists sometimes deal with serious cases that may require electroconvulsive therapy (ECT) as a treatment option;[59] however, this option is rarely used for forensic-psychiatric patients or prisoners. The question of validity of informed consent may also be an important deterrent to choosing ECT as an option for this group of patients. Witzel, et al. estimated the indication for use of ECT in forensic psychiatry as approximately 3% and 12.5% for schizophrenia and depressive patients, respectively, in forensic psychiatry units.

RACE AND ETHNICITY

Race refers to genetic heritage, in theoretical framework. In practice, it is characteristically based on biological traits that are supposed to be inherited and visibly evident, such as hair texture, skin color and eyelid folds. The genetic studies question the authenticity of the very concept of race. The average genetic variation amongst individuals of same race is similar to the genetic variation between the racial groups. Every population is considered a microcosm that recapitulates the whole human macrocosm, even if there is slight variation in the precise genetic compositions. Around one-third of white European genetic inheritance is derivative of African admixtures, and 30% of African-American genetic heritage is derived from the white American admixtures.[5] In light of these evidence, it would be imprudent to assume much about an individual's genetic make-up on the basis of racial appearance.

Ethnicity denotes cultural rather than the genetic heritage. An ethnic group can be demarcated by its shared place of origin, language, history, arts, religion, cuisine, and various other cultural factors. Research rarely differentiates among these potentially coinciding categories or recognizes how racial or ethnic obligations are made. In clinical practice, the patient is infrequently asked how he or she recognizes himself or herself. Research validity questions are there, even when a patient is probed to recognize his or her ethnic background, since degree of identification with components of his or her background can fluctuate over time.

ETHNICITY IN FORENSIC PSYCHIATRY

Forensic opinions are grounded in clinical assessment. An invalid diagnosis or clinical formulation may jeopardize the validity of the forensic conclusion. For the same reason, forensic psychiatrists are required to be mindful of the impact of ethnicity and culture can put on the diagnosis. In spite of similar illness prevalence among diverse ethnic groups, numerous studies have shown bias of clinicians in diagnosing. In a study, it was seen that therapists presented with such a scenario that rated the behavior of African American adolescents as less clinically significant.[10] Numerous study findings have revealed that African Americans are more commonly diagnosed with psychosis and whites with mood disorders in the emergency rooms and during hospitalization.[11-14] Researchers have considered the various factors that might be reasons to these discrepancies, including help-seeking patterns, illness presentation, and clinician bias.[20-22] In a study, it was seen that emergency room clinicians unsuccessful to elicit sufficient information about mood signs and symptoms in nonwhite patients. In India, some studies report anxious and avoidance behavior among minority group subjects compared with others.[60]

When diagnoses are based on a structured clinical interviews and diagnostic criteria, lesser disparities are detected.[24] Proper diagnosis may also be interfered due to language difficulties.

REFERENCES

1. Sutker P. Drug and Psychopathology. National Institute of Drug Abuse Research, Maryland. 1977, Issue No. 19.
2. Orlandi MA. Cultural Competence for the Evaluators. US Department of Health and Human Services, Rockville, Maryland, 1992.
3. Linton R. The Study of Man. Apple-tone, New York, 1947.
4. Berne E. Games People Play: The Psychology of Human Relationship. Newton Books, New York, 1964.
5. Bellah RN. Habits o the Heart. Harper and Row, New York, 1985.
6. Light D Jr, Keller S. Sociology. New York, Knopf, 1985.
7. Group for the Advancement of Psychiatry, Committee on Cultural Psychiatry. Washington: American Psychiatric Publishing; 2001. Cultural Assessment in Clinical Psychiatry.
8. Read CH. Sir Edward Burnett Tylor. Man. 1917;17(16):25-6.
9. Moore JD. Visions of Culture: An Introduction to Anthropological Theories and Theorists, 3rd ed. New York: Rowman Altamira, 2008:5.
10. Powys JC. The Meaning of Culture. Read Books, 2008.
11. Jiloha RC. Deprivation, Discrimination, Human Rights Violation and Mental Health of the Deprived. Indian J Psychiatry. 2010;52(3):207-12.
12. Kalra G, Bhugra D. Cross Cultural Psychiatry. In: Psychiatric Update, 2nd ed. Deka K, Bhuyan D (Eds). Dibrugarh: Indian Psychiatric Society, Assam State Branch; 2010 .pp. 493-525.
13. Kirmayer LJ. Cultural variations in the response to psychiatric disorders and emotional distress. Social Science & Medicine. 1989;29(3):327-39.
14. Sproston K, Nazroo J (Eds). Ethnic Minority Psychiatric Illness Rates in the Community (EMPIRIC). London: Stationery Office, 2002.
15. Stansfeld SA, Haines MM, Head JA, et al. Ethnicity, social deprivation and psychological distresss in adolescents: school-based epidemiological study in east London. Br J Psychiatry. 2004;185:233-8.
16. Ross CE, Mirowsky J, Cockerham WC. Social class, Mexican culture, and fatalism: their effects on psychological distress. Am J Community Psychology. 1983;11(4):383-99.
17. Kessler D, Lloyd K, Lewis G, et al. Cross-sectional study of symptom attribution and recognition of depression and anxiety in primary care. Br Med J. 1999;318(7181):436-9.
18. Tylee A, Freeling P, Kerry S, et al. How does the content of consultations affect recognition by general practitioners of major depression in women. Br J Gen Pract. 1995;45(400):575-8.
19. Bhugra D, Mastrogianni A. Globalisation and mental disorders. Overview with relation to depression. Br J Psychiatry. 2004;184:10-20.
20. Ebigbo PO. Development of a culture specific (Nigeria) screening scale of somatic complaints indicating psychiatric disturbance. Cult Med Psychiatry. 1982;6(1):29-43.
21. Manson SM. Culture and major depression. Current challenges in the diagnosis of mood disorders. Psychiatric Clin North Am. 1995;18(3):487-501.
22. White GM. The role of cultural explanations in 'somatization' and 'psychologization'. Soc Sci Med. 1982;16(16):1519-30.

23. Niiniluoto I. Tieteellinen paattely ja selittaminen. Helsinki: Otava, 1983.
24. Kirmayer LJ, Young A. Culture and somatization: Clinical, epidemiological, and ethnographic perspectives. Psychosomatic Med. 1998;60(4):420-30.
25. Kirmayer LJ, Looper KJ, Taillefer S. Somatoform Disorders. In: Adult Psychopathology, 4th ed. In: Turner S, Hersen M (Eds). New York: John Wiley & Sons, 2003.
26. Robbins JM, Kirmayer LJ. Attributions of common somatic symptoms. Psychol Med. 1991;21(4):1029-45.
27. Kirmayer LJ, Young A, Robbins JM. Symptom attribution in cultural perspective. Canadian J Psychiatry. 1994;39(10):584-95.
28. Gater R, de Almeida e Sousa B, Barrientos G. The pathways to psychiatric care: A cross-cultural study. Psychol Med. 1991;21(3):761-74.
29. Bhui K, Bhugra D. Mental illness in Black and Asian ethnic minorities: Pathways to care and outcomes. Adv Psychiatr Treat. 2002;8:26-33.
30. Morgan C, Mallett R, Hutchinson G, et al. Negative pathways to psychiatric care and ethnicity: the bridge between social science and psychiatry. Soc Sci Med. 2004;58(4):739-52.
31. Parkman S, Davies S, Leese M, et al. Ethnic differences in satisfaction with mental health services among representative people with psychosis in south London: PRiSM study 4. Br J Psychiatry. 1997;171:260-4.
32. Commander MJ, Sashi Dharan SP, Odell SM, et al. Access to mental health care in an innercity health district. II: Association with demographic factors. Br J Psychiatry. 1997;170:317-20.
33. Gray P. Voluntary Organizations. Ethnicity: An Agenda for Mental Health. In: Bhugra D, Bahl V (Eds). London: Gaskell; 1999 .pp. 202-10.
34. Thomas CS, Stone K, Osborn M, et al. Psychiatric morbidity and compulsory admission among UK-born Europeans, Afro-Caribbeans and Asians in central Manchester. Br J Psychiatry. 1993;163:91-9.
35. Mechanic D. Medical Sociology: A Comprehensive Text, 2nd ed. New York: Free Press, 1968.
36. Dunn J, Fahy TA. Police admissions to a psychiatric hospital. Demographic and clinical differences between ethnic groups. Br J Psychiatry. 1990;156:373-8.
37. Kleinman A. Patients and Healers in the Context of Culture: An Exploration of the Borderland between Anthropology, Medicine, and Psychiatry. Berkeley, CA: University of California Press, 1980.
38. Jiloha RC, Kishore J. Supernatural beliefs, psychiatric disorder and treatment outcomes in Indian patients. Indian J Soc Psychiatry. 1997;13(3-4):24-31.
39. Brown AS, Varma VK, Malhotra S, et al. Course of acute affective disorders in a developing country setting. J Nervous Ment Dis. 1998;186(4):207-10.
40. Jiloha RC, Kishore J. Sociodemography, personality profile and academic performance of various categories of medical students. Indian J Psychiatry. 1998;40(3):231-41.
41. Goldberg D, Huxley P. Mental Illness in the Community. London: Tavistock, 1980.
42. Burnett R, Mallett R, Bhugra D, et al. The first contact of patient with schizophrenia with psychotic services: social factors and pathways to care in a multi-ethnic population. Psychol Med.1999;II:581-99.
43. Cole E, Leavey G, King M, et al. Pathways to care for patients with first episode psychosis. A comparison of ethnic groups. Br J Psychiatry. 1995;167:770-6.
44. Moodley P, Perkins RE. Routes to psychiatric inpatient care in an Inner London Borough. Soc Psychiatry Psychiatr Epidemiol. 1991;26:47-51.
45. Maden A, Swinton M, Gunn J. The ethnic origins of women serving a prison sentence. Br J Criminol. 1992;32:218-21.

46. Coid J, Kahtan N, Gault S, et al. Ethnic differences in admissions to secure forensic psychiatry services. Br J Psychiatry. 2000;177:241.
47. O'Farrell N, Lau R, Yoganathan K, et al. AIDS in Africans living in London. Genitourinary Med. 1995;71(6):358-62.
48. Coid JW, Kirkbride JB, Barker D, et al. Raised incidence rates of all psychoses among migrant groups. Findings from the east London first episode psychosis study. Archives of Gen Psychiatry. 2008;65(11):1250-8.
49. Decuyper M, De Fruyt F, Buschman J. A five-factor model perspective on psychopathy and comorbid Axis-II disorders in a forensic-psychiatric sample. Int J Law Psychiatry. 2008;31(5):394-406.
50. Coid J, Yang M, Ullrich S, et al. Psychopathy among prisoners in England and Wales. Int J Law Psychiatry. 2009;32(3):134-41.
51. Bhui K, Brown P, Hardie T, et al. African-Caribbean men remanded to Brixton Prison. Psychiatric and forensic characteristics and outcome of final court appearance. Br J Psychiatry. 1998;172:337-44.
52. Bhui K, Stansfeld S, Hull S, Priebe S, Mole F, Feder G (Eds). Ethnic variations in pathways to and use of specialist mental health services in the UK. Systematic review. Br J Psychiatry. 2003;182:105-16.
53. Harrison G, Holton A, Nielson D, et al. Severe mental disorder in Afro-Caribbean patients: Some social, demographic and service factors. Psychol Med. 1989;19:683-96.
54. Jiloha RC. Aggression and locus of control among scheduled caste students. Indian J Soc Psychiatry. 1995;11(1-4):18-21.
55. Jiloha RC. Relative deprivation and reaction to frustration among scheduled caste students. Indian J Soc Psychiatry. 1995;11(1-4):22-6.
56. Kennedy JC, Olsson K. Health care seeking behavior and formal integration: a rural Mexican case study. Human Organization. 1996;55(1):4.
57. Parsons T. The Social System. Glencoe, IL: Free Press, 1951.
58. Grubin D. Commentary: mapping a changing landscape in the ethics of forensic psychiatry. J Am Acade Psychiatry Law. 2008;36(2):185-90.
59. Witzel J, Held E, Bogerts B. Electroconvulsive therapy in forensic psychiatry-ethical problems in daily practice. J ECT. 2009;25(2):129-32.
60. Jiloha RC. Mental Health Issues in Indian Minorities. Textbook of Postgraduate Psychiatry. In: Vyas JN, Ahuja N (Eds). Jaypee Brothers Medical Publishers (P) Ltd. New Delhi, India; 1999.

CHAPTER 11

Report Writing in Forensic Psychiatry: General Principles

> **LEARNING OBJECTIVES**
> - Structure of a forensic report
> - Characteristics of a good report
> - What not to include in a forensic psychiatry report
> - Issues to be aware of while reporting

Writing report of the assessment carried out is an important construct that helps the agency ordering assessment find a clear answer to the psycholegal question raised. Forensic reports should be designed to meet the needs of the court and the specific questions addressed or standards referenced.

STRUCTURE OF A FORENSIC REPORT

The report can be submitted in three parts
1. Covering letter
2. A brief opinion addressing the psycholegal question asked by agency ordering assessment (Court/Employer/Educational Institutes), e.g. in a psycholegal question posed by court regarding "fitness to stand trial" commenting on fitness asked, whether the client is fit or not and if unfit whether temporarily or permanently; if temporarily then when should be the next reassessment done. Additive measure, e.g. medicines or counseling or supportive family care to ensure compliance necessary to restore temporary state of not being fit
3. Details of the facts of the case and procedure used in reaching to the opinion
   - Patient details: Name, Age, Sex, Address, Hospital Registration number
   - Copy of written informed consent mentioning limitation of confidentiality and incorporating following:
     i. Person or family presenting for assessment should be informed before assessment about following and a written consent to same should be recorded.
     ii. Who ordered the examination?
     iii. Purpose of examination.

iv. Who all will have access to report? Limitations of confidentiality and duty to report to court the facts apparent during assessment process.
   a. Background of assessment:
      - Who ordered the assessment?
      - Purpose of assessment
   b. Medical board details:
      - Date and time of medical board proceedings
      - Constituent of medical board: Chairperson, members (mentioning name, designation, qualification of each)
   c. Details of assessors (if assessment team is different from medical board team):
      - Who all health professionals assessed client (for reaching on to opinion prior to medical board presentation
      - Date and time of assessments
   d. Source of information to reach on opinion:
      - Who all were interviewed?
      - Records accessed for information
   e. Clinical case summary:
      - Diagnosis and brief facts about case history
      - Current mental state examination finding
   f. Report of any psychological test used (including date, time, assessor's detail)
   g. Competency assessment details specific to case:
      - Criteria used for capacity assessment
      - Timing of different assessments
      - Details of specific questions asked and answers in verbatim
      - Who all carried out assessments
v. Opinion and recommendations
vi. Additional riders in incapacity reports: If report of "not fit" being submitted
   a. Please mention, is this temporary or permanent
   b. If temporary, what measures are needed to restore fitness? (e.g. Medication, psychosocial intervention or legal assistance)
   c. If temporary, at what time client should be sent back for re-assessment
vii. Any support measures needed during trial: For client with mental health issues, where it is anticipated that there can be effect of deposing in court on person's mental health, additional measures can be suggested to the court to prevent that likelihood, e.g. frequent breaks, daytime medicine during deposing, need of any support person or in camera hearing, etc.
viii. Any support measures needed during work place: If a fitness for job is being evaluated, and person is given fitness then to mention if any specific need that employer needs to take care of such employee who has recently recovered from a mental illness and nature of job suitable for the person.

All the reports submitted to the court are documentary evidence and psychiatrist can be called in court of law as expert evidence to corroborate their own or someone else's report submitted on the matter **(Box 1)**.

CHAPTER 11: Report Writing in Forensic Psychiatry: General Principles

Box 1: Structure of a forensic report.

1. *Covering letter*
2. A brief *opinion addressing the psycholegal question asked* by concerned agency including:
    - Opinion regarding question asked
    - If declared 'unfit', when is next fitness evaluation desirable
    - Any cautions to be exercised by concerned agency ordering investigations (e.g. support measures if any needed during trial for a fitness to trial case or any workplace accommodation needed for an employee being evaluated for fitness to resume job)
3. *Relevant case details instrumental in reaching the final opinion:*
    - Patient particulars
    - Sources of information
    - Relevant brief case summary
    - Relevant clinical findings
    - Any tests conducted (biological/psychological)
    - Assessment details (assessment done by whom, when)
    - Medical board details (board team, interview details, final opinion)

CHARACTERISTICS OF A GOOD REPORT

- *A good report must adhere to what are known as the three "Is" of ethical practice:* It will need to demonstrate 'the three Is' of being an expert witness: that is, impartiality (and the appearance of impartiality), independence and integrity.[1]
- *Focusing on target audience:* A forensic report is usually read first by legal representatives of the defendant, as well as other lawyers, judge, and paralegal professionals. These individuals do not have technical medical expertise, and therefore the report should be succinct and understandable to the lay public. The language used must not use excessive jargon, and must be explicit in descriptions for the nonmedical reader.[2]
- *Scientific evidence:* All documents that form a forensic psychiatric report are documentary court evidence to be used in the case under consideration. In addition, this report often forms the basis for the forensic psychiatrist's oral evidence to the court. It should be prepared keeping this fact in mind, and therefore must be meticulous and thorough in its contents.
- *Not just diagnosis:* The purpose of a forensic report is not simply to provide a clinical diagnosis, if one is available in the first place. It must describe all complex biopsychosocial issues, including the behavioral consequences of the diagnosis, and the legal relevance of the psychiatric findings. Above all, it should frame the narrative in a way that is organized, understandable, and as complete as possible.[1]
- *Opinions with rationale:* Mere facts or unexplained inferences do not make a good forensic report. The information should be sufficiently detailed in order to allow the reader to arrive logically at the inferences made based on the evidence provided.[1]

WHAT NOT TO INCLUDE IN A FORENSIC PSYCHIATRY REPORT[2]

- *Professional jargon:* It must be written with target audience in mind. If use of any technical word is unavoidable, it should be immediately followed by the explanation of same in parenthesis.

- *Details not directly relevant to the issue at hand:* A forensic report does not need to delve in to all the dimensions and complexities of an individual's internal or social life. It is merely an exploration of the specific legal issue at hand from a psychiatric point of view and must be limited to the task at hand.
- *Biased language:* Ethical professional conduct demands that the language used in a forensic report should remain strictly neutral, neither pejorative nor excessively sympathetic. Descriptions should be objective rather than florid.

ISSUES TO BE AWARE OF WHILE REPORTING[1]

- Be aware that the legal and medical concepts of mental illness differ significantly.
- Ensure that the purpose of the test is understood and only the relevant legal tests are applied, so as to avoid any confusion created in legal issues by use of medical language.
- Be careful in the reporting of risk assessments; the purpose of risk assessment reporting is usually different from the formulation for other purposes such as sentencing.
- Reconsider the need for a forensic psychiatric assessment if there is no diagnosed mental disorder in the evaluee.
- It is not a psychiatrist's job to recommend punishment. Refrain from doing so.
- Limit yourself to the requirements of the assessment—one must not go beyond the instructions of assessment.
- Refrain from drawing causative relationships between the presence of mental illness and the offence. It is extremely unlikely that the mental disorder can 'cause' an offence.
- All proposed associations between mental disorder and any offence must be expressed with great caution.

Specific reporting parameters for individualized civil and criminal cases and criteria used have been detailed in individual chapters

REFERENCES

1. Eastman N, Adshead G, Fox S, et al. Forensic Psychiatry. Oxford Specialists Handbooks. London: Oxford University Press; 2017.
2. Conroy MA. Report writing and testimony (Electronic Version). Applied Psychology in Criminal Justice. 2006;2(3):237-60.

CHAPTER

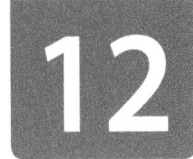

Psychiatrist as an Expert Witness in Court

> **LEARNING OBJECTIVES**
> - Role of Psychiatrist as an expert witness
> - Oral evidence
> - Types of oral evidence
> - Role of expert witness
> - Courtroom behavior

ROLE OF PSYCHIATRIST AS AN EXPERT WITNESS

Situations requiring expert testimony by psychiatrist:
1. Issues pertaining to Mental Health Act—Admission, Discharge
2. Criminal—Competence to stand trial—Criminal responsibility—Assess risk of suicide, homicide, disruptive or antisocial behavior
3. Civil— Guardianship, marriage, divorce, annulment, maintenance, custody of children—Adoption, guardianship—Testamentary capacity—Contracts—Organ donation—Fitness for employment, rehabilitation.

ORAL EVIDENCE (COURT APPEARANCES) VS DOCUMENTARY EVIDENCE (REPORTS SUBMITTED)

Oral evidence is always superior to documentary evidence in trial for the reasons that, the person has to prove on oath that the evidence is true and is cross-examined. However, a person giving documentary evidence is also supposed to do the same, exceptions being:
- Dying declaration.
- Printed opinion of experts in the form of textbooks, when author is either dead or stays at a very distant place, and to bring him/her would mean unnecessary loss of time and money.
- Evidence previously given in a judicial procedure.
- Deposition of a medical witness in a lower court, attested by the magistrate.
- Chemical examiner's report is sufficient and his/her personal attendance is usually not necessary.

All these documentary evidences are accepted by court as unsworn documents, without any oral testimony.[1]

TYPES OF ORAL EVIDENCE

Types of oral evidence could be of two types:
1. *Direct*: Refers to facts, which are seen, heard or perceived by any other sense.
2. *Circumstantial*: It proves one or more of the subsidiary circumstances or associated events.

Witness

Definition

Witness is defined as a person who provides evidence about a case in the court of law under oath and is summoned to court to attend without failure and under penalty.

Classification

Witnesses are classified into following types:
- *Common witness*: Common witness is a lay person, who narrates what he/she has heard or perceived or states the facts observed by him/her.
- *Expert witness*: Expert witness based on their special professional training and skill, can give opinion on facts observed by himself or by others, i.e. Forensic psychiatrist, Medical Men, Chemical Examiner, Fingerprint Expert, Handwriting Expert, Ballistic Expert, etc.
- *Medical witness (Doctor)*: A medical witness is generally considered as both common and expert witness.[1]

ROLE OF EXPERT WITNESS

1. State the facts and give opinion
2. Order of examination of witnesses:
    a. Examination in chief by the party that would have summoned the expert
    b. Cross examination by the opposing lawyer if the advocate so desires
    c. Re-examination by the first party.[1]

Receiving Summons for Court Appearance as Expert Witness

Summons can be issued by the Court for the psychiatrist to appear as witness before a particular court, for a given case, at a specified date, time and venue.
- Recipient must acknowledge receipt of the summons.
- The date and time of receipt must be noted while signing acceptance
- If the specified date and time are too short or otherwise unsuitable, a fresh date must be sought in writing or after personal appearance.
- One must prepare well, before testifying.
- Attending the court is mandatory. Only in exceptional circumstances can an exemption be made after these are reported at court. These circumstances are:
    – Personal indisposition
    – Professional priorities
    – Personal preoccupation.

These circumstances must be conveyed to court. Their presence may only reschedule the summons, not obviate the need for it.[1]

COURTROOM BEHAVIOR

Tips to the Expert Witness for Court Appearances[1,2]

Forensic practitioner is frequently required to testify as an expert witness. The following are guidelines for effectively fulfilling the role of an expert witness:

- *Preparation before going to court*: One should keep thorough notes, documentations, records, photographs to support the testimony. All documents and details of the case must be reviewed before delivering the testimony, and appropriate language should be used to deliver the facts and inferences of the case. On must not allow oneself to be pressured beyond the area of expertise. To fulfil this, an internal debate can be carried out with a presumed opponent who is an expert in the field, and who would be able to detect any comments beyond the expertise of the field.
- *Giving expert testimony*: Wear decent and dignified clothing. When responding to questions, address the judges/magistrate, not lawyers. Ensure eye contact when speaking. Think before you speak—it is acceptable to pause before you answer. The opposition must get a chance to object to your statements. Avoid blank spaces in the middle of an answer, including any "filler" sounds such as "uhms" and "aahs". One must present themselves in a professional manner, and non-verbal communication is vital. How one stands, the posture one naturally assumes, and body language is important in effective communication. Physical signs of nervousness such as fidgeting or swaying are off-putting to the audience, and must be avoided. Argumentation should be civil, and one must not generate animosity among opponents. One must be aware of and acknowledge the limitations in their knowledge, and appear sincere and fair. Opinions must be emphasized and jargon must be avoided. Any technical concepts must be clarified. Be aware that every statement made in court is documented. Respond directly to the question being asked.
- *Cross-examination*
Not all questions have to be answered with a yes or a no, one must take their time to explain their reasoning. Be aware of the opposition manipulating your words to give new meaning to your statements: phrases such as "is it fair to say…" must be addressed with caution. You can draw a limit on your capabilities as an expert witness. Ask lawyers for clarification if all aspects of the question are not clear to you. A second chance to explain your inferences must be asked for if there is a suspicion that your statement has been misinterpreted. Be aware of your personal biases, you are not in the court to take sides, but to present objective truths. The louder the opposition lawyer gets, the calmer you should- fear tactics are well-known in courts, and they should not phase you. Ask for clarification when things are not clear.
- *Other points*
Avoid scientific jargon.
Be objective: It is the lawyer's job to take sides, not yours.

Go over prior testimony, reports, and exhibits before the trial.
- Use visual aids, analogies, illustrations from everyday life.
- Pay attention to the judge/magistrate and follow his orders for the court proceedings.
- Do not become a victim of the line of questioning. Beware of questions that ask details about your personal practice or a possibility your past mistakes.
- Do not obfuscate. A difficult question must be answered either directly, or limitations must be clearly defined.
- Be aware of the cross-examination trick of taking an excerpt from a publication out of context or an excerpt from a nonexistent article. You can always ask the lawyer to show you the article to refresh your memory or even to read it out.
- It is okay to say 'I don't know'.
- Take the lead to meet with and talk with counsel.
- Mentor new, inexperienced prosecutors. Empathize with them and offer advise based on your experience, do not be afraid of sharing past mistakes and the lessons you learnt.

REFERENCES

1. Rao NG. Textbook of Forensic Medicine and Toxicology, 2nd edn. Jaypee Brothers Medical Publishers (P) Ltd; 2010.
2. Vahia V, Bhujan PM. Psychiatrist as an expert witness. Indian J Psychiatry Clinicals Pract Guidelines, 2009. Article 12. pp. 210-17. Available at: http://www.indianjpsychiatry.org/cpg/cpg2009/article12.pdf.last accessed on 07.02.18.

CHAPTER 13

Malingering

> **LEARNING OBJECTIVES**
> - Concept of malingering
> - Malingering and psychiatry
> - Subtypes of malingering
> - Clinical assessment of malingering in psychiatry settings
> - Psychological assessment of malingering
> - Differential diagnosis
> - Approach in assessment of malingering

■ INTRODUCTION

What is malingering?: Deception is a human behavior occurring commonly in everyday life. However, it becomes challenging when it occurs in clinical setting as it makes job of a clinician difficult who has been trained and duty bound to trust the patient and keep their interests above all. "Malingering is the deliberate production or gross exaggeration of false, physical or psychologic symptoms for a known external reward."[1]

Need of identifying: In presence of apparent specific motivation, clinicians are in a position to identify determinant phenomenological features pointing towards malingering. The task becomes more difficult, when suspicion of malingering arises in presence of comorbid genuine mental illness, because, denial of treatment in such situations become ethical violation. It is important to identify malingering in clinical settings because of medicolegal concerns associated and also more importantly for judicious allocation of already meagre health resources towards patients with genuine symptoms.

■ MALINGERING AND PSYCHIATRY

Magnitude of problem: Mental health professionals often come across cases of malingering. "Mittenberg and associates reported that in a recent study of 33,531 cases seen by members of the American Board of Clinical Neuropsychology during a 1-year period, probable malingering and symptom exaggeration were found in 30% of disability evaluations, 29% of personal injury evaluations, 19% of criminal evaluations and 8% of medical cases."[1] As compared to general psychiatry, specialized forensic settings dealing with cases concerning jail settings, court ordered evaluations and compensation seeking clients seeking treatment for post-traumatic stress disorder (PTSD), may witness higher rates of malingering.[2]

Symptoms that can be commonly malingered: memory deficits, seizure, sleep disorders, altered identity, mood symptoms, suicidal ideations and hallucinations

Malingered psychiatry conditions: It includes dissociative identity disorder, dissociative amnesia, dissociative motor disorders, amnestic disorders, PTSD, psychosis, mood disorders, suicide, "malingering by proxy" in the pediatric setting.[3]

Difficulty in diagnosing malingering: The difficulties in detecting malingering were aptly demonstrated by Rosenhan's (1973) famous study.[4] Concept of malingering is easy to define, difficult to pick and much more challenging to diagnose, even if index of suspicion in high due to following reasons:
- Ethical dilemma
- Difficulty in proving it due to lack of awareness and availability of standardized objective tests to prove it
- Fear of legal suit
- Pejorative term, fear of stigmatizing patient
- Easy access in public domain about psychiatric symptoms and easy to feign psychiatry symptoms in absence of any objective laboratory test.

Therefore, mental health clinicians should have familiarity with key points in malingering assessment.

Nosology

Malingering is not a mental disorder, in DSM-5 it is listed as "other conditions that may be a focus on clinical attention". In "V code"[5] and as "Z code" in ICD-10.[6] The term "malinger" has its origin from French idiom (malingerer) meaning either "to suffer" or "pretend to be ill". Modern connotations reflect more incriminating nuance. DSM-5 defines malingering as "...the intentional production of false or grossly exaggerated physical or psychological symptoms, motivated by external incentives". The entry goes on to state that malingering should be "strongly suspected if any combination of the following is noted".[5] It further states to suspect malingering in following contexts:

1. There is a "marked discrepancy" between the individual's "claimed stress or disability" and "objective findings and observations".
2. Medicolegal context of presentation.
3. "Lack of cooperation during the diagnostic evaluation" and in complying with the prescribed treatment regimen.
4. The presence of antisocial personality disorder.

These external incentives might include:
a. Avoiding work
b. Avoiding military duty
c. Obtaining financial compensation
d. Evading criminal prosecution
e. Obtaining narcotic drugs

Subtypes: Resnick[7] comments on following subtypes of malingering based on symptom presentation:

- *Pure malingering*: Complete fabrication,
- *Partial malingering*: Exaggeration of existing symptoms,
- *False imputation*: When an evaluee intentionally attributes symptoms to an unrelated cause.

Lipian & Mills, 2000[8] described following subtypes of malingering:
- *Positive malingering*: Feigning the symptoms of an illness.
- *Negative malingering*: Hiding or misreporting the symptoms.
- *Data tampering*: Altering diagnostic instruments, data or record to influence test results.
- *False imputation*: Ascribing actual symptoms to an unrelated cause consciously.
- *Staging events*: Carefully planning and executing events to result in an injury or an explanation for feigning disability.
- *Misattribution*: Ascribing actual symptoms to an unrelated cause erroneously believed to have caused it.

ASSESSMENT OF MALINGERING IN PSYCHIATRY SETTINGS

When to Suspect Malingering?

As per Cunnien, 1997, index of suspicion should be high in specific situations involving:[3,9]
- Motivation/Circumstances
  - Financial incentive
  - Solution to socioeconomic problems
  - Antisocial acts/Behaviors
  - Career dissatisfaction
  - Work conflict
  - End of career
  - In treatment for documentation purposes
  - History of lying, malingering or dishonesty
  - Change in diagnosis to fit policy requirements
- Symptom presentation
  - Unusual/atypical symptoms
  - Currently asymptomatic with claim of future decompensation
  - Exaggeration of symptoms/impairment
  - Symptoms incongruent with course of illness
  - Bizarre or absurd symptomatology
  - Unusual symptomatic response to treatment
  - Atypical symptomatic fluctuation consistent with external incentives
  - Marked discrepancy between subjective complaints and objective findings
  - Suspicion of voluntary control over symptoms.

For example, in patients feigning psychotic symptoms, evaluee may reports hallucinations and/or delusions, but objective signs of psychosis (e.g. negative symptoms, distraction due to hallucinations, derailment, thought blocking, clang-bang associations, loose associations, neologisms, incoherence, or perseveration) are minimal or absent. Auditory hallucinations may be continuous rather than intermittent, vague, or inaudible, or spoken in stilted language (overly formal and not paralleling the normal syntactical structure used by the evaluee). Evaluee may have no strategies to diminish auditory hallucinations. Visual hallucinations may be seen in black and white. Hallucinations may not associated with a delusion. Evaluee may claim that a delusion suddenly developed or disappeared. Content of a delusion may be bizarre, but evaluee does not exhibit disorganized thinking. None of this can be pathognomic but can be pointers in atypical presentations in a backdrop of medicolegal setting.

- Claimant interview presentation
  - Admission of malingering
  - Lack of cooperation or substantial noncompliance with assessment or treatment
  - Discrepancy between interview report and history documentation
  - Inconsistent reporting to different interviewers and during different time of day
- Activity or behavior outside interview
  - Working during periods of claim
  - Capacity for recreation, non-work activity
  - Functioning well except in particular type of work
  - Non compliance with treatment
  - Surveillance.

Obtaining History and Style of Interviewing

Obtain history from collateral sources: This may serve to refute or confirm the patient's information or provide additional information. Records of prior functioning at the work place may be reviewed to confirm or refute any evidence of claimed disability. Any history of substance abuse, psychiatric illness or antisocial acts will increase the suspicion of malingering.

Interview technique: Interview should be long and detailed as it is difficult to maintain guard for malingered symptoms for long period of time. The evaluee may be deliberately asked leading questions about an unrelated different illness to see the response. Othmer and Othmer has given an elaborate 'Cross Examination Clinical Interview' technique. It based on the principle that adversary position for lies of suspected malingerer has to be taken not against the individual. It involves following five steps:[10]

- *Listen:* Listen the evaluee and encourage elaboration by open ended questions
- *Tag*: Tag or double check the story for its consistency, accuracy, details, rehearsed statements
- *Confront*: Confront for inconsistencies in non-threatening way
- *Solve and approve*: Continue interview in yes-no questions despite resistance from evaluee and close by approval of evaluee.[2]

Observation During Interview Situation

Speech: Subjects who are lying tend to speak in high-pitched voices; make frequent grammatical errors and also hesitate and pause during interviews more than genuine subjects.

Their pauses may be filled with non-informative fillers such as "uh, er. Ah". However, changes in pitch and volume are less reliable indicators of deception.

Facial expression: Gestures and facial expression are less apt to be rehearsed since facial muscles are under both voluntary and involuntary control. In addition, false affects are 'deliberate'; 'prolonged' and lack the usual 'crescendo-decrescendo' of natural affects. The timing of affective display may be either early or late as compared to normal subjects.

Body gestures: Body movements are less frequently monitored by a malingerer and are a good source of leakage. In a malingerer, illustrators, i.e. gestures that accompany speech are used less frequently; emblems, i.e. gestures that communicate a specific meaning in a specific culture, may be discordant with the spoken language, and manipulators, i.e. movements involving self-grooming, scratching, pulling, rubbing another body part and use of props viz. a pen, are distinctly prolonged and frequently repeated by the subject.[2]

Observation Across Time and Situations

It is better to observe in different settings OPD, IPD and being interviewed by different health professionals across different cross sections to check for consistencies of symptom reporting. Admission in inpatient setting is desirable and can be supplemented with video recording and covert observations because of difficulty in maintaining feigned symptoms uniformly across time span and for prolong periods.[2]

Caution for interviewer: Clinicians to be cautious of **ABCS** during interview of:[3]
- **A**void accusations of lying.
- **B**eware of countertransference.
- **C**larification, not "confrontation."
- **S**ecurity measures.

PSYCHOLOGICAL ASSESSMENT OF MALINGERING

In medicolegal contexts, psychometric testing may provide a more objective measure of inconsistencies.

Principle: In attempt to magnify illness, claimant will perform far less adequately than predicted on even simple measure of cognition. The test batteries include validity scales to pick up:
- Exaggeration
- Defensiveness
- Untruthfulness
- Consistency in responding over time
- Tendency to excessively respond in either positive (true) or negative (false) manner.

Detail of few commonly used tests is listed in **Table 1**.

Table 1: Commonly used psychological tests for assessment of malingering.

Psychological test		Remarks
Minnesota Multiphasic Personality Inventory (MMPI-2)[11,12]	568 items 20 primary scales	Evaluating the validity of the test-taker's attitude to exaggerate *F-scale (malingering index)*: Addresses stereotypic symptoms associated with serious psychopathology but rarely found in patients. *Fake bad scale (FBS)*: Evaluating faking of physical complaints among personal injury claimants
Structured Interview of Reported Symptoms (SIRS)	172 items	Evaluating exaggerated, over-reported, atypical, or absurd symptoms Good sensitivity and specificity[13] Good for screening in correctional setting[14]
Miller-Forensic Assessment of Symptoms Test (M-FAST)[15]		Good evidence of construct and criterion validity Good for screening in correctional setting
Victoria Symptom Validity Test (VSVT)	Computerized test (15 min)	It has 48 trials, divided into 3 blocks of 16 trials. Each block containing 8 "easy" and 8 "difficult" items. It assesses total errors and compares errors and reaction time on easy versus difficult items to determine feigning.[16]
Personality Assessment Inventory (PAI)[17,18]	344 items with 22 scales	Contains 6 response distortion indicators in clinical, personality and validity scales Moderately effective with discriminant analysis yielding a hit rate above 80%
Personality Inventory for Youth (PIY)[19]	4 validity scales	It has inconsistency scale, consisting of pairs of highly correlated statements; dissimulation scale, which would expose intentional distortion Point toward minimization, malingering, and random response sets on the PIY validity scales
Structured Inventory of Malingered Symptomatology (SIMS)[20,21]	brief self-report inventory	Can be administered to 5th-grade reading level Detects manipulative and antisocial personality features Adequate test-retest reliability, internal consistency, and high accuracy limitation: Not validated in forensic settings
Rorschach Test	Projective test	Inconclusive data about the utility of this test in detecting malingering • Perry and Kinder (1990)[22] reported that no specific malingering pattern has been found • Ganellan et al. (1996)[23] reported that malingerers give less emotion laden and more dramatic responses on Rorschach Recommended to use in combination with MMPI-2
Test of Memory Malingering (TOMM)[24,25]	50 items	Identifies poor effort level Results are not affected by variables like mental disorders, language disorders, dementia, or mild intellectual impairment Validated in the forensic setting Excellent specificity and modest sensitivity

contd...

contd...

Psychological test	Remarks
Rey Auditory Verbal Learning Test (RAVLT)[26,27]	To detect symptom exaggeration Based on 'serial position patterns' concept as indicator of poor effort Serial position effect refers to better quality of recall for early (primacy) and recent (recency) material during word recall test. Simulators tend to suppress the primacy effect.
Wisconsin Card Sorting Test (WCST)[28]	Measures abstraction, planning abilities, tendency to perseverate 70.7% sensitivity, and 87.1% specificity

Limitations of Psychological Testing

Psychologic testing often provides useful information but has limitations. Approximately 40% of malingering claimants who are exaggerating symptoms will not be identified and only approximately 30% of malingering claimants will be identified on standard cognitive tests, and approximately 40% of cases that involve symptom exaggeration can be identified by validity scales on personality tests.[29] Informed clinical practice therefore requires that multiple sources of information be considered.

Six Potential Strategies to Detect Malingering

1. Floor effect—individual performing at bottom of a particular test, not being able to give even very basic information.[30]
2. Symptom validity testing—individuals given forced choice alternatives and they perform very poorly, raising the suspicion of malingering.
3. Performance curve—malingers may fail easy item and pass more difficult ones.
4. Magnitude of error—qualitative and quantitative pattern of wrong answer point towards symptom exaggeration or fabricated deficits.
5. Atypical presentations—variable performance across different time spans on similar tests. (Caution: seen at times in some head injury cases)
6. Psychological sequelae—faking symptoms unrelated to alleged complaint.

DIFFERENTIAL DIAGNOSIS

Factitious disorder: Unlike the observable external gratification that motivates a malingerer, patients with factitious disorder, especially Munchausen's syndrome, have the need to fulfill nonobservable intrapsychic needs of maintaining a sick role. These patients with factitious disorder go to extreme lengths to produce clinically convincing physical and laboratory signs of disease. They may inject their knees to produce swelling or ingest agents to distort their laboratory findings.

Somatoform disorder: With regards to somatoform disorder, they differ from malingering as here motive is not external gains, but symptoms production relieving unconscious intrapsychic conflict. According to literature, unlike in conversion disorder, suggestions or hypnosis do not influence the symptoms in malingering.[2,3]

CONCLUSION

Malingering of psychiatric disorders is easy and not so uncommon but much more difficult to detect. In absence of any gold standard investigative tool for malingering, identification of it is associated with definitive risk for clinician. Thus, a systematic approach is needed for identification and careful documentation is of utmost importance. Clinicians should be wary of their own biases and caution should be taken for not confronting the accused directly, as it may lead to hostility, undesirable lawsuits and rarely violence against doctor. More advisable is to inform the person that objective finding do not match with the standard diagnostic criteria and let the claimant be given opportunity to voice his/her opinion and further way out. It is not a psychopathological disorder to have treatment, but, given the considerable cost of malingering to society, it is vital that mental health professionals pay due attention to the presence of this condition and if required, remain equipped to deal with the same.

REFERENCES

1. Mittenberg W, Patton C, Canyock EM, et al. Base rates of malingering and symptom exaggeration. J Clin Exp Neuropsychol. 2002;24(8):1094-102.
2. Singh J, Avasthi A, Grover S. Malingering of psychiatric disorders: a review. German Journal of Psychiatry. 2007;10:126-32.
3. LeBourgeois III HW. Malingering: key points in assessment. Psychiatric Times. 2007; 24(10):21-9. Available at: http://www.psychiatrictimes.com/forensic-psychiatry/malingering-key-points-assessment.
4. Rosenhan D. On being sane in an insane place. Science 1973;179:250.
5. The diagnostic and statistical manual of mental disorders, 5th edn.;DSM-5; American Psychiatric Association, 2013.
6. ICD-10 Classifications of Mental and Behavioural Disorder: Clinical Descriptions and Diagnostic Guidelines. Geneva. World Health Organisation. 1992.
7. Resnick PJ. The detection of malingered psychosis. Psychiatr Clin N Am. 1999; 22: 159-72.
8. Mills MJ, Lipian MS. Malingering. In: Sadock BJ, Sadock VA (Eds). Comprehensive Textbook of Psychiatry, 8th edn. Philadelphia: Lippincott Williams and Wilkins, 2005; 2247-58.
9. Cunnien AJ. Psychiatric and medical syndromes associated with deception: In: Rogers R (Ed). Clinical Assessment of Malingering and Deception, 2nd edn. New York, NY: Guildford Press; 1997:23-46.
10. Othmer E, Othmer SC. Falsifying and lying. In: The clinical interview using DSM-IV, the difficult patient. Washington DC: American Psychiatric Press; 2000:349-84.
11. Berry DT, Baer RA, Harris MJ. Detection of malingering on the MMPI: A meta-analytic review. Clin Psychol Rev. 1991;11:585-98.
12. Steffan JS, Clopton JR, Morgan RD. An MMPI-2 scale to detect malingered depression (Md scale). Assessment. 2003;10(4):382-92.
13. Rogers R. Structured interviews and dissimulation. In: Rogers R (Ed). Clinical Assessment of Malingering and Deception, 2nd edn. New York, NY: Guilford Press; 1997:301-28.
14. Rogers R, Kropp PR, Bagby RM, et al. Faking specific disorders: a study of the Structured Interview of reported symptoms (SIRS). J Clin Psychol. 1992;48(5):643-8.

15. Miller HA. Examining the use of the M-FAST with criminal defendants incompetent to stand trial. Int J Offender Ther Comp Criminol. 2004;48(3):268-280.
16. Thompson G. Victoria symptom validity test: an enhanced test of symptom validity. J Forensic Neuropsychol. 2002;2:43-67.
17. Morey LC, Lanier VW. Operating characteristics of six response distortion indicators for the personality assessment inventory. Assessment 1998; 5: 203-14.
18. Morey LC. Personality Assessment Inventory: Professional Manual. Florida, USA: Psychological Assessment Resources Inc; 1991.
19. Wrobel TA, Lachar D, Wrobel NH, et al. Performance of the Personality Inventory for Youth validity scales. Assessment. 1999;6(4):367-380.
20. Smith GP, Burger GK. Detection of malingering: Validation of the structured inventory of malingered Symptomatology (SIMS). J Am Acad Psychiatry Law. 1997;25(2):183-189.
21. Cima M, Hollnack S, Kremer K, et al. The German version of the structured inventory of malingered symptomatology: SIMS. Nervenarzt. 2003;74(11):977-86.
22. Perry GG, Kinder BN. The susceptibility of the Rorschach to malingering: a critical review. J Pers Assess 1990; 54: 47-57.
23. Ganellen RJ, Wasyliw OE, Haywood TW, et al. Can psychosis be malingered on the Rorschach? An empirical study. J Pers Assess 1996; 66: 65-80.
24. Tombaugh TN. The Test of Memory Malingering: TOMM. Toronto, Canada: Multy Health Systems; 1996.
25. Weinborn M, Orr T, Woods SP, et al. A validation of the test of memory malingering in a forensic psychiatric setting. J Clin Exp Neuropsychol. 2003;25(7):979-90.
26. Rey A. L'Examen Clinique en Psychologie [Clinical Examinations in Psychology]. Paris, France: Presses Universitaire de France; 1964.
27. Powell MR, Gfeller JD, Oliveri MV, et al. The Rey AVLT Serial Position Effect: a useful indicator of symptom exaggeration? Clin Neuropsychol. 2004;18(3):465-76.
28. Grant DA, Berg EA. A behavioral analysis of reinforcement and ease of shifting to new responses in a Weiggl-type card-sorting problem. J Exp Psychol. 1948;38:404-11.
29. Harris MR, Resnick PJ. Suspected Malingering: Guidelines for Clinicians. Psychiatric Times. 2003;20(13):68-71.
30. Eastman N, Adshead G, Fox S, et al. Forensic Psychiatry. Oxford Specialists Handbooks. London: Oxford University Press, 2017.

SECTION IV

Intersection of Mental Health and Civil Law

CHAPTER 14

Testamentary Capacity

> **LEARNING OBJECTIVES**
> - Law of succession
> - Codicil
> - Essentials of Will making
> - Testamentary capacity
> - Important elements of testamentary capacity
> - Factors affecting testamentary capacity
> - Indications of undue influence
> - Behavioral clues to undue influence
> - Symptoms of testamentary incapacity
> - Law and testamentary capacity
> - Assessment of testamentary capacity
> - Evaluation of testamentary capacity
> - Process for assessing testamentary capacity
> - Common cognitive screening tests
> - Retrospective assessment
> - Documentation for assessment of testamentary capacity and undue influence

One would like to ensure that his property goes to the genuine recipients who could utilize it in a proper way after his demise. For this purpose, there has been a provision of disposing off one's property after death by making a Will. A Will is an important document which enables the individual/living person to rightfully leave his assets to whoever he chooses to, after his death. It is a legal declaration of a person's intention which he desires to be performed after his death. Often complications arise when a person dies without making a Will.

After the death of a person, his property devolves in two ways:
i. According to the respective laws of the land when no Will is made, i.e. intestate
ii. By way of Will, i.e. testamentary

LAW OF SUCCESSION

The laws of inheritance are diverse and complicated. The rules of distribution of property in case a person dies without making a Will are defined by every law of succession. These rules provide for a class of persons and percentage of property that will be inherited by such persons. When a person dies a sudden death without making a Will, there is possibility of unintended injustice to some potential beneficiaries. For example, wife and the mother of the deceased get equal shares as legal heirs despite the fact that wife never shared cordial relations with her deceased husband and he would not have given equal share had he made a Will.

India has a well developed system of succession law that governs a person's property after his death. Indian Succession Act 1925[1] applies expressly to Wills and Codicils made by Hindus, Buddhists, Sikhs, Jains, Jews, Parsis and Christians. The Muslim Personal Law is applicable to Muslims. They are not governed by Indian Succession Act, 1925.

Following are the Acts operating in India:[2]
- The Indian Succession Act, 1925
- The Hindu Succession Act (amendment) 2005
- The Muslim Personal Law
- The Indian Registration Act, 1908

Apart from these Acts, various states of India have their own amendments of Hindu Succession Act 1956, according to the local customs.

According to law of inheritance and succession, if a Hindu male passes away:
- Hindu female shares equally with the male, i.e. a son and daughter will succeed with equal shares.
- The wife as well as the mother also gets the equal share
- There is nothing to prevent a Hindu male from bequeathing his entire property to a stranger if he so desires.

Muslim male cannot will away more than 1/3 of estate and 2/3 of the property must be divided among the family members in the shares as laid down in the law.
- A Muslim wife cannot be dispossessed.
- Even though she shares with other wives (if more than one wife).
- The widow gets a definite share.
- The male heirs, sons get twice the share of daughters.

A male who makes a Will is called testator and a female testatrix. A testator (or testatrix) is a person who is executing a Will. When Will is created, the property is disposed according to the Will. The declaration should be relating to the testator's property and the testator should intend to dispose off his property after his death. All properties, movable or immovable, of which testator is the owner and which are transferable can be disposed off by a Will. Formerly, a Hindu coparcener governed by the Mitakshara law could not dispose of his undivided share in the coparcenary property he is, now entitled to do so under Section 30 of the Hindu Succession Act, 1956. Testator can also bequeath properties, incomes and interest that may be acquired by him after the execution of Will.

According to Section 2(h) of the Indian Succession Act, 1925, a Will is defined as follows:

"A Will is a legal declaration of the intention of the testator, with respect to his property which he desires to be carried into effect after his death." Important postulates of the Will are as follows:
- A Will is a legal declaration. It must be signed and attested as required.
- The declaration should relate to disposition of the person making the Will.
- A Will becomes enforceable only after the death of the testator. It has no effect during the life-time of the testator.
- It is revocable and the testator can change the Will at any time during his life-time.

Persons capable and competent to make a Will, according to Section 59 of Indian Succession Act, 1925:
- Any person of sound mind can make a Will.
- A person who has reached the age of majority can make a Will. However, as per Section 60 of the Act, a father whatever his age may be, may by Will appoint a guardian or guardians for his child during minority.
- A married woman may make a Will of her property which she could alienate by her own act during her life-time.

The following persons cannot make a Will:
- Lunatic, insane persons
- Minor, i.e. below 18 years of age.
- Corporate bodies by their very nature are incapable of making a Will, though they may benefit under the Will of an individual partner.

Other persons who can make a Will:
- Persons who are deaf or dumb or blind are not thereby, incapable in making a Will, if they are of sound mind
- Persons, who are ordinarily insane, may make a Will during an interval while they are of sound mind.
- No person can make a Will while he is in such a state of mind, whether arising from intoxication or from illness or from any other cause, so that he does not know what he is doing.

CODICIL

A codicil is a supplement to a Will when a testator intends to make any minor alterations in his Will, e.g. change in the number of trustees. According to the Section 2(b) of the Indian Succession Act, 1925, codicil means an instrument made in relation to a Will and explaining, altering or adding to its disposition and shall be deemed to form the part of the Will. Accordingly, a codicil has to be executed and attested just as a Will (Section 64, Indian Succession Act, 1925).

A codicil may be endorsed on the original Will itself, or it may be a separate document. Its nature is not substantive but adjective. A codicil may stand even though the Will to which it is supplementary is revoked. However, a codicil cannot be an independent document. When alterations are considerable, a fresh Will revoking the earlier Will should be executed.

ESSENTIALS OF WILL MAKING

- It is a legal document
- Person to be competent to make a will
- Signature of the testator on the Will
- Attestation by two or more witnesses, witness cannot be the beneficiaries
- No particular form of Will prescribed by law
- Registration not compulsory
- Safe custody of Will
- Secrecy of the Will
- It is effective only after the death of the testator
- Execution of the Will

Legal Document

Will is a legal document in conformity with the provisions of Indian Succession Act, 1925. It is in writing. Will made by a Hindu, Buddhist, Jain, Sikh, Parsi, Jew or a Christian must be in writing. However, a privileged Will by a member of armed forces in an expedition, or engaged in actual warfare and mariner at sea can be oral Will. Muslims are permitted to make an oral Will by Muslim Personal Law. Will can be made by any person competent to do it.

Competency of the Person to Make the Will

Every person of sound mind and not a minor can execute a will. Any movable or immovable property can be disposed by a will by its owner. Under Mitakshara law, a Hindu coparcener could not dispose his undivided property by will, even if other coparceners consented for it, he is, now entitled to do so under Section 30 of the Hindu Succession Act, 1956. Under Muslim Personal law every adult Muslim of sound mind can make a will. Legatee can be any person capable of holding property, and bequest can be made to non-Muslim institutions and charitable purposes, unborn persons, etc.

Persons who are deaf, dumb or blind are not incapable of making a will, if they know what they do by it. A person who is ordinarily insane may make a Will if his psychopathology does not influence his decision making or at times when he has sound mind. No person can make a Will, while he is in such a state of mind, whether arising from intoxication or from illness or from any other cause that he does not know what he is doing. The declaration takes effect only after death of the testator and it is revocable any time before the death of the testator.

Signature of the Testator on the Will

The testator shall sign or shall affix his mark to the Will, or some other person shall sign it in his presence and by his direction. The signature or the mark of the testator or the signature of the person signing shall appear clearly and should be legible. It should appear in the manner that is appropriate and makes the Will legal. It should be dated. The Will must be initialled by the testator at the end of every page and next to any correction and alteration.

Attestation

The Will shall be attested by two or more witnesses, each of whom has seen the testator sign or affix his mark to the Will or has seen other person sign the will, in the presence and by the direction of the testator, or has received from the testator. Each of the witnesses shall sign the Will in the presence of the testator. The attesting witness or his/her spouse must not be beneficiary otherwise Will in their favor will be invalid (Section 67 of Indian Succession Act, 1925).

Form of Will

There is no particular form of Will prescribed by law. Forms in vogue in England have been followed in India for the last several decades and they may be adopted. The language of the Will should be easily understandable and the wording should be such that the intention of the testator can be known there from (Section 74). A Will can be made on any plain paper of durable quality no stamp paper is needed for this purpose.

Registration

Under Section 18 of the Registration Act, the registration of a Will is not compulsory but it must be proved duly and validly executed, as required by the Indian Succession Act. A Will has to be registered with the registrar/sub-registrar with a nominal registration fee for which the testator must be personally present at the registrar's office along with the witnesses. The endorsement of the registrar is sufficient to prove the execution of the Will, Will need not be made in stamp paper and there is no formal prescribed form of a Will. Will can be registered by the testator during his life time or by the executor or legatee after the testator's death.

Safe Custody of Will

The Will may be deposited in some safe custody, such as with a banker, or a solicitor. After the registration it can be kept with the registrar's office in a sealed cover bearing the name of the testator and that of his agent.

Secrecy of Will

Once the Will is made, it should be kept secret and not to disclose to the beneficiaries. The Testator, after making the Will should inform about it to some persons in whom he has confidence and trust. In case, husband making a Will may inform his wife. The Will thus made shall takes effect only after the death of the testator.

Execution of the Will

On the death of the testator, an executor of the Will or an heir of the deceased testator can apply for probate. The court will ask the other heirs of the deceased if they have any objection to the Will. If there are no objections, the court will grant probate. A probate is a copy of a Will, certified by the court. A probate is to be treated as conclusive evidence of the genuineness of the Will. In case any objections are raised by any of the heirs, a citation has to be served, calling upon them to consent. This has to be displayed prominently in the court. Thereafter, if no objection is received, the probate will be granted. It is only after this that the Will comes into effect.

Capacity of an individual to make a Will is testamentary capacity. Testamentary capacity is a construct rooted in both the legal and medical domains thus inviting a collaborative approach to its definition and assessment.[3]

TESTAMENTARY CAPACITY

Testamentary capacity refers to person's full sense and mental sanity to have confirmed and signed the Will after understanding what his assets comprised and what he is doing by making a Will. He understands in full mental capacity who he is naming the assets to and how are they related to him and what repercussions it may have later. Testamentary capacity is the legal status of being capable of executing a Will.

Testamentary capacity is defined in common law and US, Canada and English jurisdictions, addresses its task-specific nature as opposed to the global status of the mental illness. It means that a person suffering from mental disorder can make a Will provided he is capable of required competency for making a Will.

In *Banks vs. Goodfellow*,[4] a commonly cited English case, John Banks, the testator clearly suffered from a chronic and serious mental disorder but was deemed capable with respect to the execution of his Will because his delusions did not affect the distribution of his assets. This judgment remains the test in most common law jurisdictions today.

The Banks vs. Goodfellow Criteria

- Understanding of the nature of the Act (Will making) and its effects.
- Knowledge of the nature and extent of one's assets.
- Knowledge of persons who have a reasonable claim to be beneficiaries.
- Understanding of the impact of the distribution of the assets of the estate.
- A confirmation that the testator is free of any delusions that influence the disposition of the assets.
- Ability to express wishes clearly and consistently in an orderly plan of disposition.

In the US jurisdictions, the definition of testamentary capacity is similar except that the doctrine of insane delusion is distinct from general testamentary capacity. Thus, it is possible for a testator to possess general testamentary capacity and yet suffer from an insane delusion that invalidates the Will.

According to Indian Succession Act, 1925, a person is said to have testamentary capacity only if he is in a sound disposing state of mind. It is essential that the testator should have sufficient capacity to comprehend perfectly the conditions of his property, his relations to the persons who were or should or might have been object of his bequest and the scope or the bearing of the provisions of his Will.

IMPORTANT ELEMENTS OF TESTAMENTARY CAPACITY

Important elements in testamentary capacity are as follows:
- It is a voluntary Act on the part of the testator.
- Testator should have a sound disposing mind.
- Testator should know what he is doing by making a Will.
- Testator should have sufficient capacity to know the extent of his/her property.
- Testator should be aware of potential beneficiaries.
- Testator should be aware of the consequences of his/her decision.
- Testator should be free from undue influence/fraud/coercion.
- Testator must know the contents of the Will.

1. Making a will is a voluntary act on the part of the testator and there should be no compulsion or force on the testator to make the Will. It is his own decision to dispose off his property.
2. The testator should have a sound disposing mind while making the Will. He should not be suffering from any mental disorder which could possibly interfere in his decision making. He should not be in a state of intoxication due to alcohol, drugs or disease at the time of making the Will.

   Testamentary capacity is task-specific, a person suffering from mental illness can make a will provided his psychopathology is not interfering in his decision making.

   Testamentary capacity is also situation-specific. Clinician should explore the circumstances under which the testator is making the Will.
3. The testator should know what he is doing by making a Will. The testator should be in full senses to appreciate the nature of the act.
4. The testator should have sufficient capacity to know the extent of his property; he should also know the nature and extent of his assets which he is going to distribute with approximate value of his property.
5. The testator should be aware of the potential beneficiary, should have the knowledge about the legal heirs of his property. He should also know the potential beneficiaries whom he is likely to distribute his property and the relationship with them. He should be able to rationalize his decision.
6. The testator should be aware of the consequences of his decision and he should be aware of the possible consequences of the distribution of his assets.
7. The testator should be free from undue influence, fraud, or coercion Under Section 61 of Indian Succession Act, 1925, a Will or any part of a Will, the making of which has been caused by fraud or coercion or by such importunity as takes away the free agency of the testator is void. However, sound mind the testator may be having, if it has been the subject of undue influence, the soundness of mind will not help the will to be declared valid.
8. The testator must have the knowledge of the contents of the Will. If the testator does not know the contents of his Will it cannot be said to be a valid Will. However, such knowledge and approval of the testator may be presumed on the proof of signature of the testator.

FACTORS AFFECTING TESTAMENTARY CAPACITY

There are several factors that can impact someone's capacity to create a Will that accurately reflects his or her true wishes. These factors include:
1. Physical factors
2. Psychiatric disorders
3. Undue influence

The conditions discussed below may affect cognition, perception, which in turn may have effect on individual's ability to understand relevant facts related to testamentary capacity. These conditions affect the person's appreciation of consequences of specific actions or his interpretation of situation-specific factors.

Physical Factors

Factors which lead to brain dysfunction either due to certain diseases, trauma or medication may have impact on the client's ability to think clearly. Physical factors include a wide range of medical disorders, including head trauma, systemic diseases, i.e. metabolic, endocrine, infectious and other disorders that affect brain functioning and mental state. Certain drugs may have effect on cognition and perception and hence may interfere in decision making.

Alcohol

Alcohol abuse can have both acute and chronic effects on cognition, judgment and behavior. In the acute phase of alcohol consumption even the small amounts of alcohol may affect perception, judgment and impulsiveness. These mental changes could affect testator's decision regarding the execution of a Will. The effects of chronic alcohol abuse are similar.

Psychiatric Disorders

Dementia

Dementias such as Alzheimer's disease, Lewy body dementia, and vascular cognitive impairment are characterized by diffuse cognitive deficits. In cases of obvious and severe cognitive impairment, there will be little need for subtle interpretations of brain function, and the lawyers or the courts can assess the impact of the impairment without the help of experts. However, in many disputed cases, the level of cognitive impairment is relatively mild or subtle. Some individuals with dementia maintain their social graces and appear perfectly normal to a lay person. Therefore, probing and documentation of the rationale disposition, particularly in suspicious circumstances, are especially important to demonstrate that the individual is capable. In dementia, executive impairment is particularly important, as it can affect insight, perception and judgment and impulse control. Mild forms of memory impairment can be associated with suspiciousness or even paranoid delusions as testators attempt to compensate for their memory deficits. In retrospective assessments, evidence for progression of dementia after the last Will was executed can help to support hypotheses about impaired thinking, perception, or judgment at the time of the execution of the Will. While there is some evidence that courts have developed principles relevant to dementias, a deeper and wider knowledge base among jurists surely will enhance law's ability to adjudicate Will contents.[5]

Mood Disorders

Mood disorders, including depression and bipolar disorder, may produce cognitive distortions (delusions), compromise judgment, and cause irritability or impulsiveness. These acute and sub-acute changes may affect testamentary capacity and vulnerability to undue influence. Usually these changes in mental state can be identified during a specific episode, but in some cases they can become chronic.

Delusions

Paranoid delusions may be secondary to a number of clinical syndromes, including schizophrenia, delusional disorders, and other forms of neurological disease, such as dementia, delirium, acquired brain injury, and other brain lesions. According to the Banks vs. Goodfellow criteria, the testator must be free of any delusions that directly affect the distribution of the estate. Changes made in the Will on the basis of false belief make the Will invalid. Even if such beliefs do not reach delusional intensity, they can make the testator vulnerable to undue influence. Careful questioning and probing by the assessor will help to elicit the impact of these beliefs on the distribution of assets.

Undue Influence

Historically, the notion of undue influence emphasized the concept of coercion, whereas subversion of Will seems a more appropriate term for testamentary capacity. Subversion allows for a continuum of influence depending on the extent of the cognitive impairment. The lower the cognitive capacity of an individual, the lesser influence would be required to determine that the individual was incapable or unduly influenced. On the other hand, an individual with no cognitive impairment would have to be subjected to a severe level of influence to the point of coercion or containment before that influence would be considered undue. Undue influence has been defined by one of the courts as: " ...the opportunity of the beneficiary of the influenced bequest to mould the mind of the testator to suit his or her purpose" (Hyatt vs. Wrote, 1937).[6] Undue influence is a strictly legal concept; the onus of proof is on those claiming undue influence[7,8] have delineated the indications which are as follows:

Indications of Undue Influence

- A confidential relationship existed between testator and the influencer that created an opportunity for the latter to control the testamentary act.
- The influencer used the relationship to secure a change in the distribution of the testator's estate.
- There were unnatural provisions in the Will.
- The change in distribution did not reflect the true wishes of the testator.
- The testator was vulnerable to being influenced either because of a neurological or psychiatric disorder or because of specific emotional circumstances.
- The beneficiary actively participated in or initiated the procurement of the Will.
- There was undue benefit to the beneficiary.

The doctrine of undue influence allows the courts to maintain a relatively low threshold for testamentary capacity and hence to preserve the principle of autonomy and individual freedom with respect to the distribution of one's assets.[7] In such a situation, a testator with moderate cognitive impairment could still be considered to have testamentary capacity. However, if the circumstances are more complex or there is a suggestion of undue influence, the legal threshold becomes higher and calls for more careful probing of rationale at the time of the execution of the Will. Regan and[9] suggest behavioral clues to undue influence.

Behavioral Clues to Undue Influence

- The individual who asks for the examination states the evaluation is merely "routine" owing to the testator's age.
- Someone other than the testator (or his lawyer) makes the appointment for the evaluation.
- The person transporting the testator to the appointment is reluctant to permit him to be interviewed privately.
- Details about the Will are absent, or the testator appears vague about specific items in the Will.
- The testator is hesitant about providing information about the potential heir and his relationship to that person.

Section 61 of the Indian Succession Act, 1925 says that, a will is avoided when it is affected by coercion or fraud because the person otherwise capable does not have a free mind. At times it is difficult to differentiate between the undue influence on the part of the potential beneficiary and expression of gratitude and desire on the part of testator. If an elderly testator becomes infatuated with a young woman who is suggestive or providing sexual favors to entice his interest, and he then revises his Will in her favor—it is not likely to be undue influence. If a nurse serving an ailing testator asks for some incentive to serve him better—is undue influence. However, the influence of wife over her husband may not be undue influence. When a wife persuades the testator husband to execute a Will in supersession of a former Will less favorable to her, but the influence she exercised was not such as to deprive the testator of the exercise of his judgment and volition, the conduct of wife would not amount to undue influence.[10]

SYMPTOMS OF TESTAMENTARY INCAPACITY

- Difficulties in attention and information processing
- Language difficulties
- Memory difficulties
- Impairment of higher executive functions
- Persecutory delusions
- Delusions of poverty

There have been certain symptoms which make an individual incapable of making a Will. Following symptoms are the potential signs of incapacity:

- Difficulties in attention and information processing
- Language difficulties.
- Memory difficulties.
- Impairment of higher executive functions.
- Persecutory delusions about a family member causing the testator to exclude the person from the Will.
- Delusions of poverty – the testator does not realize the worth of his own or of his estate which may influence his decision making and distribution of property.

A person displaying these symptoms at the time of giving instructions to prepare the Will or signing of the Will may be suffering from some form of mental incapacity.

LAW AND TESTAMENTARY CAPACITY

Testamentary capacity like other capacities is both task-specific and situation-specific. The law does not require that a person, in order to be capable of making a Will, must be possessed of his mental powers at their best and unimpaired in any degree by old age or disease. What is required for the validity of Will is that the testator should have been able, at the time of making it, to comprehend the nature and the effect of disposition, should have sufficient memory and intelligence to form a proper judgment regarding it, and should have freely decided to make it. Whether or not a testator had the required capacity has naturally to be ascertained with reference to the disposition in question. Testamentary capacity has to be judged not by an absolute standard but as relative to a particular testamentary Act (Krishna Kumar Sinha vs. Kayasha Pathak, 1966).[11]

A person of unsound mind can make a Will during lucid interval. A mentally disordered person can also make a Will through his guardian. Delusions may not affect validity of Will. Superstitious terrors may be sufficient to set aside a Will where they deprive a person of exercise of his free judgment. A Will made by a person of full capacity is not revoked by the fact that he has subsequently become incapable of making a Will.

The law of making a Will is contained in the para VI of Indian Succession Act, 1925. All the provisions of part VI do not apply to Hindus, Buddhists, Sikhs and Jains. The Will made by a Muslim is governed by Muslim Personal Law.

ASSESSMENT OF TESTAMENTARY CAPACITY

At the time of drafting the Will, lawyers make an initial assessment of testamentary capacity but may call upon experts to assist in specific circumstances. Experts may include neuro-psychiatrists, geriatric psychiatrists, neuro-psychologists and others. Expert's role involves confirmation of testamentary capacity when cognitive and mental state is concerned. Expert may also be asked to assess the potential role of undue influence. He may also be asked to give retrospective opinion regarding capacity or undue influence after the death of the testator when the Will is challenged. A careful review of the available medical records and interview with the testator when alive are important inputs to form an opinion.

The assessment of environment (situation-specific factors) is important in the ultimate determination of capacity and impact of the influence. When there is suspicion of undue influence, the assessor must inquire into specific areas and higher levels of cognition by probing testator's rationale for decision as well as testator's appreciation of his circumstances and the impact of the distribution of his assets.

Doctors are often asked for an opinion whether a person has or did not have the mental capacity to make a will. This question is important and relevant in the context of Will making, as only persons of sound mind, memory and understanding are able to make a valid Will. The testamentary capacity of a testator is not always apparent to a non-medically trained legal professional, and hence the need for an expert opinion on the testamentary capacity of a testator.

Evaluation of Testamentary Capacity

When a solicitor requests a doctor to make assessment of testamentary capacity of his client, the doctor must insist for a letter of instruction from the solicitor confirming that the client has consented to examination and disclosure of results. The solicitor should also provide the doctor at the outset with verifiable information about client's family and assets and confirm in writing the legal test for capacity. The doctor should not assess the client in hurry; enough time should be given for assessment. Consent of the testator is essential before proceeding for evaluation of testamentary capacity. Assessment of a testator's testamentary capacity in a single interview is not sufficient. An assessment will be more accurate if it occurs over a period of time rather than one interview.

Process for Assessing Testamentary Capacity (*Jacoby and Steer 2007*)[12]

- Get a letter from the solicitor detailing legal tests
- Set aside enough time for evaluation
- Assess (in the standard way) whether the client has dementia
- Thorough physical and neurological examination
- Psychiatric examination, presence of delusions, hallucination, thought disorder, mood state, cognitive functions and their effect on decision making
- Record the answers verbatim
- Check facts such as extent of assets, with the solicitor
- Ask about and review previous Wills
- Ask why potential beneficiaries are included or excluded.
- Check that client understands each of the Banks vs. Goodfellow points
- If in doubt about mental capacity seek second opinion.

The testator should be examined over at least two separate consultations. There are two distinct times in Will-making process where a lawyer might insist on a doctor's assessment. Usually, these times are:
- Prior to the lawyer taking the instructions from the testator, and
- Prior to the execution of the completed Will.

The second consultation should be ideally on the day testator executes the Will. These two times are crucial, however in circumstances in which testator has declined mentally since giving instructions, it may be sufficient that he had capacity at the time he gave instructions. One should keep four criteria in mind used for determining whether a person has testamentary capacity:

1. The testator understands that he is giving instructions for the disposal of his property after his death.
2. The testator can recollect the extent and character of his property and dispose it off with understanding and reason.
3. The testator can recall and understand the claim of potential heirs such as his family; and
4. The testator is not suffering from any disorder of mind such as delusions and hallucinations which influence his decisions.

One may proceed with a semi-structured questionnaire asking a series of questions including:
1. Asking the testator to explain the effects of a Will, and asking whether he understands what would happen to his property if he does not make one.
2. Asking the testator to give a general estimate of his property and its value.
3. Asking the testator to describe the reasoning behind his decision to include or exclude potential heirs.
4. Asking the testator whether he understands that the Will revokes all previous Wills.

Specific questions posed to the testator may help in elucidating and probing the relationship between task-specific and situation-specific factors:
1. Can you tell me the reasons that you decided to make changes in your Will?
2. Why did you decide to divide estate in this particular fashion?
3. Do you understand how individual A might feel, having been excluded from the will or having been given significantly less amount than previously expected or promised.
4. Do you understand economic implications for individual B for this particular distribution in your Will?
5. Can you describe the nature of any family or personal disputes or tensions that may have influenced your decision?
6. Can you tell me about the important relationships in your family and others close to you?

If the client has the possibility of suffering from dementia, Mini-Mental State Examination (MMSE) should be administered. The examination of the client should be conducted in the absence of anyone who stands to benefit or might exert influence.

COMMON COGNITIVE SCREENING TESTS

Clinicians tend to use a small number of cognitive screening tests that may be referred to in medical records or expert reports. These tests assess high level brain functions that control initiative, motivation, planning, impulse control, capacity for abstract thinking and exercise of the judgment. The identification of subtle impairment of these functions in the context of a complex environment could easily produce a vulnerability to undue influence and affect testamentary capacity.[13] Evaluators of testamentary capacity, undue influence and the courts essentially be able to deduce the significance of these tests which are commonly used. Both clinicians and legal experts should appreciate that these cognitive tests do not have diagnostic power for dementia and can only be used to measure capacity. Their importance lies in the ability to screen any cognitive impairment and to reveal changes in cognition over period of time. Two most commonly used cognitive screening tests are the Mini-mental State Examination (MMSE) and Clock-draw Test.[3]

The Mini-mental State Examination

The mini-mental state examination (MMSE) is the most commonly used test for cognitive screening throughout the world. This test includes many cognitive domains of functions,[7] with a total possible score of 30: orientation to time (5 points), orientation to place (5 points), registration of 3 word (3 points), attention and calculation (5 points), recall of 3 words (3 points), language (8 points) and visuospatial ability (1 point).

Limitations of MMSE include the fact that it does not test specifically for frontal lobe or executive brain functions. The MMSE is heavily weighted towards orientation, short-term memory, and language skills. Nonetheless, the MMSE score has come to be used as a shorthand for severity of cognitive dysfunction, and thus it is important that the lawyers and clinicians understand the use and limitations of the instrument and its scoring. The score alone is not necessarily a reflection of dementia or clinically significant cognitive impairment (Landmark Trust vs. Goodhue 2001).[14] The scores below 26 suggest impairment. However, the MMSE score may be significantly influenced by factors such as native language, education and pre-morbid IQ.

The Clock-drawing Test

The Clock-drawing Test which has been widely used as a cognitive screening instrument,[15] consists of a standardized circle with the instruction, "This is a clock face; please put in the numbers so that it looks like a clock." The patient is then instructed to "set the time to 10 past 11." This test is useful as a cognitive screening because it subsumes many different brain functions covering a wide range of intellectual and perceptual skills: comprehension; planning; visual memory and construction of a graphic; visuospatial ability; motor planning and execution; numerical knowledge; abstract thinking; inhibition of tendency to be pulled by perceptual features of the stimulus (i.e. the "frontal pull" of the hands to "10" in the instruction "10 past 11"); concentration and frustration tolerance.

The mix of visuospatial ability as well as executive control function makes the clock-drawing test particularly useful as a cognitive screening instrument. Although various methods of scoring and interpretation have been proposed, the test's qualitative merits and simple global assessment are considered more important than complex scoring systems (Shulman 2000).[15]

RETROSPECTIVE ASSESSMENT

- Obtaining the relevant document
- All medical records
- Results of any neuropsychological examination
- Neuroimaging results
- References to the testator's mental state or behavior
- Relevant financial documents
- Other personal documents such as cheque books, diaries, business records or contracts
- Obtaining corroborative information about deceased's behavior from:
  - The surviving spouse
  - Relatives
  - Friends and business associates
  - Informed assessment

Often medical professionals are asked to give a retrospective assessment of whether a testator did or did not have testamentary capacity at the time of making his Will after that person has died. Where some medical conditions existed, questions may be raised after testator's death about his competence at a particular time.

When asked to make a retrospective assessment, a physician should carefully attempt to obtain following documents:
- All medical records (which may contain formal diagnoses)
- Results of any neuropsychological examinations
- Neuroimaging results
- References as to the testator's mental state or behavior
- Relevant financial documents
- Other personal documents such as:
  - Cheque books
  - Diaries
  - Business records
  - Contacts

The Will itself and any contemporaneous notes made by the legal practitioner preparing the Will may offer additional insight into the mental state of the testator. In addition to this, the physician should attempt to gather corroborative information about the deceased's behavior and functioning from:
- The surviving spouse
- Relatives
- Friends and business associates

After the receipt of the above information, a physician can make an informed assessment as to whether the testator had or was likely to have had testamentary capacity at the time of making the Will.

DOCUMENTATION FOR ASSESSMENT OF TESTAMENTARY CAPACITY AND UNDUE INFLUENCE[16]

The following issues should be addressed and documented in a forensic assessment:
1. Rationale for any dramatic changes or significant deviations from the pattern identified in prior wills or previous consistently expressed wishes regarding disposition of assets.
2. The appreciation of the consequences and impact of particular distribution especially if it deviates from or excludes "natural" beneficiaries such as close family members and spouses.
3. Clarification of concerns about potential beneficiaries who are excluded from the Will or bequeathed lower amounts than might have been expected – that is, ruling out the presence of a specific delusion or overvalued ideas that influence the distribution.
4. Evidence of the presence of a specific neurological or mental disorder that may affect cognition, judgment or impulse control.

5. Evidence of behavioral disturbances or psychiatric symptoms at the time of execution of a Will, such as agitation, impulsiveness, disinhibition, aggression, hallucinations or delusions.
6. The emotional/psychological milieu in which the testator lives, with specific reference to conflict or tension within the family.
7. The testator's understanding and appreciation of any conflicts or tensions in his environment.
8. Evidence of pathological or dependent relationship with a formal or informal caregiver, such as a younger woman who gives comfort and reassurance or plants seeds of suspiciousness towards family and friends.
9. Evidence of inconsistency in expressed wishes or an inability to communicate a clear, consistent wish with respect to distribution of assets; for example, frequent will changes are sometimes made in a desperate attempt to garner care, support or comfort at a time when testator feels increasingly vulnerable or threatened.
10. Any of the indications of undue influence.

Documentation for assessment of testamentary capacity and undue influence:
- Rationale for making changes
- Appreciation of consequences and impact
- Clarification of concerns about potential beneficiaries
- Evidence of presence of specific neurological or mental disorders
- Evidence of psychiatric symptoms at the time of execution of Will
- Emotional/psychological milieu
- Testator's understanding and appreciation of any conflicts
- Evidence of pathological or dependent relationship with a formal or informal caregiver
- Evidence of inconsistencies in expression
- Any indication of undue influence.

Where there is a Will, there is law suit. It is expected that in the times to come challenges to testamentary capacity in the courts of law are going to increase. The increasing complexity of modern families, where asset disposition is sensitive, complicated, may lead to feeling of rejection and injustice and result in more challenges. Number of elderly people is increasing and prevalence of cognitive impairment and dementia in older adults creates a fertile environment for challenge to Wills. It therefore behooves psychiatrists and other experts to be aware of the legal, medical and psychological issues that underlie the assessment of testamentary capacity and the role of undue influence.

REFERENCES

1. Indian Succession Act, 1925. Bare Act, Nabhi Publications, New Delhi.
2. Jiloha RC. In: Gautam S, Avasthi A. Mental Capacity/Testamentary Capacity. In Clinical Practice Guidelines on Forensic Psychiatry. Indian Psychiatric Society; 2009. p. 20-34.
3. Shulman KI, Cohen CA, Kirsch FC, et al. Assessment of testamentary capacity and vulnerability to undue influence. Am J Psychiatry. 2007;164:722-7.
4. Banks vs. Goodfellow, 5 LR QB.1870;549.
5. Gorman WF. Testamentary capacity in Alzheimer's disease. Elder Law Journal.1996;4:225-46.

6. Hyatt vs. Wrote 43SW 2d 726 (Ark.1931) as quoted in the article by Gutheil TG. Common pitfalls in the evaluation of Testamentary Capacity. Journal of American Academy of Psychiatry and Law. 2007;35: 514-17.
7. Folstein MF, Folstein SE, McHugh PR. Mini-Mental State a practical method for grading the cognitive state of patients for clinician. Journal of Psychiatric Research. 1975;12:189-98.
8. Frolik LA. The strange interplay of testamentary capacity and the doctrine of undue influence: are we protecting older testators or overriding individual preferences? International Journal of Law and Psychiatry. 2001;24:253-66.
9. Spar JE, Garb AS. Assessing competency to make a Will. Am J Psychiatry. 1992;149: 169-74.
10. Nabhi. How to make a Will. A Nabhi Publication; New Delhi, 1999.
11. Krishna Kumar Sinha vs. Kayasha Pathak (Pryag) Allahbad AIR. All. 1966;570.
12. Jacoby R, Steer P. How to assess capacity to make a Will. Practice British Medical Journal. 2007;335:155.
13. Royall DR, Lauterbach EC, Cummings JL, et al. Executive control function: a review of its promise and challenges for clinical research. Journal of Neuropsychiatry and Clinical Neurosciences. 2002;14:377-405.
14. Landmark Trust vs. Goodhue, 782A 2d 1219, 1226-27 (vt 2001).
15. Shulman KI. Clock-drawing: is it ideal cognitive screening test? International Journal of German Psychiatry. 2000;15:548-56.
16. Shulman KI, Hermann N, Brodaty H, et al. Survey of brief cognitive screening instruments. International Psychogeriatrics. 2006;18:281-94.

CHAPTER 15

Marriage and Divorce-related Issues with Regard to Mental Illnesses

> **LEARNING OBJECTIVES**
> - Indian laws concerning marriage and divorce
> - Discriminatory practices for persons with mental illness
> - Legal aspects of impotence and assessment

▓ INTRODUCTION

Marriage is one of the oldest social institutions and forms the basis of civilization, social structure and cohesiveness of a society. The traditional Indian view that the 'marriages are performed in the heaven', is contrasted with the current concept of contractual agreement that formalizes and stabilizes the social relationship to raise the family.[1] Marriage is defined as "a union between a man and a woman such that children born to the woman are the recognized legitimate offspring of both partners."[2] Leach offered a list of 10 rights associated with marriage, with specific rights differing across cultures, which are:[3]

- To establish a legal father of a woman's children
- To establish a legal mother of a man's children
- To give the husband a monopoly in the wife's sexuality
- To give the wife a monopoly in the husband's sexuality
- To give the husband partial or monopolistic rights to the wife's domestic and other labor services
- To give the wife partial or monopolistic rights to the husband's domestic and other labor services
- To give the husband partial or total control over property belonging or potentially accruing to the wife
- To give the wife partial or total control over property belonging or potentially accruing to the husband
- To establish a joint fund of property–a partnership–for the benefit of the children of the marriage
- To establish a socially significant "relationship of affinity" between the husband and the wife's brother.[4]

In the traditional Indian society, marriage is viewed as a sacrosanct life event in a individual's life, and every person is thought to get married, have a family and raise children to continue his progeny. The traditional Hindu belief that marriage is vital not only for begetting a son to liberation his dues to the lineages but also for enactment of other spiritual and religious duties, is anchored in the concept of series of births. A person having a daughter is expected to marry her off at the marriageable age in order to fulfill his religious commitment. In Indian society, for a woman marriage is one of the utmost vital phases of her life, and the social position of the women augments after marriage, while after a certain age if remain unmarried is considered stigmatizing for her.[5] Parents frequently cough up their life investments, take loans or dispose immovable possessions to organize ample dowry to get married their daughters.[6] Concept of divorce is not usually acceptable in society which is traditional. After marriage, there is even a sturdier social and moral pressure to carry on the relationship in spite of facing troubles/problems in the marriage.[5]

INDIAN LAWS CONCERNING MARRIAGE AND DIVORCE

In the legal spheres marriages in Hindu society are regulated by Hindu Marriage Act, 1955 which prescribes both the preconditions of marriage and grounds for divorce related to mental disorders. Under Hindu Marriage Act, 1955,[7] conditions in respect to mental disorders [Section 5(ii)], which must be met before the marriage is solemnized, are as follows:
- Neither party is incapable of giving a valid consent as a consequence of unsoundness of mind.
- Even if capable of giving consent must not suffer from mental disorders of such a kind or to such an extent as to be unfit for marriage and the procreation of children.
- Must not suffer from recurrent attacks of insanity.

The original provision was "neither party is an idiot or a lunatic," which was changed to the present provision by Marriage Laws (Amendment) Act, 1976. "Recurrent attacks of epilepsy" was also a disqualification for marriage, which was removed by the Marriage Laws (Amendment) Act, 1999. Supreme Court perceived that to label the wife as unfit for marriage and procreation of children on reason of the mental illness, it is necessary to establish that the disorder grieved by her is of such a kind or such an extent that it is impossible for her to lead a normal married life (R. Lakshmi Narayan vs. Santhi, AIR 2001 SC 2110).[7]

Marriages in contravention to the provision with respect to mental disorders come under voidable category. Voidable marriages (Section 12) are those which may be annulled by a decree of nullity on the given grounds but may continue to be legal until the time it is annulled by a competent court.

According to the Section 13 of the Act, divorce or judicial separation can be obtained if the person has been "incurably of unsound mind", or has been suffering continuously or intermittently from "mental disorder of such a kind and to such an extent that the petitioner cannot reasonably be expected to live with the respondent." The expression "mental disorder" means mental illness, arrested, or incomplete development of mind, or psychopathy, or any other disorder or disability of mind and includes schizophrenia. In Sharda vs. Dharmapaul (2003, 4 SCC 493) case, Supreme Court held that each case of schizophrenia has to be considered on its own merits. The medical evidence concerning the required degree of mental disorder is pertinent though not conclusive. Supreme Court also observed that when there was sufficient evidence for the court to conclude that the slight mental disorder of the wife was not of such a kind and to such an extent that the husband could not reasonably be expected to live with her, divorce could not be granted (AIR, 1982 CAL 138).[7] These judgments are significant because of the importance given to the effects and the influence rather that to the simply categorizing of mental illness.

The Special Marriage Act, 1954, is meant for any person in India and Indian nationals abroad, irrespective of the faith that the individual may profess. A marriage solemnized in any other form can be registered under this Act.[8] The Section 4(a) of the Act has provisions identical to the Section 5(ii) of Hindu Marriage Act as conditions for solemnizing marriage. Similarly, Section 27 lists identical provisions in respect to ground for divorce as in Section 13 of the Hindu Marriage Act.[8,9]

The Muslim Law regard marriage as a contract. A Muslim is considered qualified to marry who is of sound mind and has attained puberty. In cases involving a person of unsound mind, if the guardian of the person involved considers that such marriage is in the benefit of society and is ready to take up all the financial obligations of the marriage, such marriages can be accomplished. Divorce (Talaq) has to be for a rational cause and must be followed by attempts for settlements by two arbiters. A woman can obtain a verdict of divorce under "The Dissolution of Muslim Marriage Act, 1959", if her husband has been insane for 2 years.

In the Christian Law, marriage is considered voidable if either party is a lunatic or idiot. Christians can get divorce under the Indian Divorce Act 1869 (amended in 2001) on grounds of unsoundness of mind provided: (i) disease is incurable (ii) present for at least two years immediately preceding the petition.

Under the Parsi Marriage and Divorce Act, 1936 divorce cannot be admissible on ground of mental illness. However, divorce can be obtained if the defendant, at the time of marriage was of unsound mind, provided the plaintiff was ignorant of the fact and the defendant has been of unsound mind for two years upward and immediately preceding the application.[9]

Women suffer the most on account of mental disorders. When major disorders occur in young girls, parents are worried about her marriage. The widespread conviction that marriage is a remedy for all evils and lack of awareness prompt certain parents to get their daughters married even when the person is symptomatic.[6] However, when facts come out, a grave situation of mutual distrust, animosity, and hostility occurs between the two parties. Women suffering from major mental disorders, whether developed before or after the marriage are often abandoned by their husbands. As an outcome, lives of these women are traumatized beyond repair and nearly all these women come to live with their parents, several of whom are aged already.[10] These women face immense hardships and are left to fend for themselves with few options open. They are ostracized on three counts, namely female status, having severe mental disorder, and the marital status of divorce or separation. Thus, the woman has to face the "triple tragedy."[6] Divorced or separated women with major mental disorders become unwanted persons everywhere, and their plight becomes quite pitiable. Things are not so grave for male persons in Indian context. If a man with major mental disorder is married by concealing the fact, the woman in most of the cases has to reconcile with the situation and is burdened with taking care of her husband and sometimes has to be the breadwinner for the family. The stigma of living separated or divorced more acutely sensed by patients and their families than the stigma of being mentally ill *per se*.[11]

DISCRIMINATORY PRACTICES FOR PERSONS WITH MENTAL ILLNESS: AMENDMENT IS NEEDED

Time has considerably changed since the marriage laws were framed. Effective treatment of all types of mental disorders is now available. Therefore, it is felt that it is now high time that the phrases demonstrating mental disorder and referring the disorders are detached from the Hindu Marriage Act and the Special Marriage Act. The reason for this is summarized as following:

- The first ground of disability for marry is the incapability to give a valid consent as a consequence of being of unsoundness mind. If the valid consent is considered necessary in marriage, why single out only the unsoundness of mind. The incapability due to any reason must be considered a disability. The reference to "unsoundness of mind" is quite unnecessary as it stigmatizes the mental disorders. It must be pointed out that most people with major mental disorders are able to give their consent except when they have acute symptoms. Moreover, in Hindu rituals of marriage, in most of the cases, consent is hardly taken from the girl at any stage of marriage. In such instances, it is actually the proxy consent by the girls' parents/guardians. If the provision of valid consent is considered necessary, it can be retained without any reference to unsoundness of mind.
- The second point is "mental disorders of such a kind or to such an extent as to be unfit for marriage." It is quite a vague term and difficult to decide how the person with mental disorder is unfit for marriage. There are many physical illnesses also which are quite disabling and on account of these the person may be considered unfit for marriage. However, these are not listed under the condition of disability. Hence, why is there discrimination against mental disorders? Incurability of mental disorders is emphasized as a main factor of its inclusion in the list. However, with advancement in the field of psychiatry, it is now possible to treat almost all cases of mental disorders and almost all persons with mental disorders, except a tiny fraction, are able to live a normal life. Therefore, it is quite irrational and discriminatory to consider mental disorders as a disability to marriage.
- The third point is unfitness to procreation of a child. Disorders involving procreation of children are intricate subject including not some psychological disorders but several genitourinary, gynecological, endocrinal, and neurological disorders. When the involvement for this unfitness due to mental disorders is only a small part, why should only mental disorders be included as disability omitting many physical illnesses? It is worth mentioning that sterility is not a ground for divorce under Section 13 of the Hindu Marriage Act. Therefore, it is unreasonable to put restriction on inability of procreation of child only due to mental disorders.
- For nullity of marriage one of the grounds is recurrent attacks of insanity. It must be mentioned that the word insanity is now not used medically, though still in vogue in

legal dialect. Recurrent attacks include remissions and relapses and also lucid intervals. In psychiatry, most common type of such recurrent nature is the mood disorders. The mood disorders vary from mild spells of sadness to ones with severe psychotic episodes. However, these disorders are potentially curable, and almost all patients of mood disorders are able to lead a normal life. The course of schizophrenia is also characterized by remission and relapse. However, the course and prognosis of schizophrenia have considerably improved, and most of them are able to live a normal life. Therefore, there is no sense of including these in condition of disability to marry. The inclusion of insanity under the list results in further stigmatization of mental disorders.

- Previously, the reference was to recurrent attack of insanity and epilepsy. Epilepsy was removed from this list by an Act of Parliament in the year 1999. During the debate on the concerned Bill, it was pointed out that it is inhuman to compare epilepsy with insanity together as nearly 80% of the epilepsy cases are curable. However, it is forgotten that even greater percentage of the cases of mental disorders are treatable, and patients are able to live a typical life with proper treatment. If it is considered inhuman to consider epilepsy as a disability in case of marriage, the same yardstick should also apply to mental disorders and it is highly unfortunate that "insanity" continues to be a disability to marry.
- "Mental disorder" is a general term and includes many disorders ranging from minor anxiety disorders to major disorders such as schizophrenia. The course of prognosis of all is quite variable. Including the general term of mental disorder frequently causes problem to those suffering from minor disorders of anxiety or depression. If animosity develops between the parties, attempts are made to frame any type of psychiatric treatment as a ground for divorce. It causes hardship for the person having minor psychiatric ailments and seeking psychiatric treatment remains stigmatizing. Parents frequently shy away from consulting psychiatrists for their daughters with minor or major psychiatric disorders though the girl might be having a potentially curable psychiatric problem. A host of psychiatric disorders such as recurrent depression, dysthymia, conversion disorders, and obsessive compulsive disorders are frequently made the ground for divorce. The government as well as the society has a duty to take steps for reducing stigma attached to the mental disorders. Therefore, it is necessary to remove mental disorders from the list of disability to marry.
- In the condition of divorce/judicial separation, there is mention of "incurability of unsound mind." The first point is that most of the mental disorders are now curable. The second point is that anyone may also acquire a physical illness whether before or after the marriage, which may be incurable and the person so afflicted may be unable to live a normal conjugal life. However, no illness other than "incurably of unsound mind," leprosy, and venereal diseases is listed under the ground for divorce/judicial separation. Thus, the provision is quite discriminatory for persons with mental disorders, and it denies them the right to remain married.
- Other ground for divorce is the "person has been suffering continuously or intermittently from mental disorder of such a kind and to such an extent that the petitioner cannot reasonably be expected to live with the respondent." It is pertinent to note that the disability

under Section 5 was "of such a kind or to such an extent." However, here it is "of such a kind and to such an extent." Therefore, should be understood that the ground for divorce should a severe mental disorder with a severe degree of disability. There may be host of reasons, other than mental disorders, due to which a person cannot be anticipated to reasonably live with the other people. Making only mental disorders as a ground for divorce is very unfortunate. It burdens the person affected with mental disorders with unnecessary stigma, and they are hesitant to seek psychiatric treatment. Stigma of having mental disorders proves to be a major hazard to them.

- All persons with mental disorders have a right to marry and live with dignity. Putting legal restriction on this right is discriminatory. The real problem is negative attitude of the society, and the stigma attached to mental disorders. Many persons with mental illnesses execute better than those without such disorders. Marriage is one of the important support systems for many persons with mental disorders and being unmarried or getting divorced/separated denies them this support. Siblings of persons with mental disorders hardly support them.
- The UN Convention on the Rights of Persons with Disabilities (UNCRPD), 2006, has been signed and ratified by India. The purpose of UNCRPD is to promote, protect, and ensure the full and equal enjoyment of all human rights and fundamental freedoms by all persons with disabilities and to promote respect for their inherent dignity.[12] Mental illness comes under the categories of disability under the UNCRPD. Right to marry may be regarded as a basic human right. Thus, denying the persons with mental disorders the right to marry is not in accordance to the UNCRPD.

The fact of mental illness, especially in cases of girls, is frequently concealed at the time of marriage. This is mostly due to the distress that disclosure will not only result in rejection of the girl, but the crusading of the fact in the marriage market would be extremely detrimental and would prevent her from getting a suitable match.[5] Parties do not convey all the facts about the prospective bride, or the groom and camouflaging of every fact about the person is not thought as a fraud. It has been advocated that an express provision should be made in the statute to the effect that a past history of having mental disorder would be no bar to marriage and failure of disclosing that history or fact of treatment would not lead to suppression of material fact.[1] However, in the author's opinion, if all reference to mental disorders is removed from the condition of disability of marriage and from the grounds for divorce; such express provision would hardly be required.

The basic reason of inclusion of mental disorders in the conditions of disability to marry at the time of framing the laws six decades back was the incurability. However now, with remarkable advancements in the field of psychiatry, most of the mental disorders are now curable, and the persons so affected are able to lead a normal life. Therefore, mental disorders should be removed from the disability under the marriage laws. We should aim to change the negative societal attitude toward mental disorders which play important role in their stigmatization. Mention of words like "recurrent attack of insanity," "inability to live normal life or procreation of child" is derogatory and stigmatizing. It is necessary to change all these. The law should perform a facilitative role in the society, and it should not dishearten individuals from looking for treatment of mental disorders. Marriage is an important event in one's life and in Indian context, it is also a religiously sanctioned necessity. It is unreasonable to deny this right to persons with mental disorders.

Husband's inability to perform adequate and satisfactory sexual intercourse with his wife is often a cause of marital discord and many marriages become victim of divorce, separation and other marital disputes because of this. Such disputes land up in the courts of law where the question of sexual potency is often raised.

LEGAL ASPECTS OF IMPOTENCE

Impotence is the inability of a man to achieve or maintain a penile erection that is sufficient to complete sexual intercourse. Impotence is a common condition that may temporarily affect most men at some time in their lives. If impotence is short-lived and does not recur frequently, it is generally considered normal. If impotence persists, impotence can result in complications, such as male infertility and mental health issues, marital discord and legal complications.

Family is man's basic and important component, around which his life revolves. Marriage invests in every married couple to make way for procreation and nurturing of future generations and influences the social and cultural growth of society. Procreation is possible provided both the partners are sexually healthy.

EXAMINATION OF A PERSON WITH IMPOTENCE

Following are the depends for examination:
- A thorough sexual and medical history
- Look for occurrence of risk factors for various vascular disease, i.e. diabetes mellitus (DM), hypertension, smoking, serum lipid abnormalities and history of IHD, chronic renal failure (CRF), history of penile trauma, pelvic or genital surgery and Peyronie's disease.
- A detailed physical examination.
- Associated laboratory investigations, which includes serum glucose level, testosterone levels, and serum lipid profile.
- In absence of contraindication (e.g. nitrate use), a trial of oral PDE-5 inhibitors is a reasonable diagnostic (and potentially therapeutic) approach for a middle-aged man.
- Intracavernosal injection with a vasoactive agent (e.g. PGE1) can be an important step to differentiate organic from psychogenic impotence.
- The intracavernosal injection can be combined with penile duplex Doppler sonography to evaluate the vascular system of the penis.
- Abnormalities in the vascular system usually involve referral to a urologist.

There are several cultural variations in the practices marriage in Indian society. Hinduism and Islam, the two main religions of the country, have their on traditions related to marriage. While polygamy is outlawed in Hindu society, Islam gives religious sanction for polygamy.

In the recent years, following its judgment invalidating *'triple talaq,* the Supreme Court of India has now set up a Constitution bench to examine the practices of polygamy and *nikah halala*. A custom by which a woman has to marry and consummate a marriage with someone else before remarrying her previous husband. The Quran does not encourage these practices, contrary to common perception, but patriarchy gives them social sanction among a few Indian Muslims. In these provisions woman is always at the receiving end. The codified family and customary laws favor the men in various ways in marriage, divorce, property, etc. Provisions on conjugal rights and adultery and division of matrimonial assets continue to harm women.

Either way they have no place in our constitutional republic. Whatever form our family laws have, marriage is a formal union between two individuals with certain rights and obligations, and it must be fair to both partners.

Irrespective of the religious practices, both the partners should be ensured equal rights by the law without making a binding on the unwilling partner. There may be cultural differences but the individual rights are the sacrosanct.

REFERENCES

1. Nambi S. Marriage, mental health and the Indian legislation. Indian J Psychiatry. 2005;47:3-14.
2. Royal Anthroplogical Institute of Great Britain and Northern Ireland. Notes and queries on Anrhroplogy. London: Royal Anthroplogical Institute; 1951. p. 110.
3. Narayan CL, Narayan M, Shikha D, et al. Indian marriage laws and mental disorders: is it necessary to amend the legal provisions? Indian J Psychiatry. 2015;57:341-4.
4. Leach E. Polyandry, inheritance and the definition of marriage. Man. 1955;55(12):183.
5. Srivastava A. Marriage as a perceived panacea to mental illness in India: reality check. Indian J Psychiatry. 2013;55(Suppl 2):S239-42.
6. Sharma I, Pandit B, Pathak A, et al. Hinduism, marriage and mental illness. Indian J Psychiatry. 2013;55(Suppl 2):S243-9.
7. Hindu Marriage Act; 1955. Available from: http://www.indiankanoon.org/doc/590166/. [Last accessed on 2015 Jul 21].
8. Special Marriage Act; 1954. Available from: http://www.indiankanoon.org/doc/4234/. [Last accessed on 2015 Jul 21].
9. Narayan CL, Shikha D. Indian legal system and mental health. Indian J Psychiatry. 2013;55(Suppl 2):S177-81.
10. Sathyanarayana Rao TS, Nambi S, Chandrashekhar H. Marriage, Mental Health and Indian Legislation. In: Forensic Psychiatry: Clinical Practice Guidelines for Psychiatrists in India. Indian Psychiatric Society; 2009. p. 113-28.
11. Thara R, Srinivasan TN. Outcome of marriage in schizophrenia. Soc Psychiatry Psychiatr Epidemiol. 1997;32:416-20.
12. UN Convention on the Rights of Persons with Disabilities (UNCRPD); 2006. Available from: http://www.un.org/disabilities/. [Last accessed on 2015 Jul 21].

SECTION V

Intersection of Mental Health and Criminal Law

CHAPTER 16

Courts in India and Judicial Process

> **LEARNING OBJECTIVES**
> - Types of law
> - Different types of courts in India
> - Procedures in criminal courts

INTRODUCTION

Law relating to any criminal proceedings is applicable to entire India except Jammu and Kashmir. It is contained in Indian Penal Code (IPC), 1860 which defines offenses as well as punishments and *Criminal Procedure Code (CrPC), 1973* which contains the procedural aspect of the law encoded in IPC.[1-4] The entire law is covered in *484 sections* in *two schedules*. These two complement one another for punishment of offenders against the substantive criminal law.[5-7] *CrPC* is procedural law and covers *constitution, structure, classification and powers of criminal courts and prescribes procedure* of criminal proceedings.[4,8-11]

Law can also be divided into the following:[12]
- *Statute or codified law*: Law enacted by State and the Parliament
- *Common law or law of torts*: Law made by judges, which usually is about wrongs caused by one human being to another.[4] They are not covered by statute law.

COURTS IN INDIA

Courts of law in India are of two types:[4]
1. *Civil Courts* and
2. *Criminal Courts*.

Civil courts try only *civil cases*, whereas criminal courts try only *criminal cases*.

The criminal courts further belong to different categories, namely, *Supreme Court, High Court, Sessions Court,* and *Magistrates Court*. Recently, Government of India has set up certain *Fast Track Courts* for the speedy disposal of cases. These courts have the status of additional session courts.[1,4,13] Supreme Court can try both civil and criminal cases. A medical man may be deposed in both *civil* and *criminal courts,* but mostly in the latter **(Table 1)**.

Supreme Court

Supreme Court is the *highest judicial tribunal of the country* and is located at New Delhi, the Capital of India.

Table 1: Hierarchy and powers of courts in India.

Hierarchy of courts in India	Powers of courts
1. Supreme Court (highest judicial tribunal, located at New Delhi)	Powers of Supreme Court: • Court of appeal • Supervises and interprets law in the country • Law declared by it is binding on all other courts • Usually takes cases referred from State High Courts • Cases can also be filed directly here • Can pass any sentence stated in law
2. High Court (Highest judicial tribunal in the State)	Powers of High Court: • Court of appeal • Can take up all cases of criminal offenses • Can pass all sentences authorized by the law
3. Sessions Court (District Sessions Court) (Highest judicial tribunal for district) • Presided over by the Sessions Judge • Additional Sessions Judges and Assistant Sessions Judges may also be appointed to exercise jurisdiction	Powers of Session Courts: • It takes up only the cases of criminal offenses referred by Magistrates' courts • Can pass all sentences authorized by the law; however, the death sentence passed by it has to be confirmed by the High Court
4. Magistrates' Court • Criminal courts presided over by the Judicial/Metropolitan Magistrates	• *Judicial magistrates:* Appointed by and are under the control of High Court • *Executive magistrates:* Appointed by and are under the control of the State Government

Powers of Supreme Court

- It is a court of appeal.
- It supervises and interprets law in the country.
- Decisions of the Supreme Court are binding on rest all courts of the country.
- It usually takes the cases referred from State High Courts. However, cases can also be filed directly in the Supreme Court.
- It can pass any sentence.

High Court

High Court is the highest judicial tribunal in the State and is located usually in the State Capital. *However, some of the High Courts not located in the State Capital, and they are: Kerala—Cochin, MP—Jabalpur, Assam—Guwahati, Orissa—Cuttack, and UP—Allahabad.*

Powers of High Court

- It is also a court of appeal.
- It can take-up all cases of criminal offenses.
- It can pass all sentences authorized by the law.

Session's Court (District Session's Court)

This is the highest judicial tribunal for district and is located in the district headquarters. The court has a *Sessions Judge*, appointed by the High Court. High Court may also appoint *Additional Sessions Judges* and *Assistant Sessions Judges* to exercise jurisdiction in the court of sessions.

Powers of Session Courts
- It takes up only the cases of criminal offenses referred by the Magistrate's courts.
- It can pass all sentences authorized by the law; however, the death sentence passed by it has to be confirmed by the High Court.

Magistrates' Court

Magistrate's courts are criminal courts presided over by the *Judicial/Metropolitan Magistrates*. The state government in liaison with High Court may establish many Judicial Magistrate Courts in each district, as per need. Based on functions, magistrates can be divided into following categories:
- Executive Magistrates
- Judicial Magistrates
- Special Magistrates

Executive Magistrates

As per Section 20, CrPC, executive magistrate in a district could be—district magistrate, additional district magistrate (wherever necessary), subdivisional magistrate, or subordinate executive magistrate.

Special executive magistrate (Section 21, CrPC). Executive magistrates are usually officers of *revenue department*, like *District Collector, Subcollector* or *Tehsildar*, and placed *in charge* of a district, subdivision or *taluk* and have all the powers of a district or *subdivisional magistrate*.

Judicial Magistrates

On the judicial side, magistracy differs according to the population figures. Cities with a population of less than one million are considered nonmetropolitan cities, while those with more than one million are considered as metropolitan areas.

According to Sections 11, 12, CrPC, judicial magistrates in an order of hierarchy in a nonmetropolitan area are Chief Judicial Magistrate, Additional Chief Judicial Magistrate, Subdivisional Judicial Magistrate, and Judicial Magistrate First Class. As per Section 13, CrPC, the High Court in consultation with the Central/State Government may appoint *Special Judicial Magistrates*.

According to Sections 16, 17, CrPC, judicial magistrates in a metropolitan area in an order of hierarchy are—Chief Metropolitan Magistrate, Additional Chief Metropolitan Magistrate, and Special Metropolitan Magistrate. As per Section 18, CrPC, the High Court in consultation with the Central/State Government may appoint *Special Metropolitan Magistrates* also.

Cases Tried by Judicial Magistrates
All judicial magistrates can try cases such as:[1,4,13,14]
- *Warrant case:* It means a case relating to the commission of a *cognizable offense*. Thus, a case which makes one liable for arrest without warrant, e.g. homicide, rape, etc. Such cases are usually instituted upon police report, but that can also be done on private complaint.
- *Summons case:* It means that in cases of *noncognizable offenses* and being not a warrant case, a police officer has no authority to arrest without warrant. Usually, these cases are instituted on complaint and being simple case, punishment will usually be imprisonment of one year or less.

Special Magistrate

He or she could be a *metropolitan, judicial* or *executive magistrate*, appointed for special purposes, as for example to try cases of *rioting* when a number of people are arrested. They are also appointed whenever a regular magistrate cannot cope up with the *extra load of work* or the *enquiry* has to be completed within a certain time limit. These magistrates could be of *any class*.[4,13]

Railway Magistrate: He or she will be of the rank of *First Class*.
Judicial Magistrate and is appointed to try cases of offenses under *Railway Act*.[1,4,13,14]

Magistrate in Juvenile Court (Juvenile Magistrate): This is a principal magistrate/a chief judicial magistrate and usually a *woman* and she presides over a *Juvenile Court* and tries *juvenile offenders*,[15] who are children less than eighteen years of age (Juvenile Justice Act, 2000) and are accused of having committed a crime. These offenders are tried in juvenile courts under the *Children Act, 1960*, and if found guilty are usually not imprisoned or punished as an adult offender but, sent to a *Child Reformation Centre* called *Borstal or Juvenile homes*.[1,4,14]

Public Prosecutor

He or she being a *public servant* under *Section 24, CrPC*, is a legal expert, appointed by the Central or State Government for conducting court prosecutions or other proceedings like *appeal*, etc. on behalf of the government. *Doctors when summoned to give evidence can approach him/her for the case file or other such help.* Public prosecutors could be of two ranks: *Additional Public Prosecutor*, and *Assistant Public Prosecutor*.

Legal Sentences that can be Passed under Law

As per *Section 53, IPC*, on conviction, criminals are punished by:
- Death sentence, which is to be passed by court of sessions, subject to confirmation by the High Court.
- Life imprisonment is to be passed by court of sessions, the time usually comprises 20 years, which can be *reduced* to 14 years for *good behavior* of the prisoner.
- Imprisonment types:
  - Rigorous imprisonment with hard labor—all courts and First Class Magistrate can pass this order.

- Simple imprisonment—all courts and magistrates can pass this order.
  - Solitary imprisonment—all courts and First Class Magistrates can pass this order.
- *Monetary fine:* High Court and Sessions Court can impose any amount of the fine. But First Class Magistrate and Second Class Magistrate cannot impose more than ₹ 5000/- and ₹ 1000/- respectively.
- *Attachment of movable property:* This can be done by the High Court, Sessions Court, and Chief Judicial/Metropolitan Magistrate as per court's direction and power.
- *Detention in reformatories:* This can be ordered by the Chief Judicial Magistrate or Judicial Magistrate of Juvenile Court, where the offender is below 18 years and sent to Reformatory Centers/Borstal Schools.[14]
- **Usually court can order detention till rise of court for contempt of court.**

PROCEDURES IN CRIMINAL COURTS

There are several court procedures, which a doctor may have to know in attending the criminal court and tender his evidence[1,7,8,13,14,16-20] and they are:
- Attendance in court
- Subpoena (summons)
- Warrant
- Conduct money
- Oath taking
- Recording of evidence.

Attendance in Court

Most of the medical reports/medical certificates are not acceptable in the court of law, unless testified in the presence of the accused. Thus, the medical officer as an expert witness will have to attend the court on a particular day, during the trial, for deposition and cross-examination of the contents in the report issued by him to the court.

Subpoena (Summons)

Definition

Subpoena is defined as a document compelling the attendance of a witness on a particular day and time in the court of law under penalty.

Explanation

Subpoena is a written document issued in duplicate by the presiding officer of the court with proper seal and signature, to be served to the witness demanding his/her presence in court punctually at the specified date and time for giving evidence in connection with a particular case and with a warning to not to be absent without prior permission of the court. It can be served also to produce any official document or any paper before the court of law. However, the summons is a milder form of process.

Procedure of Serving the Summons

Usually, it is issued by the Presiding Officer of the court, delivered by a court official or a police constable. Person receiving should sign on the original and keep the duplicate with him. If the person summoned to is not available, it may be served to:
- The other major member of the family/relatives, but not to a servant.
- If the person is a government servant, it may be served through the head of the office in which he or she is employed.
- It may be even affixed on some conspicuous part of the house in which the person summoned ordinarily resides.
- *Summons by post:* It can even be sent by registered post.

However, on these occasions, the court may not consider this as being served. If the postal authority returns the cover stating, he or she is refusing to receive the same, the court considers that it has been served in spite of not receiving it.

Rules of Summons

If a medical officer is summoned to attend two courts on a particular time and day, following *rules* may be opted:
- *Criminal cases* should be given preference over civil cases.
- If both are criminal cases, *higher courts* should be given first preference. However, the medical officer should *inform* the other court which he or she is not attending.
- If both cases are of the same ranking courts, summons received *earlier* should be attended first.
- *Noncompliance to summons* in a civil case, may render one liable to an action for *damages*, but in a criminal case, fine or even imprisonment (unless some satisfactory excuse is given) may be ordered.
- He or she cannot leave the court without the permission of the magistrate or the judge.
- If he or she fails to attend the summons in time, a warrant can be issued to compel his or her attendance.[4,13,14]
- An attendance certificate will be issued by the court on demand.

Warrant (Witness Warrant)

Definition

Warrant is an authority under the seal and signature of the presiding officer of a court to a person to be arrested and produced before the court to be dealt with according to law. It is a written order from a court, commanding police to perform specified acts/arrests to produce the witness in the court of law.

Types

Warrant could be *bailable warrant (BW)* or *nonbailable warrant (NBW)*, issued through police by a court to compel attendance of the witness in court on a fixed date.[3,4,12,13] A court may issue this in lieu of or in addition to the summons for appearance in the court for following reasons:

- If there is reason to believe that he or she will abscond or will not obey the summons.
- If the witness has failed to appear before without prior reasonable excuse, though clearly served with summons.
- In a case of *breach of bond of security* for appearing (*vide Section 90, CrPC*).

Conduct Money

Definition

Conduct money is the *fee* offered to a *witness* in a *civil case*, at the time of serving of summons to cover the *traveling expenses* for attending the court.

In the civil cases: A Government Medical Officer gets the *conduct money* when he or she serves a summons.

In the criminal cases: Where state is the prosecuting party, Government Medical Officer will *not* get conduct money, but *as per law (Section 312, CrPC)*, he or she will be paid the *travel allowances (TA) by the court*. This is also called *Witness* Officers will get a fee, private practitioners will get a fee from the *state* or the *private party* concerned.

Oath Taking

Before deposition of evidence begins, the witness must take an *oath* or *affirmation*. Unoathed evidence is not admissible to the court of law, except when a person is *below 7 years of age*.[18,20]

As per *Section 191, IPC*, a witness who willfully makes a false statement after taking an oath is considered as guilty of the crime of *perjury* (giving false evidence under oath) and may be prosecuted. Punishment for perjury is dealt with as per Section 193, IPC.

Recording of Evidence

After taking the oath, the recording of evidence will be done by following four steps:[1]
1. Examination-in-Chief
2. Cross-examination
3. Re-examination
4. Court questions.

REFERENCES

1. Rao NG. Legal Procedures for Medical Doctors, 2nd edn. HR Publication Aid, Manipal, India, 2002.
2. Mathiharan K, Patnaik AK. Modi's Medical Jurisprudence and Toxicology, 23rd edn. Lexis Nexis Butterworth's; 2005
3. Dogra TD, Lt Col. Abhijith Rudra (Eds). Lyon's Medical Jurisprudence and Toxicology for India, 11th edn. Delhi Law House, New Delhi (India), 2005.
4. Ratanlal and Dhirajlal's—The Code of Criminal Procedure, 18th edn. Wadhwa and Company, Nagpur, 2006.
5. Dikshit PC (Ed). HWV Cox, Medical Jurisprudence and Toxicology, 7th edn. Lexis Nexis Butterworths, 2002.

6. Lyon. Commentary on Medical Jurisprudence for India, 10th edn, 2002.
7. Nandy A. Principles of Forensic Medicine. New Central Book Agency, Kolkata, 2000.
8. Parikh CK. Parikh's Textbook of Medical Jurisprudence and Toxicology for Classrooms and Courtrooms, 7th edn, 2001.
9. Patil S Hemalatha. The Coroner, 1st edn., NM Tripathi Pvt Ltd:Mumbai, 1989.
10. Salwan SL, Narang U. Academic's Legal Dictionary, 9th edn., Academic (India) Publishers: New Delhi, 1994.
11. Rao NG. Practical Forensic Medicine, 3rd edn. Jaypee Brothers Medical Publishers, New Delhi, 2007.
12. Mehta HS. Medical Law and Ethics in India, 1st edn. The Bombay Samachar Pvt. Ltd., 1963.
13. Rao NG. Legal Procedure and Ethics for Doctors, 2nd edn. HR Publication Aid, Manipal, 2002.
14. Singh A. Principles of Law of Evidence, 10th edn. Central Law Publication, Allahabad, India, 1996.
15. The Juvenile Justice (Care and Protection of Children) Act, 2000 (30 Dec. 2000) (Short Notes) Choudhary Publications, Meerut, India, 2000.
16. Fisher B AJ. Expert Witness Tips, in Techniques of Crime Scene Investigation, 6th edn, 2001.
17. Vanessa. Churchill's Medicolegal Pocketbook. Churchill Livingston, London, 2003.
18. Mukherjee JB. Textbook of Forensic Medicine and Toxicology, Vol 1, 2nd edn, 1994.
19. Davis JH. The Future of Medical Examiner System. Am J Forensic Med Pathol. 1995;16:265-69.
20. Rao NG. Principle and Practice of Forensic Medicine. HR Publication Aid, Manipal, India, 2002.

CHAPTER 17

Principles and Procedures of Trial of Cases in India

> **LEARNING OBJECTIVES**
> - Types and stages of trial
> - Rights of accused during different stages of trial
> - Role of psychiatrist during different stages of trial

Crime: Any act committed or omitted which is prohibited and punishable by law constitutes crime. Punishment for crime and procedure of prescribing, it is decided by codified law of the land. Trials in India have a well-established statutory, judicial and administrative framework.

Trial: The term is not defined in CrPC, however, it usually refers to coming together of two or more parties to settle a dispute in legal sense. It starts after charges are framed and ends with final legal verdict given by presiding officer, usually a judge.

Tribunal: It refers to a formal setting with presiding officer and other authority figures to adjudicate or resolve a trial case. It can be review boards as mentioned in Mental Healthcare Act or Courts.

TYPES OF TRIALS

Civil Trial

It is a trial to settle dispute involving two individuals or organizations. Any of the party can be appellant and punishment is usually in form of compensation paid to redress the loss of another party. The rules for civil trial are encoded in **code of civil procedure**.[1]

Stages in a Civil Trial[1]

1. **Appearance**
    - Summons to defendant
    - Appearance of defendant
    - Filing of written statement by defendant
    - Filing of Replication/Rejoinder by plaintiff
    - Admission/denial of documents

2. **Framing of issues**
   - Issues framed
   - Application for additional issues
3. **Evidence**
   - Plaintiff evidence
   - Filing of evidence by way of affidavit by plaintiff
   - Cross examination by defendant
   - Defendant evidence
   - Filing of evidence by way of affidavit by defendant
   - Cross examination by plaintiff
4. **Final argument**
5. **Decree/judgment**
6. **Execution of decree.**

Criminal Trial

It is a trial where crime is committed against state, i.e. society in general. Only government can file the case against accused and onus is on state (prosecution) to prove guilty beyond reasonable doubt, this is termed as 'adversarial system'. Punishment usually is in form of incarceration or fine to state or death penalty.[2] Criminal law or Indian Penal law constitutes of three main laws:

I. **Substantive Criminal Law or Real Criminal Law**
   1. Indian Penal Code, 1860
II. **Procedural Criminal Law or Adjective Criminal Law**
   2. *"Code of Criminal Procedure (CrPC), 1973:* It is the procedural law for conducting a criminal trial in India. The procedure includes the manner for collection of evidence, examination of witnesses, interrogation of accused, arrests, safeguards and procedure to be adopted by Police and Courts, bail, the process of criminal trial, a method of conviction, and the rights of the accused of a fair trial by principles of natural justice."[2,3]
   3. *"Indian Evidence Act, 1872:* IEA is a detailed treaty on the law of "evidence", which can be tendered in trial, manner of production of the evidence in trial, and the evidentiary value, which can be attached to such evidence. IEA also deals with the judicial presumptions, expert and scientific evidence."[2,3]

Stages in a Criminal Trial[2,3]
I. **Pre-trial stages**
   1. Registration of FIR
   2. Investigation
II. **Trial stages**
   1. Filing of charge sheet
   2. Framing of charges/serving the notice

3. Recording of the prosecution evidence
4. Statement of the accused
5. Evidence of defense
6. Final arguments of both the sides
7. Delivery of judgment
8. Arguments on sentence
9. Judgment with punishment

III. Post-trial stages
1. Punishment as per judgment
2. Imprisonment and or fine
3. Capital punishment in rarest of rare cases.

RIGHTS OF ACCUSED DURING STAGES OF TRIAL

To ensure implementation of principles of "natural justice", every accused is accorded with following rights during different stages of trial. Trial rights as mentioned in landmark judgement by Justice Sri T Mallikarjuna Rao based on CrPC are as follows:[4,5]

I. Pre-trial Rights

The CrPC endows an individual with certain rights during course of any trial or enquiry of any offence charged.
1. *Knowledge of the accusation:* Accused should be informed of the charges and should get due opportunity of defending one self.
2. *Right to open trial:* Hearing should be conducted in public and orally, without endowing any special favours to any party.
3. *Aid of counsel:* For conducting fair trial every accused should be provided counsel of choice and it is duty to ensure that counsel is provided in all cases to accuse as per fundamental right enshrined in Article 22(1) of Constitution of India.
4. *Expeditious trial.*
5. *Protection against illegal arrest:* Section 50 CrPC states that any person arrested without warrant must be informed immediately of the grounds of same.
6. *Proceedings in the presence of the accused:* All case proceedings should take place in presence of accused or his counsel.
7. *Right to bail:* Bail refers to release from police custody. CrPC Section 436 gives accused right to claim bail in bailable offences as mentioned in First schedule of the Code.
8. *Prohibition on double jeopardy:* It means a person cannot be tried again of an offence for which he/she has already been acquitted or convicted, its termed as principle of 'autrefois acquit' and 'autrefois convict'.

9. *Right against self-incrimination:* Clause (3) of Article 20 provides: "No person accused of any offence shall be compelled to be a witness against himself." This Clause is based on the maxim nemo tenetur prodere accussare seipsum, which means that "no man is bound to accuse himself."[4,5]

II. Post-trial Rights

1. *Lawful punishment:* Article 20(1) explains that a person can be convicted of an offence only if that act is made punishable by a law in force. It gives constitutional recognition to the rule that no one can be convicted except for the violation of a law in force.
2. *Right to humane treatment:* A prisoner does not become a non-person. Prison deprives liberty. Even while doing this, prison system must aim at reformation. In prison, treatment must be geared to psychic healing, release of stress, restoration of self-respect apart from training to adapt oneself to the life outside.
3. *Right to appeal:* Section 389(1) empowers the appellate court to suspend execution of sentence, or when the convicted person in confinement, to grant bail pending any appeal to it.
4. *Proper execution of sentence.*[4,5]

ROLE OF PSYCHIATRIST DURING DIFFERENT STAGES OF TRIALS

During these different stages, role of psychiatrist can be in following areas:
1. Competence assessment for various civil responsibilities
2. Competence assessment and management issues in criminal cases.

Pre-trial Stages

- Assessment of fitness for interrogation
- No person with mental illness should be detained unlawfully in prisons on name of "preventive detention"
- Screening for mental illnesses in accused and offering appropriate treatment
- Assessment of fitness for standing trial (if invoked during enquiry stage).

Trial Stages

- Assessment of fitness for standing trial (if noticed or invoked during trial stage)
- Insanity defense assessment
- Appearing as expert witness
- Screening for mental illnesses in accused and offering appropriate treatment in prison setting for under trials.

Post-trial Stages

- Screening for mental illnesses and offering appropriate treatment in prison settings for convicts
- Assessment of fitness for execution.

REFERENCES

1. Process flow in a civil suit in India—Legal Service India. Available at: www.legalserviceindia.com/lawforum/index.php?topic=2069.0. Last accessed on 07.02.18.
2. Dalmia VP. Process of trial of criminal cases in India. Vaish associates advocates, 2014.
3. Furtado R. All about the various stages of criminal trial in India. Available at: https://blog.ipleaders.in/all-about-the-various-stages-of-criminal-trial-in-india/ Last accessed on 07.02.18.
4. Duggal S. Concept of a Fair Trial. Available at: https://www.lawctopus.com/academike/concept-fair-trial/ 2/24. Last accessed on 07.02.18.
5. http://ecourts.gov.in/sites/default/files/1st%20Topic.pdf.

CHAPTER

Role of Forensic Psychiatrist during Different Stages of Trial

> **LEARNING OBJECTIVES**
> - Violation of rights of persons with mental illness during trial
> - Psychiatry assessment during different stages of trial
> - Relevance of psychiatry assessment in legal trials
> - Legal insanity vs. medical insanity

VIOLATION OF RIGHTS OF PERSONS WITH MENTAL ILLNESS DURING TRIAL

An important goal of criminal justice system should be to ensure that no one with a mental disability is inappropriately held in judicial custody or prison. Very often persons with mental disabilities are prosecuted and imprisoned, in some cases for relatively minor offenses, but end up spending much more time in the process of incarceration than the punishment due to prolonged trial phase because of inability to stand trial, lack of formal mental health assessment at any point and poor social support by family members.

Indian case laws: Violation of Rights of Persons with mental illness in conflict with criminal law during trial stages.

- *Prolonged detention of mentally ill due to administrative lapses:* Few of the persons who were mentally ill at the time of trial but had subsequently recovered could never be released due to inaction of state authorities (Veena Sethi vs. State of Bihar, 1982).[1]
- *Prolonged detention of mentally ill due to perpetual inability to become fit for trial:* Few under trials persons were found languishing in jail for years much more than the actual punishment because of perpetual inability to stand trial on grounds of mental illness (Hussainara Khatoon vs. State of Bihar, 1980),[2] [Charanjit Singh and National vs. Government of National Capital Territory of Delhi (GNCTD) and others, 2005].[3]
- *Shortage of mental health professional in jail:* Non availability of mental health professionals in jail for periodic evaluation and treatment of mental health problems for prison inmates was responsible for not being able to detect people with mental health issues at any stage of trial and being offered appropriate help.[4]

Role of Mental Health Professionals

Mental health professional can play important role in assessment and treatment for such individuals. Psychiatrist are often called at various stages for certain assessments by court of law, ones of special relevance during trial phases (arrest and prosecution state) are as follows:
1. *Pretrial:* Assessment of Fitness for interrogation
2. *During trial:* Assessment of Fitness for standing trial, assessment of insanity defense/criminal responsibility assessment
3. *Post-trial:* Assessment of risk factors/mitigating factors, fitness for execution.

RELEVANCE OF PERFORMING THESE FORENSIC PSYCHIATRY ASSESSMENT BY MENTAL HEALTH PROFESSIONALS

As per Richard Bonnie, forensic psychiatry assessments of various competencies during different stages of trial will serve following purpose:[5]
1. *Accuracy of criminal process:* Participation of a defendant in judicial process is very important to have a fair outcome. An incompetent defendant may not understand the nature and process of trial and may not be in a state to convey relevant details to assist the counsel in one's defense and may lead to erroneous convictions, jeopardizing the accuracy of criminal trial process.
2. *Protecting defendants' decision-making autonomy:* Law endows every accused with certain rights like to take decision regarding presence during trial, to aid counsel in preparing self-defense, to appeal against a decision of court of law if not satisfied. So, if the client is not competent enough to understand the process and take relevant decisions, it will be violation of decision-making autonomy of individual.
3. *Preserving the dignity of the criminal process:* Purpose of trial is redressal and retribution, not merely punishment. Hence, to preserve dignity of the criminal process that it is ensured that defendant should be competent enough to understand process of trial and rationale of punishment than just being a petty object to serve punishment.

Fair trial from rights' perspective: Every individual has a "right for fair trial" as safeguarded by following statutes:[6]
1. Article 14 of the International Covenant on Civil and Political Rights, which was ratified by India and subsequently paved way for enactment of Protection of Human Rights Act (PHRA). PHRA recognizes right to fair trial as an important human right.
2. It is constitutionally recognized in Articles 14, 21, 22 and 39-A.
3. The Code of Criminal Procedure (CrPC) 1973 (Procedure to be followed in case of accused being or suspected to be of unsound mind, CrPC Sections 328 to 335).

Fair trial from natural justice's perspective: For effective justice to be delivered, principle of natural justice has to be followed as based on following two legal maxims:
1. That nobody should be a judge in his own cause
2. Nobody should be condemned unheard.

Difference Between Legal and Medical Terminology

In subsequent chapters, there will be frequent use of word **"unsound mind"** or **"insanity"** as **mentioned in substantive and procedural criminal laws of India**. It has only been used in legal context with the clear understanding that such terms are **obsolete from perspective of** current **clinical psychiatry** literature or **mental health related statues of India**.

Legal insanity: Refers to the concept of 'mental state at time of crime'. It refers to "presence of mental disorder" as well as "loss of reasoning"

Medical insanity: Only refers to presence of mental disorder **(Table 1)**.

Table 1: Difference between legal and medical insanity.

	Medical insanity	Legal insanity
What it is	Though 'insanity' word is no more used in mental health practices. In closes parlance to legal concept of insanity, it refers to presence of mental disorder	It is the 'mental state at time of crime'. Thus, it refers to "presence of mental disorder" as well as "loss of reasoning" to be present together which rendered individual incapable of knowing right or wrong
Purpose of concept	Diagnosing and treating the individual	"Welfare of public" and simultaneously 'not penalizing the innocent individual who committed the crime due to disturbed mental faculties'
Nature and degree of insanity	It can range from mild anxiety disorders to severe schizophrenia or dementia	It only refers to conditions substantially affecting cognitive faculties to the extent that person was incapable of knowing nature and quality of act or its wrongness at time of committing crime, irrespective of diagnosis or severity
Time factor	It takes into account historical evidence and course of illness in future to reach on a diagnosis	It refers to mental state 'only at the time of committing crime'

REFERENCES

1. Veena Sethi vs. State of Bihar. Writ Petition (Criminal) No. 73 of 1982. Available at:http://www.manupatrainternational.in/supremecourt/1980-2000/sc1982/s820089. [Last accessed on 02.10.18].
2. Hussainara Khatoon vs. State of Bihar. 1980-(001)-SCC -0091 -SC. Available at: http://www.bprd.gov.in/writereaddata/mainlinkfile/File713.pdf. [Last accessed on 02.10.18].
3. Writ petition (Cr) 729/2002 and 1278/2004. Available at: https://indiankanoon.org/doc/1230647. [Last accessed on 02.010.18].
4. Murthy P, Kumar S, Desai N, et al. National Human Rights Commission. Report of the technical committee on mental health; 2016. Available from: http://www.nhrc.nic.in/Documents/Mental_Health_report_vol_I_10_06_2016.pdf. [Last accessed on 02.010.18].
5. Bonnie RJ. The competence of criminal defendants: a theoretical reformulation. Behavioral Sciences and the Law. 1992;10:291-316.
6. Kumar K, Kaul M, Mittal DR, et al. Legal status of mentally ill patient. Journal of Dental and Medical Sciences. 2017;16(2):49-52.

CHAPTER 19

Pretrial Assessment: Fitness for Interview by Police

> **LEARNING OBJECTIVES**
> - Fitness for interview by police
> - Suggestibility and reliability of confessions

'Fitness for interview' though is not a definitive term appearing in any of the legal statutes of the country, but in recent years, demand for forensic examination of 'fitness for interview' by mental health professionals from police stations or defense attorneys is on rise.

NEED OF ASSESSMENT

- Reduce possibility of false confession due to inability to understand interview
- Erroneous conviction: Silence or refusal to answer or uncooperativeness due to underlying mental illness may sometimes be inferred inadvertently against the defendant and erroneous conclusions are drawn on its basis
- Violation of fair trial principles
- Identifying potential persons in need of mental health care and diverting them for treatment timely than incarceration
- Identifying resources and support persons needed to facilitate interview.

AIMS OF ASSESSMENT

Assessment of any person with mental illness with regard to fitness to be interviewed by police is aimed at following:[1,2]
- To determine capacity of person to understand interview as assessed by assessment of following parameters:
  - Concentration ability
  - Ability to understand interview
  - Ability to process interview.
- Any effect of process of interview on person's mental state in case of individuals with known mental illness.
- Assess and anticipate what resources or support will be necessary to aid the interview so as to reduce any detrimental effect of interview on person and increase productivity of interview.

Also equally important to understand that aim of this assessment is not at all to check truthfulness of content of interview.

Relevant Legislation

There is no specific legislation that covers the situation of fitness for interview by police. However, fitness for police interview implies the ability:[3]

- To understand the nature of the questioning (i.e. questioning to ascertain involvement in the commission of an offence)
- To be able to follow the course of questioning
- To be able to give instruction to a legal representative
- To be able to understand when the person is cautioned that he or she does not have to say anything, but anything that he/she say may be given in evidence
- To not be in an excessively suggestible state
- To be aware of the surroundings.

FORENSIC PSYCHIATRY ASSESSMENT OF FITNESS TO BE INTERVIEWED BY POLICE[2-5]

This is a functional test of capacity, not dependent on any particular mental disorder or diagnosis. Factors such as tiredness, emotional arousal or distress, physical pain or intoxication may constitute mental vulnerability and delay interviewing.

Before Seeing the Patient

- Obtain written information from the custody officer about his/her presentation in the police station, particularly level of intoxication, agitation, confusion, bizarre behavior, loss of consciousness or head injury
- Obtain prior written records of mental health assessment of alleged accused
- Consider potential risk of harm towards you or others during the assessment, and take appropriate measures.

On Seeing the Patient

- Obtain consent for the assessment, unless the person does not have capacity (in which case it is necessary to be satisfied that proceeding is in their best interests) and disclose limits of confidentiality
- Attempt to take a full psychiatric history, concentrating on identifying evidence of mental disorder, learning disability, personality disorder, drug and alcohol use
- Undertake a full mental state examination, including assessment of cognitive functioning as appropriate.

Consider the Capacity of the Individual to Understand
- Why he/she is in the police station, and why he/she is to be interviewed
- The police caution and his/her rights
- The questions that are likely to be asked at interview, and their significance
- The significance of his/her answers, and the potential consequences.

Consider whether the Person's Mental State could Influence His/Her Ability to Give an Accurate Account of Events
For example:
- Delusional beliefs or altered mood could lead to an exaggeration of actions
- Auditory hallucinations, thought disorder or confusion could lead to the person being unable to follow conversations or to misunderstand questions
- A confession might be unreliable—look particularly for a high degree of suggestibility with a relatively low intelligence quotient (IQ) and emotional distress.

Consider whether the Interview Process Itself might Lead to a Significant Deterioration in His/Her Pre-existing Mental Health Condition
Form a judgment based upon the assessment as to the impact of any symptoms of a mental (or physical) disorder upon the police interview, and the risks that this could pose (to individual's health, or to reliability of evidence given). Communicate your decision to the custody officer, and document in custody record.

Consider other Recommendations
- If the individual is currently deemed unfit for interview, would a reassessment be helpful and, if so, when?
- Do further safeguards need to be considered for the interview, such as more frequent breaks, simple language being used, or a mental health professional being present in the interview to monitor the person's mental health?
- Do further assessments need to be carried out, such as a psychological assessment, or by a specialist in old age or learning disability?

ASSESSING SUGGESTIBILITY AND RELIABILITY OF CONFESSIONS
In addition, you need to formulate the interviewee's suggestibility, considering:
- Historical evidence of a tendency to lie, exaggerate, seek attention in other maladaptive ways—you will need a collateral history for this
- Personality style, especially inadequate or histrionic types
- Intelligence and strategies for coping with stress—consider a formal IQ assessment
- Social skills and competence.

Additional Considerations

From past interviews by police or any judicial appearance, ask if any of the following happened:
- Any evidence of confusion or misunderstanding
- Record of biological functions or odd behavior in jail observation reports
- Any evidence of 'suggestibility' or 'undue compliance'
- Any evidence of quick change in response to oppressive technique.

Mode of Assessment

- Detailed clinical interview
- Gathering collateral information
- Assessing police transcript if possible
- Jail psychiatrist or medical officer's general or behavior report
- Psychological assessment (Gudjonsson Compliance Scale).

REFERENCES

1. Gudjonsson GH. Detention: Fitness to be interviewed. Encyclopedia of Forensic and Legal Medicine 2016 .pp. 214-9.
2. Eastman N, Adshead G, Fox S, et al. Forensic Psychiatry. Oxford Specialists Handbooks. London: Oxford University Press; 2017.
3. Ventress MA, Rix KJ, Kent JH. Keeping Pace. Fitness to be interviewed by the police. Advances in Psychiatric Treatment. 2008;14:369-81.
4. https://www2.health.vic.gov.au/about/key-staff/chief-psychiatrist/chief-psychiatrist-guidelines/police-interview-or-court-attendance.
5. Clark T, Rooprai DS. Practical Forensic Psychiatry. Taylor and Francis; 2011.

CHAPTER

During Trial Assessment: Fitness to Stand Trial

> **LEARNING OBJECTIVES**
> - Concept of fitness to stand trial
> - Criteria of fitness to stand trial
> - Clinical assessment
> - Psychological assessment
> - Report writing for courts

'Fitness to stand trial' refers to a legal construct which means mental ability of an individual to participate in legal proceedings. It is known as various similar names in different countries as detailed in **Table 1**.[1,2]

Table 1: Legal terms for fitness to stand trial in use globally.

Similar legal constructs	Used in
'Fitness to plead'	United Kingdom
'Fitness to stand trial'	India
'Competence to stand trial'	United States
'Adjudicative competency'	Legal books

■ NEED OF ASSESSMENT OF FITNESS TO STAND TRIAL

As per Richard Bonnie, forensic psychiatry assessments of fitness to stand trial serves following purpose:[3]

1. *Accuracy of criminal process:* Participation of a defendant in judicial process is very important to have a fair outcome. An incompetent defendant may not understand the nature and process of trial and may not be in a state to convey relevant details to assist the counsel in one's defense and may lead to erroneous convictions, jeopardizing the accuracy of criminal trial process.
2. *Protecting defendants' decision-making autonomy:* Law endows every accused with certain rights like to take decision regarding presence during trial, to aid counsel in preparing self-defense, to appeal against a decision of court of law if not satisfied. So, if the client is not competent enough to understand the process and take relevant decisions, it will be violation of decision making autonomy of individual.

3. *Preserving the dignity of the criminal process:* Purpose of trial is redressal and retribution, not merely punishment. Hence, to preserve dignity of criminal process that it is ensured that defendant should be competent enough to understand process of trial than just being a petty object to serve punishment.

HISTORICAL EVOLUTION OF FITNESS TO STAND TRIAL CONSTRUCT (TABLE 2)

Case laws from United Kingdom: Pritchard Criteria
They were formulated in case of ***R vs Pritchard (1836)***, a deaf and dumb, illiterate defendant. They involve assessing whether defendant has following abilities:[4]
- Sufficient intellect to comprehend the course of trial to make defense,
- Ability to challenge or object a juror, and
- Ability to understand details of evidence

In case of ***R vs John M***, the Court of Appeal further gave more **explication of *Pritchard criteria***. It required to assess ability of defendant to:[4]
- Understand charges and deciding whether to plead guilty or not
- Exercise their right to challenge jurors
- Instruct counsel, which means ability to understand the lawyers' questions and being able to answer them intelligibly
- Follow the course of proceedings, i.e. being able to understand what is being said by witnesses or counsel to jury, to communicate with their lawyers
- Give evidence in their defense, i.e. being able to understand questions asked and being able to answer them intelligibly.

Table 2: International statutes and criteria for fitness to stand trial.[6,7]

Country specific legal statutes	Criteria for fitness		
	Criteria 1	Criteria 2	Criteria 3
United States **(Dusky standard)**	Factual understanding of case and charges	Rational understanding of case and charges	Ability to consult with counsel for defense in case
Criminal Procedure **Rules of Florida**	Defendant's appreciation of charges	Defendant's appreciation of range and nature of possible penalties	Defendant's capacity to disclose offense related pertinent facts to attorney
Criminal **Code of Canada**	Accused must understand nature or object of the proceedings	Accused must understand possible consequences of proceedings	Accused must be able to communicate with counsel
Australian legal system	Understanding of charges made	Understanding of court process	Ability of accused to instruct legal advisors for proceeding in relation to the charges
Common elements of all systems	a. Ability to **understand and communicate legal** charges framed b. Ability to **understand and communicate consequences of charges** if proven guilty c. Ability to **assist lawyer in defending** the case d. Ability to **understand and follow court room procedures**		

CHAPTER 20: During Trial Assessment: Fitness to Stand Trial

Case laws from United States: Dusky Criteria
Famous case of Milton Dusky (1960) constitutes standards of adjudicative fitness for United States legal parlance. Dusky was diagnosed with schizophrenia and was charged with unlawfully transporting a girl across state and sexually assaulting her. Lower Circuit Court found him competent but Supreme Court over ruled the decision and said mere orientation to time and place doesn't make one competent to stand trial. It further elaborated that more important was whether individual had rational understanding of factual details of proceeding against him and had sufficient ability to assist counsel to prepare his defense or not.[2,5]
For further details refer to **Table 2**.

Assessing Fitness to Plead and Stand Trial[8,9]

I. *Understanding the right purpose of assessment*
- Read the court order for assessment to ascertain what the purpose of assessment is
- In case of vague instructions like 'medical examination', please feel free to clarify from court in writing to clarify the focus or purpose of assessment

II. *Informed consent and limitation of confidentiality*
Person or family presenting for assessment should be informed before assessment about following and a written consent to same should be recorded:
- Who ordered the examination?
- Purpose of examination
- Who all will have access to report?
- Limitations of confidentiality
- Duty to report to court the facts apparent during assessment process

III. *Clinical examination*
- Dependent on detailed psychiatric examination, this is a cross-sectional assessment of a specific capacity
- Report of unfitness must be followed up by serial assessments and opinion should be based on assessment as close as possible to trial of issue in the court
- It is always best to have assessment done by different mental health professionals at different time periods
- In difficult cases, it is advisable to do evaluation as inpatient
- Assessments should have details mentioned of entire process of interview preferably in question answer format and to be reported also to the judiciary with all process determinants detailed and then impression mentioned at the end.

Consider these questions for assessing fitness to stand trial
1. Can the defendant explain to you the charges against them in simple terms and consequence if proved guilty? If client is not aware, you can explain an aspect of this to them, and assess if they can assimilate it?
2. Can they give an account of what factors would lead them to decide on a guilty or not-guilty plea?
3. Do they have a basic understanding of the people who will be in the court room and their roles? If client is not aware, you can explain an aspect of this to them, and assess if they can assimilate it?

4. Can they discuss the events that led to their charges, and give an account of themselves?
5. How well can they participate during the course of a psychiatric interview? Is there any evidence of distractedness or distractibility, poor short-term memory, agitation or other impairment?

Cognitive deficits also to be assessed
1. Simple objective tests of cognitive ability, such as a serial 7s and registering and recalling a name and address, may be helpful. But they are not determinative, being rather different to the task required in a court room.
2. Where dementia or other cognitive disturbance is suspected, an MMSE is useful but remember that this is a screening test for dementia, not a capacity test for the courtroom. Similarly further cognitive testing or brain imaging may support a conclusion that they are unfit, but are not essential to the capacity assessment.
3. In suspected learning disability formal IQ assessment may be important supportive evidence, but a low IQ does not necessarily lead to being under disability.

The following psychiatric symptoms commonly interfere with fitness to plead:
1. Auditory hallucinations may distract the patient, preventing them from following evidence or giving evidence—consider the frequency, intensity and degree of insight. Look for objective evidence that the patient is distracted, during your examination, for example. Less commonly, somatic hallucinations or passivity may have a similar impact.
2. Psychotic disorganization symptoms, such as perplexity and thought disorder, are likely, if present, to render a defendant under disability.
3. Depression may affect the patient's ability to attend to, concentrate on and remember the evidence. Such cognitive deficits may be evident on simple testing. Evidence of psychomotor retardation, irrepressible tearfulness or an intense preoccupation with depressive cognitions may be important.
4. Hypomania may affect attention and concentration, and short-term memory. A patient who is sufficiently disturbed to be considered manic will almost certainly be under disability.
5. Delusions are only likely to affect fitness to plead when they relate to the court procedure. So if a patient is deluded that, for example their defense team is conspiring against them, or that the court is in some other way fixed, they may not be able to instruct council and participate in the trial properly.
    - Try not to adopt too dichotomous an approach to the clinical decision-making. You should consider what measures might be put in place to enable a fair trial to take place. This might include measures such as:
        a. More frequent than usual breaks
        b. Having a friend or intermediary with them as support person to facilitate interview minimally
        c. Giving evidence by video link rather than in person or in camera hearings
        d. Pointing out to the court how any further deterioration in mental state might be recognized and managed.

IV. *Structured assessment using standardized psychological instruments* (Table 3).[7]

Table 3: Psychological instruments for fitness to trial assessment.

Standardized instrument	Author	Description of instrument	Remarks about clinical utility of instrument
Competency screening test (CST)	Lipsitt et al. 1971	• Screening measure	*Advantage:* Short screening measure *Disadvantage:* Not much in use due to high false positive rate
Competency assessment instrument (CAI)	McGarry	• Structured interview • 2 stage screening • **Domains assessed:** Contains 13 items – Appraisal of available legal defenses – Quality of relating to attorney – Capacity to disclose pertinent facts • **Scoring:** 1–5 from total capacity to incapacity	*Advantages:* • Good inter-rater reliability • Good instrument as screening and as interview *Disadvantage:* Does not focus on the nexus between psychopathology and psycholegal impairment
Interdisciplinary fitness interview (IFI)	Golding et al. 1984	• Structured interview schedule • Assess both the legal and psychopathological aspects of competency • Domains assessed: Contains 3 major sections: – Legal issues (5 items) – Psychopathological issues (11 items) – Overall evaluation (4 items)	*Advantages:* • Good inter rater reliability • Good psychometric property as an interview schedule • Focuses on the nexus between psychopathology and psycholegal impairment
Interdisciplinary fitness interview-revised (IFI-R)	Golding et al. 1993	• Structured interview schedule • Assess both the legal and psychopathological aspects of competency • Domains assessed: Contains 3 major sections – Legal issues – Psychopathological issues – Overall evaluation – Issue of the iatrogenic effects of psychotropic medications – Defendant's decisional competency to engage in rational choice about trial strategies, – Proceeding pro se or pleading guilty – Competency to confess.	*Advantage:* Focuses on the nexus between psychopathology and psycholegal impairment *Disadvantage:* Not many studies available for psychometric property

Contd...

Contd...

Standardized instrument	Author	Description of instrument	Remarks about clinical utility of instrument

The fitness interview test, revised (FIT-R)	FIT: Roesch, Webster, and Eaves, 1984
	FIT-R: Roesch, Webster, and Eaves, 1994
		• Structured interview schedule
		• Based on Criminal Code of Canada.
		• Focuses on the psycholegal abilities of the individual
		• Domains assessed: Contains 3 sections
		  – Ability to understand nature or object of the proceedings, or factual knowledge of criminal procedure
		  – Ability to understand the possible consequences of the proceedings, or the appreciation of personal involvement in and importance of the proceedings
		  – Ability to communicate with counsel, or to participate in the defense.
		• Scoring: 3-point scale, score of "0" meaning definite impairment, "1" possible or mild impairment, and "2" meaning No impairment
			Advantages:
			• Less time consuming (takes approx 30 minutes)
			• Good inter rater reliability
			• Good psychometric property as an interview schedule
			• Focuses on the nexus between psychopathology and psycholegal impairment

MacArthur Competence Assessment Tool-Criminal Adjudication (MacCAT-CA) Poythress et al., 1999			
Evaluation of Competency to Stand Trial-Revised (ECST-R) Rogers et al. 2004			
Competence Assessment for Standing Trial for Defendants with Mental Retardation (CAST-MR) Everington and Luckasson, 1992			

REPORT WRITING FOR COURTS

The report can be submitted in two parts:
1. A brief **opinion addressing the question asked** by court of law
   - Declared fit (Fit/Fit with legal assistance) or unfit
   - If unfit reported, is it temporary or permanent unfitness?
   - If temporarily unfit, interval after which next assessment should be offered

   Fit with legal assistance: It refers to capacity to stand trial otherwise being intact as assessed for mental faculties but person is not able to answer the questions related to fitness to stand trial due to poor legal literacy. It can be improved by legal counselling regarding process of trial, sections levied against them and punishments prescribed in law for same, role of lawyer and other court room personnel, process of pleading guilty/not guilty, how to assist lawyer in defense and planning of hearings)

2. *Details of assessment which helped to arrive at the stated opinion*
   A. **Patient details:** Name, Age, Sex, Address, Hospital Registration number
   B. **Copy of written informed consent mentioning limitation of confidentiality**
   C. **Background of assessment:**
      - Who ordered the assessment?
      - Purpose of assessment
   D. **Medical Board details:**
      - Date and time of medical board proceedings
      - Constituent of medical board: Chairperson, members (mentioning name, designation, qualification of each)
   E. **Details of assessors (if assessment team is different from medical board team):**
      - Who all health professionals assessed client (for reaching on to opinion prior to medical board presentation
      - Date and time of assessments
   F. **Source of information to reach on opinion**
      - Who all were interviewed?
      - Records accessed for information
   G. **Clinical case summary**
      - Diagnosis and brief facts about case history
      - Current mental state examination finding
   H. **Report of any psychological test used (including date, time, assessors detail)**
   I. **Fitness to stand trial assessment:**
      - Criteria used for assessment
      - Timing of different assessments
      - Details of specific questions asked and answers in verbatim
   J. **Opinion and recommendation**
   K. **Additional riders in incapacity reports:** If report of "not fit" being submitted
      - Please mention is this temporary or permanent
      - If temporary, what measures are needed to restore fitness? (e.g. Medication, psychosocial intervention or legal assistance)
      - If temporary, at what time client should be sent back for re-assessment

L. **Any support measures needed during trial:** For client with mental health issues, where it is anticipated that there can be effect of deposing in court on persons mental health, additional measures can be suggested to the court to prevent that likelihood e.g. frequent breaks, daytime medicine during deposing, need of any support person or in camera hearing, etc.

All the reports submitted to the court are documentary evidence and psychiatrist can be called in court of law as expert evidence to corroborate their own or someone else report submitted on the matter.

Under the new Mental Health Act 2017, as per Section 105—If during any judicial process before any competent court, proof of mental illness is produced and is challenged by the other party, the court shall refer the same for further scrutiny to the concerned mental health review Board and the Board shall, after examination of the person alleged to have a mental illness either by itself or through a committee of experts, submit its opinion to the court.[10]

CONCLUSION

Fitness to stand trial is an important legal construct, it safeguards the right to fair trial of individual and helps in diverting needy clients towards therapy than languishing in prisons for inability to become fit and denied opportunity of a fair trial. It is the most common assessments asked from mental health professionals in respect to criminal cases. Thus, an informed mental health professional can discharge the duties in ethically, legally and scientifically correct way.

REFERENCES

1. American Psychiatric Association 2002. A Psychiatric Services in Jails and Prisons, 2nd edn, Washington, DC: American Psychiatric Association.
2. Mossman D, Noffsinger SG, Ash P, et al. AAPL Practice Guideline for the forensic psychiatric evaluation of competence to stand trial. J Am Acad Psychiatry Law. 2007;35:S3-72.
3. Bonnie RJ. The competence of criminal defendants: A theoretical reformulation. Behavioral Sciences and the Law. 1992;10:291-316.
4. Akinkunmi AA. The MacArthur competence assessment tool – fitness to plead: a preliminary evaluation of a research instrument for assessing fitness to plead in England and Wales. Journal of the American Academy of Psychiatry and the Law. 2002;30:476-82.
5. Dusky vs. US. 362 U.S. 402 (1960).
6. Badamath S, Murthy P, Parthasarthy R, et al. Mind Imprisoned: Mental health care in prisons. NIMHANS 2011.
7. Roesch R, Zapf PA, Golding SI, et al. Defining and assessing competency to stand trial. Available at: https://www.justice.gov/sites/default/files/eoir/legacy/2014/08/15/Defining_and_Assessing_Competency_to_Stand_Trial.pdf Last accessed on 07.02.18.
8. Eastman N, Adshead G, Fox S, et al. Forensic Psychiatry. Oxford Specialists Handbooks. London: Oxford University Press 2017.
9. Clark T, Rooprai DS. Practical Forensic Psychiatry. Taylor and Francis, 2011.
10. The Mental Health Care Act 2017, Gazette of India, 07.04.2017. Available at: http://www.prsindia.org/uploads/media/Mental%20Health/Mental%20Healthcare%20Act,%202017.pdf. [Last accessed on 02.010.18].

CHAPTER 21

Prisoners with Mental Illness not Fit to Stand Trial

> **LEARNING OBJECTIVES**
> - Violation of human rights and illegal detention
> - Criminal Procedure Code and Prison Act relevant sections
> - Acquittal on grounds of unsoundness of mind
> - Legal responsibility of psychiatry hospital
> - Legal responsibility of jail psychiatrist
> - Supreme Court guidelines
> - MHCA Provisions

Problem statement concerning persons with mental health issues found unfit to stand trial: When any client is found unfit to stand trial on grounds of mental illness, it leads to suspension of trial process for time being and patient is diverted to psychiatric treatment. But in certain instances, it has happened that these persons have spent decades either in prison or mental hospital without having faced the trial even, one patient from Kerala spent 38 years and another one from Uttar Pradesh spent 34 years in psychiatry hospital for alleged offences of punishment less than 7 years in both cases. One famous case of Mr Machal Lalung from Assam who spent 38 years in a psychiatric hospital just as an under trial prisoner despite being declared fit by hospital, brought attention of Supreme Court to the matter and led to guidelines being laid in this regard.[1]

Reasons for such prolonged illegal detention of persons with mental illness in past:
- No formal mechanism for screening of under trial being uniformly followed across prisons for mental health assessment due to dearth of mental health professionals in all prisons
- No formal mechanism of regular reporting to judicial officer and appropriate redressal of clients declared unfit to stand trial
- No regular mechanism of reporting from hospital to court for such cases at regular intervals being followed uniformly across all hospitals
- No regular mechanism form prison department regarding taking review of such clients from psychiatry hospitals
- Administrative delays
- Refusal of family members to some forth for taking patient on surety for treatment purposes.

1. **Legal statutes of relevance for under trial prisoners found unfit to stand trial due to mental illness:**
    A. **Accused of unsound mind in custody pending investigation or trial is dealt with following provisions under Chapter XXV of CrPC Sections 328-335 (Flowchart 1):**[2]

Procedure to be followed if an under trial person appears to be of unsound mind	
s. 328: Procedure in case of accused being lunatic	When during *enquiry stage*, if a *Magistrate has reason to believe* that an accused is of unsound mind, he shall inquire into the fact of such unsoundness of mind and shall *cause such person to be examined* by the civil surgeon of the district or such other medical officer as the State Government may direct, and pending such examination *shall postpone further proceedings* in the case
s. 329: Procedure in case of person of unsound mind tried before Court	When *during trial stage*, if *Magistrate or Court is satisfied* that the person being tried is of unsound mind, on such evidence, the Magistrate *shall postpone further proceedings*. In practice judge relies on psychiatrist's report for same, however, judges have to satisfy themselves with independent examination also. Psychiatry evaluation can be challenged by defense like any other evidence as per CrPC
<ul><li>Where the accused is determined to be of unsound mind, the magistrate has to, nonetheless, determine whether a *prima facie* case against the accused is made out. The decision to discharge or postpone the trial/inquiry is a subsequent one.</li><li>However, in cases of mental retardation, the accused is discharged. This distinction between a person of unsound mind and mental retardation, as also the determination of a *prima facie* case, were introduced by way of amendments to the CrPC in 2008.</li><li>Sections 328 and 329 were amended in 2008 to incorporate the reality of accused persons with mental retardation. The amendments make a distinction between persons who can be treated and resume fitness to stand trial (persons of unsound mind), and persons with mental retardation, whose mental condition will not alter to enable them to enter a defence. This distinction was made on the basis of the recommendations of the 154th Law Commission of India Report, 1996. The recommendations were made in consonance with the fundamental right of individuals to not only free and fair trials, but also to speedy trials, procedurally recognized in *s.428 of the CrPC which provides for the release of under trial prisoners who have served more time than they would have, had their trials resulted in conviction*.</li></ul>	
Procedure to be followed for diversion or release or under trial person found to be of unsound mind	
s. 330: Release of person of unsound mind pending investigation or trial	Whenever a person is found, under Section 328 or 329, to be of unsound mind and incapable of making his defense, the Magistrate or Court, as the case may be order: 1. *In Bailable offences: May order release with a relative on sufficient security* being given that accused shall be properly taken care of and shall be prevented from doing injury to himself or to any other person, and can appoint a person for court appearances 2. *In Nonbailable offences: May order the accused to be detained in safe custody* in such place and manner as he or it may think fit, and shall report the action taken to the State Government

Contd...

Contd...

Procedure to be followed for resumption of trial an under trial person regains soundness of mind	
s. 331: Resumption of inquiry or trial when the person ceases to be of unsound mind	**Ss. 331 and 332:** These provisions enable the resumption of an inquiry or trial when an accused regains capacity to stand trial. If the judge finds that the accused is still incapable of making defence, recourse must be sought to s.330. However, despite the recommendation of the Law Commission in its 154th Report, *no time limits have been prescribed for the trial where the accused is repeatedly found to be of unsound mind, which might lead to trials being extended even beyond the period of the prescribed punishment, had the accused been found guilty*
s. 332: Procedure on accused appearing before Magistrate or Court for resumption of trial	
s. 333: When accused appears to have been of sound mind	
s. 337: Procedure where lunatic prisoner is reported capable of making his defense	It describes the procedure where a prisoner of unsound mind is reported capable of making his defense. It provides that if the Inspector General of Prisons (in case where prisoner is in jail) or two visitors of an asylum (where the prisoner is in a lunatic asylum) certify that the prisoner is capable of making his defense such certificate shall be received as evidence and the Court/Magistrate will deal with such persons as provided under Section 332 by proceedings with the inquiry or trial
s. 338: Procedure where lunatic detained is declared fit to be released	Section 338 provides the procedure where a person of unsound mind detained, is declared fit to be released. The said section provides that if a person of unsound mind is detained under the provisions of sub-Section (2) of Section 330 and the Inspector General or visitors certify that, in his or their judgment, he may be released without danger of his doing injury to himself or any other person. The State Government may order him to be • released, or • to be detained in custody, • or to be transferred to a state psychiatric hospital (may appoint a Commission, consisting of a judicial and two medical officers, which shall make a formal inquiry into the state of mind of such person for periodic reporting to state government, which may order his release or his detention as it thinks fit)
Procedure to be followed for acquittal on grounds of unsoundness of mind or discharge regarding under trial person found to be of unsound mind	
s. 334: Judgment of acquittal on ground of unsoundness of mind **s. 335:** Person acquitted on such ground to be detained in safe custody **s. 336:** Power of State Government to empower officer-in-charge to discharge	
s. 339: Delivery of lunatic to care of relative or friend	State government may order a person to be delivered to any relative or friend of any person detained under the provisions of Section 330 or 335 if they give application and security to the satisfaction to ensure that the person delivered shall: • be properly taken care of and prevented from doing injury to himself or others; • be produced for the inspection at times and places directed by State Government
Under the new Mental Health Act 2017, as per Section 105—If during any judicial process before any competent court, proof of mental illness is produced and is challenged by the other party, the court shall refer the same for further scrutiny to the concerned mental health review Board and the Board shall, after examination of the person alleged to have a mental illness either by itself or through a committee of experts, submit its opinion to the court.[3]	

Flowchart 1: Procedure to be followed if an under trial person with mental illness appears to be unfit to stand trial.

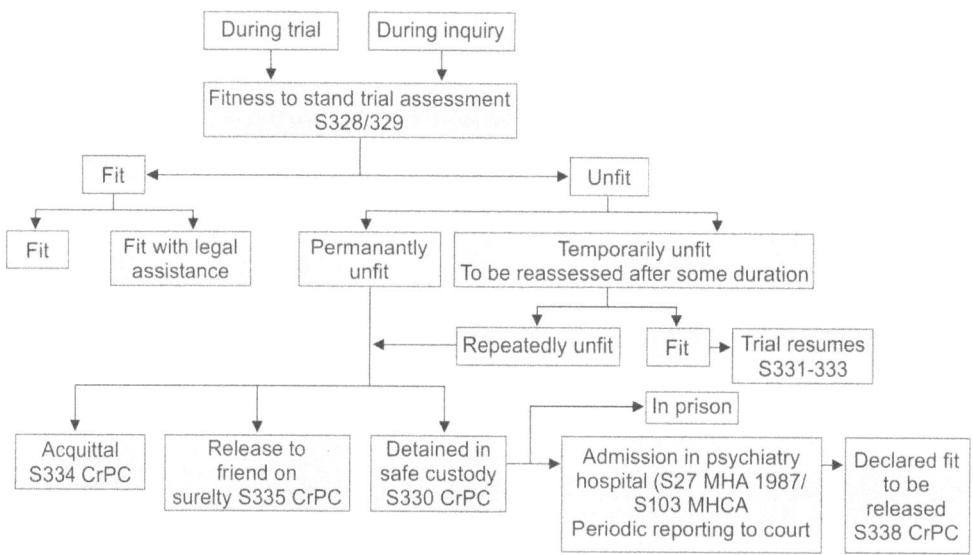

B. Legal statutes of relevance for *convicted prisoners* found unfit to stand trial due to mental illness:

Convicted persons in jail who become mentally unsound are dealt under provisions of Section 30 of Prisoners Act, 1900 (3 of 1900) which are as follows[4]:

At any point of time during imprisoned, if a convict prisoner is found to have developed 'unsoundness of mind', then following are the responsibilities of State Government in this regard:

- *When prisoner becomes of unsound mind:* Where it appears to the State Government that any person detained or imprisoned under any order or sentence of any Court is of unsound mind, the State Government may, by a warrant order his removal to:
  – A state psychiatry hospital or
  – Other place of safe custody within the State
  Till when person of unsound mind to be kept at abovementioned places:
  – For the remainder of the term for which he has been ordered or sentenced to be detained or imprisoned or,
  – If on the expiration of that sentenced term it is certified by a medical officer that it is necessary for the safety of the prisoner or others that he should be further detained under medical care or treatment, then until he is discharged according to law.
- *When prisoner ceases to be of unsound mind or becomes of sound mind:* Where it appears to the State Government that the prisoner has become of sound mind, the State Government shall, by a warrant directed to the person having charge of the prisoner to:

CHAPTER 21: Prisoners with Mental Illness not Fit to Stand Trial

- Remand him to the prison from which he was removed, or to another prison within the State, if still liable to be kept in custody, or
- Order him to be discharged, if the prisoner is no longer liable to be kept in custody.

2. **Medicolegal responsibilities of psychiatrist for monitoring of prisoners with mental illness unfit to stand trial admitted in "psychiatry hospital"**
    A. **Relevant provisions for admission, monitoring and discharge of prisoners with mental illness unfit to stand trial admitted in psychiatry hospital as per Mental Health Act (MHA 1987)**[1,5]
        I. **Admission in psychiatry hospital**
            Section 27 of the Act provides that an order under section 30 of the Prisoners Act, 1900 or an order under section 330 of the Code directing the reception of a mentally ill prisoner into any psychiatric hospital/nursing home shall be sufficient authority for the admission of such person in such hospital/nursing home.
        II. **Procedures to be followed for regular monitoring during inpatient stay**
            Provision of assessment by Board of visitors
            Section 37 requires the concerned government to appoint not less than five visitors to each psychiatric hospital/nursing home.
            Frequency of assessment by Board of visitors
            Section 38 provides for *monthly* inspection by the visitors and authorizes them to make remarks in regard to the management and condition of the psychiatric hospital/nursing home and of the inpatient thereof.
            Frequency of reporting by Board of visitors
            Section 39 sub-section (1) of the Act provides that *any three of the visitors* shall *once in every three months* visit to assess the state of mind of such person and make a report thereon to the authority under whose order such person is detained.
            Frequency of assessment by Board of visitors
            Sub-section (3) provides that the *medical officer in charge* of a psychiatric hospital/nursing home where any person is detained under the provisions of section 330 shall *once in six months*, make a special report regarding the mental state of the person detained.
        III. **Discharge from psychiatry hospital:**
            Section 40 of the Act empowers the medical officer in-charge of a psychiatric hospital/nursing home to discharge any mentally ill prisoner, on recommendation of two medical practitioners one of whom shall preferably be a psychiatrist in the manner.
    B. **Relevant provisions for admission, monitoring and discharge of prisoners with mental illness unfit to stand trial admitted in psychiatry hospital admission in psychiatry hospital as per Mental Health Care Act, 2017 (MHCA)**[1,3]**:**
        I. *Admission in psychiatry hospital: Section 103 of the Act* provides that an order under Section 30 of the Prisoners Act, 1900 or an order under Section 330 or 335 of the CrPC directing the reception of a mentally ill prisoner into any psychiatric hospital/

nursing home shall be sufficient authority for the admission of such person in such hospital/nursing home for lawful care and treatment.

II. *Standard of care:* The mental health establishment shall be registered under this Act with the Central or State Mental Health Authority, as the case may be, and shall conform to such standards and procedures as may be prescribed.

III. *Procedures to be followed for regular monitoring during inpatient stay:* Section 103 MHCA sub-section (5) states that the medical officer in-charge of a mental health establishment wherein any person referred to in sub-section (1) is detained, shall *once in every six months,* make a special report regarding the mental and physical condition of such person to the authority under whose order such person is detained.

IV. *Transfer of persons with mental illness from one mental health establishment to another mental health establishment:* Section 93 MHCA sub-section (1) states that A person with mental illness admitted to a mental health establishment under Section 103 may be subject to any general or special order of the Board or state government be removed from such mental health establishment and admitted to another mental health establishment or other place of safe custody within the State or with the consent of the Central Authority to any mental health establishment in any other State.

V. *Absence without leave or discharge:* Section 92 of MHCA states that if any person to whom Section 103 applies absents himself without leave or without discharge from the mental health establishment, he shall be taken into protection by any police officer at the request of the medical officer or mental health professional in-charge of the mental health establishment and shall be sent back to the mental health establishment immediately.

VI. *Discharge planning:* Whenever a person undergoing treatment for mental illness in a mental health establishment is to be discharged into the community or to a different mental health establishment or where a new psychiatrist is to take responsibility of the person's care and treatment, the psychiatrist who has been responsible for the person's care and treatment shall consult with the person with mental illness, the nominated representative, the family member or care-giver with whom the person with mental illness shall reside on discharge from the hospital or the psychiatrist expected to be responsible for the person's care and treatment in the future, and such other persons as may be appropriate, as to what treatment or services would be appropriate for the person.

C. **Supreme Court guidelines for psychiatry hospitals and courts with regard to mentally ill under trial prisoners:**[1]

In a writ petition filed for illegal detention of mentally ill under trial prisoner, it was found that regular reporting of these cases was not happening in line with Sections 38 and 39 of MHA 1987 as prescribed, So, Supreme Court issued following guidelines for psychiatry hospitals with regard to mentally ill under trial prisoners admitted in psychiatry hospital in 2005:

CHAPTER 21: Prisoners with Mental Illness not Fit to Stand Trial

(i) Whenever a person of unsound mind is ordered to be detained in any psychiatric hospital/nursing home under Section 330(2) of the Code, the reports contemplated under Section 39 shall be submitted to the concerned Court/Magistrate periodically.

(ii) The Court/Magistrate shall also call for such reports if they are not received in time.

(iii) When the reports are received, the Court/Magistrate shall consider the reports and pass appropriate orders wherever necessary. In regard to prisoners covered by sub-section (1) of Section 30 of the Prisoners Act, 1900, the procedure prescribed by sub-sections (2) and (3) of that section read with Section 40 of the Mental Health Act, 1987 shall be followed.

(iv) Wherever any undertrial prisoner is in jail for more than the maximum period of imprisonment prescribed for the offence for which he is charged (other than those charged for offences for which life imprisonment or death is the punishment), the Magistrate/Court shall treat the case as closed and report the matter to the medical officer in-charge of the psychiatric hospital, so that the medical officer in-charge of the hospital can consider his discharge as per Section 40 of the Act.

(v) In cases where, the under trial prisoners (who are not being charged with offence for which the punishment is imprisonment for life or death penalty), their cases may be considered for release in accordance with sub-section (1) of Section 330 of the Code, if they have completed five or more years as inpatients.

(vi) As regards the under trial prisoners who have been charged with grave offences for which life imprisonment or death penalty is the punishment, such persons shall be subjected to examination periodically as provided in sub-sections (1), (3) and (4) of Section 39 of the Act and the officers named therein (visitors, medical officer in charge of the hospital and the examining medical officer respectively) should send the reports to the court as to whether the under trial prisoner is fit enough to face the trial to defend the charge. The Sessions Courts where the cases are pending should also seek periodic reports from such hospitals and every such case shall be given a hearing at least once in three months. The Sessions Judge shall commence the trial of such cases as soon as it is found that such mentally ill person has been found fit to face trial.

3. **Medicolegal responsibilities of psychiatrist for monitoring of prisoners with mental illness unfit to stand trial detained in "jail"**[6]
   A. **Current legal provisions as per Section 30 of Prisons Act, 1900 and Section 39 of Mental Health Act, 1987**[1,4,5]
      - *Monitoring by inspector general:* Inspector General of Prisons or any officer empowered by state government shall *once in every three months* visit to assess the state of mind of such person and make a report thereon to the authority under whose order such person is detained.
      - *Medical/psychiatry review:* Every such person who is detained in jail under Section 330 of the Code, shall be visited *at least once in every three months by a psychiatrist or* where a psychiatrist is not available, *by a medical officer* empowered by the State

Government, and such psychiatrist/medical officer shall make a special report regarding the mental and physical conditions of such persons to the authority under whose order such person is detained.

B. **Legal provisions as per Section 30 of Prisons Act, 1900 and Section 103 Mental Health Care Act 2017**[1,3,4]
- **Provision of psychiatry wing in prisons medical wing:** Sub-section(6) of Section 103 of the MHCA states that appropriate Government shall setup mental health establishment in the medical wing of at least one prison in each State and Union territory and prisoners with mental illness may ordinarily be referred to and cared for in the said mental health establishment.
- **Regular reporting by jail medical wing:** Sub-section (3) of Section 103 of the MHCA states that medical officer of a prison or jail shall send a quarterly report to the concerned Board certifying therein that there are no prisoners with mental illness in the prison or jail.
- **Provision of monitoring by mental health review board:** Sub-section (4) of Section 103 of the MHCA states that Board may visit the prison or jail and ask the medical officer as to why the prisoner with mental illness, if any, has been kept in the prison or jail and not transferred for treatment to a mental health establishment.

CONCLUSION

Any prisoner whether under trial or convict rendered unfit on grounds of mental disability has to be treated in accordance with correct legal provisions detailed into ensure appropriate mental health services being offered, regular reporting to judicial agencies and preventing undue prolonged illegal detentions.

REFERENCES

1. Supreme Court of India. Record of proceedings, Writ petition (crl.) No(s), 296 of 2005.
2. Code of Criminal Procedure Act, 1973, Bare Acts.
3. The Mental Health Care Act 2017, Gazette of India, 07.04.2017. Available at: http://www.prsindia.org/uploads/media/Mental%20Health/Mental%20 Healthcare%20Act,%202017.pdf. [Last accessed on 02.010.18].
4. Indian Prisons Act 1900. Available at: https://indiankanoon.org/doc/5955 1850/. Last accessed on 07.02.18.
5. The Mental Health Act 1987, Gazette of India. Available at: ncw.nic.in/acts/THEMENTALHEALTHACT1987.pdf. Last accessed on 07.02.18.
6. Government order No.V-17014/4/2007-PR. Government of India/Bharat Sarkar Ministry of Home Affairs/Grinh Mantralaya, 13.12.07. Available at: mha1.nic.in/Prison Reforms/pdf/DetentionMentally13Dec2007.pdf. Last accessed on 07.02.18.

CHAPTER 22

During Trial Assessments: Assessment for Insanity Defense

> **LEARNING OBJECTIVES**
> - Conflicting positions of law and medical sciences
> - Evolution of insanity defense criteria
> - Diminished responsibility
> - Substantive law concerning insanity and criminal responsibility in India
> - Important case laws from Indian Courts
> - Degree of insanity
> - Role of psychiatrist in Insanity defense assessments

What is insanity defense: It is a legal concept used in criminal cases, based on the assumption that at the time of crime, defendant was suffering from such a severe mental illness that, he/she was not having the 'guilty intent' to commit crime, as he/she was incapable of appreciating the nature of the crime and differentiating right from wrong behavior, hence making them not legally liable for the crime.

Conflicting positions of law and medical science: Against the common notion prevalent in masses, every person with mental illness is not absolved of his/her criminal liability on prima facie. Legal and medical construct of insanity differs remarkably from each other in their definition of concept, degree and standards. Medical science sees insanity as a medical disorder affecting human mind and behavior including an entire range from mild anxiety disorders to severe dementia, with the sole purpose to diagnose and treat. However, law views **insanity only as the** 'mental state at time of crime'. Although legal and medical unanimously believe any person with severe disturbance of mind and behavior should be protected but views about how to reach this conclusion is discordant as insanity of insanity defense is itself difficult to define and in which circumstances to exercise is difficult to characterize.[1] The difference between medical and legal insanity as different concepts is detailed in **Table 1**.

Evolution of insanity defense criteria: **Table 2** is the review from International Case laws that helped in establishing insanity defense criteria.[1]

Table 1: Legal terms for fitness to stand trial in use globally.

	Medical insanity	Legal insanity
What it is	Though 'insanity' word is no more used in mental health practices. In closes parlance to legal concept of insanity, it refers to presence of mental disorder	It is the 'mental state at time of crime'. Thus, it refers to "presence of mental disorder" as well as "loss of reasoning" to be present together which rendered individual incapable of knowing right or wrong
Purpose of concept	Diagnosing and treating the individual	"Welfare of public" and simultaneously 'not penalizing the innocent individual who committed the crime due to disturbed mental faculties'
Nature and degree of insanity	It can range from mild anxiety disorders to severe schizophrenia or dementia	It only refers to conditions substantially affecting cognitive faculties to the extent that person was incapable of knowing nature and quality of act or its wrongness at time of committing crime, irrespective of diagnosis or severity
Time factor	It takes into account historical evidence and course of illness in future to reach on a diagnosis	It refers to mental state 'only at the time of committing crime'

SUBSTANTIVE LAW CONCERNING INSANITY AND CRIMINAL RESPONSIBILITY IN INDIA[1]

- **Insanity defense** (Section 84 of the Indian Penal Code, 1860): The defense of insanity in criminal cases in India is based on McNaghten's rule and is mentioned in section 84 of the Indian Penal Code, 1860, which states that "Nothing is an offence which is done by a person who at the time of doing it, by reason of unsoundness of mind, is in capable of knowing the nature of the act, or that he is doing what is either wrong or contrary to law."[2]
- **Test of insanity devised by the Calcutta High Court in *Ashiruddin Ahmed v. The King*[1,3]**

  The Court laid down that in order to get the benefit of Section 84 the accused should establish any one of the following three elements:
  1. That the nature of the act was not known to the accused.
  2. That the act was not known to him to be contrary to law.
  3. That the act was not known by him to be wrong.

  Thus, mere abnormality of mind or partial delusion, irresistible impulse or compulsive behavior of a psychopath affords no protection under Section 84 IPC and burden of proof is on accused.[1,3]

- *Defense on ground of diminished responsibility and irresistible impulse does not exist in India*
- **Defense for involuntary intoxication**[2]
  1. Section 85 of the Indian Penal Code, 1860 is about **"Act of a person incapable of judgment by reason of intoxication caused against his will"**. It states that nothing is an offence which is done by a person who, at the time of doing it, is, by reason of

Table 2: International case laws showing evolution of insanity defense criteria.

Name of the test/case	Case background	Verdict	Concept used in judgment	Principle evolved for insanity defense
Wild Beast Test (R v *Arnold*)	Edward Arnold was tried for homicide attempt of a British Lord and there was evidence to support severe mental illness.	Not guilty by reason of insanity	"A mad man must be totally deprived of his understanding and memory. He is no more than *a brute, or a wild beast*, such a one is never the object of punishment."[1]	A person should be 'totally deprived of understanding and memory' to be given benefit of insanity defense than a specific capacity
In *Lord Ferrers*	Earl Ferrers acting on his persecutory delusions shot his steward to death.	Guilty	The House of Lords had replied "that total want of reason will acquit the prisoner, but that if there be a partial degree of reason and a competent use of it "sufficient to have restrained those passions which produced crime, if there be thought and design and faculty to distinguish between moral good and evil" responsibility attaches".[1]	A person to get insanity defense benefit should be **'totally deprived of understanding and memory'** and should be unable to discern the **differences between moral good and evil**
Hadfield test of delusion	Hadfield acting under a delusion tried assassinating King George III publicly. He was charged for treason and homicide attempt	Not guilty by reason of insanity	The prosecutor argued based on previous test that defendant must have lost all sense, however planned shooting attempt contradicts same. But the defense counsel argued that delusional disorder is not always accompanied by loss of all other faculties. Moreover, accused developed disorder due to a head injury and his crime was direct result of his delusions.	Discarded two previous concepts of 'presence of total loss of all intellectual faculties" and subjective "inability to distinguish moral good and evil". It brought out the concept that though defendant had not lost all understanding and memory, he could tell right and wrong, but **due to fixed delusion, he had lost ability to exercise control over his acting out behavior**
Irresistible impulse test	It brought a medical view that mind is not compartmentalized and insanity not only affects thought, planning, understanding but also emotion and will. Thus, despite having adequate understanding one is irresistibly impelled to commit a task under influence of mental illness for which he/she should be absolved of criminal liability.			

Contd...

Name of the test/case	Case background	Verdict	Concept used in judgment	Principle evolved for insanity defense

McNaughten	Daniel M'Naghten, a Scotsman in 1843 was tried for the murder of Edmond Drummond, Private Secretary to Sir Robert Peel, then Prime Minister of England. Daniel M'Naghten was under an insane delusion that Sir Robert peel had injured him and mistaking Drummond for Sir Robert peel he shot and killed him.	Acquitted	"The Chief Justice in his charge to the jury said that the question for them to be determined was whether at the time of committing the act he had or had not the use of his understanding so as to know that he was violating the laws of God and man. The jury said
			1. Every man is presumed to be sane and is responsible for his crimes, until the contrary be proved to the satisfaction of the jury or the court.
			2. To establish defense of ground of insanity it must be clearly shown that at the time of committing the act, the accused was laboring under such a defect of reason from disease of mind, as not to know the nature and quality of the act he was doing, or he did not know it, that he did not know that what he was doing was wrong.
			3. If the accused was conscious that the act was one which he ought not to do and if that act was at the same time contrary to the law of the land, he is punishable.
			4. A medical witness who has not seen the accused before trial should not be asked whether on evidence he thinks that the accused was insane.
			5. Where the Criminal Act is committed by a man under some insane delusion as to the surrounding facts, which conceals from him the true nature of the act he is doing, he will be under the same degree of responsibility as he would have been on the fact as he imagined them to be."[1]
				It brought out new concept for claiming insanity defense, following should be present:
				• **Defect of reason** from disease of mind
				• **Disease of mind rendered** accused **incapable of:**
				  – **distinguishing nature of act**
				  – **wrongness of act**
				  – **act being against law**

Contd...

Contd...

Name of the test/case	Case background	Verdict	Concept used in judgment	Principle evolved for insanity defense
Durham's test	Durham was charged of house breaking and he pleaded insanity in his defense.		In this case the court evolved a new test, namely, "simply that an accused is not criminally responsible if his unlawful act was the product of mental disease or mental defect".[1]	It brought forth the concept that mere presence of mental disease is not sufficient, **more important is to find out the casual connection between unlawful act and mental disease**. Insanity defense to be given only in cases where act was direct product of mental illness.
Diminished responsibility	It is a legal term which is a partial defense and states that emphasis should be on "substantial incapacity", then 'total incapacity required by the M'Naghten Rules' to make the trial more pragmatic. The doctrine of diminished responsibility posits a reduction of culpability (and punishment) because of a reduced capacity to form all the required mental elements.			

intoxication, incapable of knowing the nature of the act, or that he is doing what is either wrong, or contrary to law. Provided that the thing which intoxicated him was administered to him without his knowledge or against his will.

2. Section 85 of the Indian Penal Code, 1860 is about **"Offence requiring a particular intent or knowledge committed by one who is intoxicated".** It states that in cases where an act done is not an offence unless done with a particular knowledge or intent, a person who does the act in a state of intoxication shall be liable to be dealt with as if he had the same knowledge as he would have had if he had not been intoxicated, unless the thing which intoxicated him was administered to him without his knowledge or against his will.

Ingredients: The ingredients of Sections 85 and 86 are that a person will be exonerated from liability for an act done while in a state of intoxication, if he, at the time of doing it, by reason of intoxication, was:

a. Incapable of knowing the nature of the act; or
b. That he was not in a state of mind to know that the act was either wrong or contrary to law; and
c. That the thing which intoxicated him was administered to him without his knowledge or against his will;
d. And that voluntary drunkenness is not excuse for the commission of a crime;
e. Burden of proof lies upon the accused.

IMPORTANT CASE LAWS FROM INDIAN COURTS[1]

Test of Insanity as Assessed by Calcutta High Court

Ashiruddin Ahmed vs. The King: Accused in his dream was commanded by someone in paradise to sacrifice his five years old son. On the next morning the accused took his son, to a nearly mosque and killed him by the thrusting a knife in his throat. Then he went straight to his uncle, but finding a village chowkidar nearby, took to the uncle to a tank at some at some distance, and then narrated the whole story to him. On trial, the accused retracted his confession but the evidence was not seriously challenged. The court held on evidence that he believed that his dream was a reality; though he knew the nature of the act and knew that, it was contrary to law. This was evident from his conduct of not saying what he did in front of the chowkidar. According to the court, the accused was clearly of unsound mind because acting under delusion of his disease, he made this sacrifice believing it to be right.[1]

Degree of Insanity

It may be said that between the normal and the abnormal there is only difference of degrees but not of kind. The mind may be unsound, affected by disease, disorderly or disturbed or abnormal. These factors must be of such degree, which renders the accused capable of knowing the nature of his act or that what he is doing is either wrong or contrary to law. It should be obliterate the perceptional or volitional capacity.

In *Hazara Singh vs. The State:* The Punjab High Court said: *"In order to earn immunity from criminal liability the disease, disorder or disturbances of mind must of degree, which should obliterate perceptual or volitional capacity. A person may be a fit subject for confinement in a mental hospital, but that fact alone will not permit him to enjoy exemption from punishment. Crotchetiness of cranks, feeble mindedness, any mental irresponsibility, mere frenzy, emotional imbalance, heat of passion, uncontrollable anger or jealously, fits of insensate hatred, or revenge, moral depravity, dethroning, reason, incurable perversions, hypersensitive excitability, ungovernible fits of temper, stupidity, obtuseness, lack of self-control, gross eccentricity and idiosyncrasy and other similar manifestations, evidencing derangement of mental functions, by themselves, do not offer relief from criminal responsibility".*[1]

Impairment of Cognitive Faculties

The cognitive faculties of mind are very much responsible for human conduct. Therefore, exemption from liability affects the cognitive faculties of the accused. In other words, exemption is available when the insanity affects the faculty of understanding the significance of his act in its bearing on the victims and in relation to the accused person's own responsibility for the act.

In *Sarka Gundusa vs. State:* Accused came out of his house brandishing an axe and gave a blow to a 3-year-old boy playing outside, on his neck. The boy died instantaneously and the accused ran over to the jungle close by and returned only the next day. Convicting the accused Justice GK Mishra said, *Any and every type of insanity recognized in medical science is not legal insanity. Every minor mental aberration is not insanity. There can be no legal insanity unless the cognitive faculty of mind is destroyed as a result of unsoundness of mind to such an extent as to render the accused in capable of knowing the nature of the act or that what he is doing is wrong or contrary to law.*[1]

Role of Psychiatrist in Insanity Defense Assessments[4,5]

A. **Focus of assessment:** Any mental health professional dealing with insanity defense case must go beyond making just a diagnosis. It is a difficult retrospective determination of likely state at time of actus reus or 'guilty act'. More important is to have retrospective assessment of a specific capacity at that time than mere presence of illness.
B. **Limitation of assessment**: *It has to be kept in mind that in most cases **it is a retrospective** assessment until **unless accused** is a follow up case of a particular mental health facility where crime has been **seen very near the crime** and a mental state to that regard is documented. However, **that is also not likely to be conclusive as it can only be a clinical assessment done at that time from therapeutic need and no capacity assessment** would have been done or documented. Before undertaking any such assessments, it is always prudent to **honestly inform the Court about limitation of this assessment or even citing these as reasons of not taking up this assessment in certain cases.***
C. **Locus of assessment:** It is advisable to admit the patient for comprehensive evaluation.
D. **Collateral information and records**. Court can be requested to be make following available to assessor prior to evaluation:

E. **Accompanying legal documents**: FIR, postmortem and autopsy report, photographs of the crime scene, behavior observational report, interview with the family members.
F. **Medical documents:** Defendant's all relevant medical and psychiatric records.
G. **Clinical assessment:** Evaluation should address following issues:
   I. **History of psychiatric illness**
      1. Nature of illness
      2. Duration of illness
      3. Severity of illness
      4. Treatment and assessment records
      5. Past violent aggressive behavior
      6. History of substance use
      7. Personality assessment
      8. Any significant legal history in past
   II. **Details concerning alleged crime**
      1. Account of patient's behavior, emotion and cognition prior to event
      2. Incidence as mentioned in legal documents as narrated by defendant
      3. Presence of motive
      4. Behavior immediately after the incidence
      5. Defendant's view about event being nature and quality of act
      6. Defendant's view about event being right or wrong
      7. Defendant's view about seriousness of predicament
      8. Defendant's legal knowledge about the crime
      9. Defendant's description about the degree of intent, willfulness, or premeditation for the alleged act.
   III. **Current mental status examination**
   IV. **Assessment of cognitive functions**
   V. **Psychological assessment of personality and malingering**
   VI. **Ward behavior observation report** (If needed, can do a continuous assessment of ward behavior thru CCTV camera through court's permission).

Insanity Defense Seen from Prism of Modern Legal and Mental Health Field

"Substantive law in India is based on the McNaghten rules where only the impairment of the defendant's faculties is taken into consideration. No enquiry is made into the degree to which the defendant's self-control is impaired. Despite proved severe mental illness, the defendant will be convicted if he is aware of the nature of the act and its wrongfulness or illegality. Illustrative cases reveal an immense gulf between psychiatric knowledge on mental illness and the legality recognized criteria for exonerating a person from punishment. Present day psychiatry recognizes gradation of mental disturbances in a wide range from normalcy to abnormality. Juristic thinking is yet to fall in line with this development. Caught in the web of obsolete McNaghten rules the Indian law on insanity still harps on the notions of the early 19th century psychology which conceived brain as bundles of functions, each working independently. This conception neglects volitional and emotional aspects of the mind. According to modern psychology and psychiatry the mind cannot be split into water tight, unrelated and autonomously functioning compartments. The mind and body are one continuum in which each part influences, and is influenced by the whole. Every case of unsoundness of mind cannot therefore be fitted into the straight jacket of an old age old legal definition. The legal conundrum of "right and wrong" test of insanity is one of the most striking instances of conservatism of the law. These concepts distinctly belong to ethics and present no scientifically cognizable categories. There is no universal standard of right and wrong, and hence of responsibility. It is a more difficult for an individual to distinguish right from wrong in the complex social context of today than it was in a simple, homogenous society of the past when cultural values were relatively uniform. Except in cases of gross moral turpitude where there could be said to be social consensus on ethical evaluation, there is a still a large part of human conduct in which the ethical assessment by the society is not clearly defined. It is felt that by looking to the magnitude of the problem a commission consisting of members of all three branches of law and the medical profession and behavioral scientists should be set up to examine the possibility of introducing such changes in the existing law of insanity as would make it reflect the modern advances of medical knowledge".[1]

REFERENCES

1. Rajan S. Facets of insanity. Available at: http://www.lawyersclub india.com/articles/article_display_list_by_member.asp?member_id=169.Last accessed on 07.02.18.
2. Gandhi BM. Indian Penal Code (Paper Back) (2013 ed.). EBC. pp. 1–832 ISBN 81-7012-892-7.
3. Available at: https://indiankanoon.org/doc/1101879/ Last accessed on 07.02.18.
4. Math SB, Kumar CN, Moirangthem S. Insanity Defense: Past, Present, and Future. Indian Journal of Psychological Medicine. 2015;37(4):381-7. doi:10.4103/0253-7176.168559.
5. Nigel Eastman, Gwen Adshead, Simone Fox, Richard Latham, and Sean Whyte. Forensic Psychiatry. Oxford Specialists Handbooks. London: Oxford University Press, 2017.

SECTION VI
Medicolegal Responsibilities Concerning Management of Cases of Sexual Offence

Medicolegal Approach for Management of Adult Victims of Sexual Violence

> **LEARNING OBJECTIVES**
> - Health consequences of sexual assault
> - Relevant IPC and CrPC sections for sexual offences
> - Role of health professionals
> - Legal responsibilities of health professionals
> - Treatment guidelines and professional support
> - Documentation
> - Patient information
> - Role of family, friends and community
> - Mental health assessment for fitness to give statement
> - Assessment for capacity to consent to a sexual relationship
> - Interface with social welfare

INTRODUCTION

The World Health Organization (WHO) defines sexual violence as "any sexual act, attempt to obtain a sexual act, unwanted sexual comments or advances, or acts to traffic, or otherwise directed against a person's sexuality using coercion, by any reason regardless of their relationship to the victim, in any setting, including but not limited to home and work." The circumstances of sexual violence or sexual assault may range from rape by strangers to rape within any established relationships, sex trafficking, child marriage and violent sexual acts.[1]

MAGNITUDE OF THE PROBLEM

Magnitude of the problem is alarmingly disturbing, globally, nearly 7–36% women and 5–10% children of male sex report having experienced sexual violence in some form.[2] National statistics of India is also equally gruesome, according to National Crime Record Bureau Data 2015, sexual offences account for 1.3 lac sexual offences per lac female population per year, which amounts to 21.4% of all the crimes committed annually, including rape, attempt to rape, outraging modestly of women and insult to modesty of women.[3] Of these, rape accounts for 26.6% of total sexual offences. In the states, maximum cases were reported from Uttar Pradesh nearly 10.9% cases followed by West Bengal (10.1%) and in Union Territories, Delhi soars the chart.[4]

Despite huge magnitude of problem, globally, rates of health services utilization after sexual violence are only 25–40%.[2] Reasons behind are two-fold, first, at individual level, trauma related psychological distress in form of severe anxiety and depression provokes self-guilt and reduces active help seeking. Secondly, societal attitude and secondary victimization at the hand of family, legal agencies and healthcare providers discourages victims from disclosure and help seeking ("Secondary victimization refers to the victimization that occurs not as a direct result of the criminal act but through the response of institutions and individuals to the victim").[5]

Responses related to sexual violence are highly variable and complex. Some of the survivors may experience insurmountable distress, whereas others could have little or no distress depending on attributes related to survivor's resilience and coping strategies, past negative life experiences, societal reaction, and available societal support. Thus, mental health professionals can encounter such victims as direct presentation with a psychological distress following the aftermath or being brought by law enforcement agencies for some legal opinion. In resource constrained settings like ours, there is wide gap between needs of clients with sexual assault and existing provision of services. For example, a victim being subjected to multiple examinations, absence of sufficient number of trained medicolegal healthcare professionals, absence of sexual assault resource centers equipped with team of concerned medical, social, legal personnel. Most of the available services are more inclined towards medicolegal angle for collecting evidence for punishing perpetrator than being victim friendly. Sexual assault victims are often handled in an insensitive manner by health professionals due to clinical overload or inexperience or lack of training for handling such situations. So, there is need for developing training modules for sensitization of health professionals and imparting their skills to handle such situations.[6]

HEALTH CONSEQUENCES OF SEXUAL ASSAULT

Sexual assault is violation of one's life and dignity and is a crime against humanity. It is associated with detrimental consequences to victim's physical and mental health and undesirable devastating social consequences to victim and family.

Physical consequences: Individuals who have experienced sexual assault may suffer from:[6]
- Unwanted pregnancy
- Unsafe abortion
- Sexually transmitted infections (STIs), HIV/AIDS
- Pelvic pain/pelvic inflammatory disease
- Urinary tract infections
- Genital injuries
- Sexual dysfunctions.[6]

Psychological consequences: Psychological effects vary from individual to individual. It also depends on age of victim; time elapsed since the assault, relationship with perpetrator, circumstances surrounding assault, victim's life situation, and reaction of supporting people, one's own coping skills and self-appraisal of assault. It may present as:[6]

- Acute stress reaction
- Adjustment disorder
- Post-traumatic stress disorder
- Depression
- Social phobias (especially in marital or date rape victims)
- Anxiety
- Increased substance use or abuse
- Suicidal behavior.[6]

In the longer-term, victims may develop eating disorders, sleep disturbances (i.e. nightmares, flashbacks), sexual dysfunctions, fear and anxiety, irritability, social phobia, chronic headaches, multiple unexplained somatic symptoms, occupational decline, school refusal, poor academic performance, low self-esteem and suicidal behavior. Childhood sexual trauma is also associated with post-traumatic stress disorder (PTSD), depression, suicide, alcohol problems, eating disorders, enduring personality changes and altered view about sexuality.

UNDERSTANDING LEGAL PROVISIONS CONCERNING SEXUAL OFFENCES

From legal point of view, prevailing laws for child and adult sexual offences are different. Adult has been defined as any individual >18 years of age for sexual offences. Indian Penal Code defines sexual offences against adults as follows along with the punishments mentioned in "Criminal Law Amendment Act, 2013 (Any of the following listed sexual assault is said to be 'aggravated' when committed by a person in a position of trust or authority)"[7,8] **(Table 1)**:

Table 1: Relevant IPC and CrPC sections for sexual offences and punishments.

S.No.	Offence and description	Punishment
1.	Section 354: Assault or criminal force to woman with intent to outrage her modesty	Imprisonment not less than 1 year but which may extend to 5 years and fine.
2.	Section 354A(1): Sexual Harassment: A man committing any of the following acts: (i) Physical contact or advances which include unwanted sexual overtures (ii) Request for sexual favors (iii) Showing pornography against will (iv) Making sexually colored remarks	Section 354A (2): An offence specified in clause (i), (ii) or (iii) of subsection (1) shall be punished with imprisonment, which may extend to three years and/or fine. Section 354A (3): An offence specified in clause (iv) of subsection (1) Shall be punished with imprisonment, which may extend to 1 year and/or fine.
3.	Section 354B: Assault or use of criminal force to any woman or abetment to such act with the intention of disrobing or compelling her to be naked	Section 354B: Imprisonment for a term not less than 3 years but which may extend to seven years, and shall also be liable to fine

Contd...

Contd...

4.	*Section 354C:* Voyeurism: Any man who watches, captures or disseminates the image of a woman engaging in a private act in circumstances where she would usually have the expectation of not being observed.	*Section 354 C:* On first conviction: imprisonment for a term not less than 1 year, but which may extend to 3 years, and fine. On a second or subsequent conviction: imprisonment of for a term not less than 3 years, but which may extend to 7 years, and fine. *On a subsequent conviction:* With imprisonment for a term which may extend to 5 years, and fine.
5.	Section 354D: Stalking (1) Any man who: (i) follows a woman and contacts, or attempts to contact such woman repeatedly despite a clear indication of disinterest or (ii) monitors the use by a woman of the internet, email or any other form of electronic communication. Such conduct shall not amount to stalking if (i) it was pursued for the purpose of preventing or detecting crime by a man entrusted with such responsibility by the State (ii) it was pursued under any condition or requirement imposed by any person under any law; or (iii) in the particular circumstances such conduct was reasonable and justified	*On first conviction:* With imprisonment for a term which may extend to 3 years, and fine. *On a subsequent conviction:* With imprisonment for a term which may extend to 5 years, and fine.
6.	Section 375 - Rape: A man is said to commit "rape" if he— (a) Penetrates his penis, to any extent, into the vagina, mouth, urethra or anus of a woman or makes her to do so with him or any other person; or (b) Inserts, to any extent, any object or a part of the body, not being the penis, into the vagina, the urethra or anus of a woman or makes her to do so with him or any other person; or (c) Manipulates any part of the body of a woman so as to cause penetration into the vagina, urethra, anus or any part of body of such woman or makes her to do so with him or any other person; or (d) Applies his mouth to the vagina, anus, urethra of a woman or makes her to do so with him or any other person, under the circumstances falling under any of the following seven descriptions:— First—Against her will. Secondly—Without her consent. Thirdly—With her consent, when her consent has been obtained by putting her or any person in whom she is interested, in fear of death or of hurt Fourthly—With her consent, when the man knows that he is not her husband and that her consent is given because she believes that he is another man to whom she is or believes herself to be lawfully married Fifthly—With her consent when, at the time of giving such consent, by reason of unsoundness of mind or intoxication or the administration by him personally or through another of any stupefying or unwholesome substance, she is unable to understand the nature and consequences of that to which she gives consent.	*Section 376 (1):* Anyone who commits rape shall be punished with rigorous imprisonment which shall not be less than 7 years, but which may extend to imprisonment for life, *Section 376 (1):* Anyone who commits rape shall be punished with rigorous imprisonment which shall not be less than 7 years, but which may extend to imprisonment for life, and shall also be liable to fine.

Contd...

Contd...

	Sixthly—With or without her consent, when she is under eighteen years of age. Seventhly—When she is unable to communicate consent. Explanation 1.—For the purposes of this section, "vagina" shall also include labia majora. Explanation 2.—Consent means an unequivocal voluntary agreement when the woman by words, gestures or any form of verbal or nonverbal communication, communicates willingness to participate in the specific sexual act: Provided that a woman who does not physically resist to the act of penetration shall not by the reason only of that fact, be regarded as consenting to the sexual activity. Exception 1—A medical procedure or intervention shall not constitute rape. Exception 2—Sexual intercourse or sexual acts by a man with his own wife, the wife not being under fifteen years of age, is not rape	
7.	*Section 376(A):* If in the course of commission of an offence under 376 (1) and (2), the man inflicts an injury which causes the death of the woman or causes the woman to be in a persistent vegetative state.	*Section 376(B):* Imprisonment for a term not less than 2 years but which may extend to 7 years, and fine.
8.	*Section 376(C):* Whoever, being in a position of authority or in a fiduciary relationship; or a public servant; or superintendent or manager of a jail, remand home or children's institution; or on the management or staff of a hospital abuses such position or fiduciary relationship to induce or seduce any woman under his charge or present to have sexual intercourse with him, such sexual intercourse not amounting to the offence of rape.	*Section 376(C):* Rigorous imprisonment for a term not less than 5 years, but which may extend to 10 years, and fine.
9.	*Section 376(D): Gang Rape:* Where a woman is raped by one or more persons constituting a group or acting in furtherance of a common intention, each of those persons shall be deemed to have committed the offence of rape.	*Section 376(D):* Rigorous imprisonment for a term not less than 20 years, but which may extend to life which shall mean imprisonment for the remainder of that person's natural life, and fine.
10.	*Section 376(E): Repeat Offenders:* Whoever has been previously convicted of an offence punishable under section 376 or section 376A or section 376D and is subsequently convicted.	*Section 376(E):* Imprisonment for life or death.

ROLE OF HEALTH PROFESSIONALS (BASED ON GUIDELINES ISSUED BY THE MINISTRY OF HEALTH AND FAMILY WELFARE)

Health professionals have to play the simultaneous role of treating and facilitating evidence collection for justice. But, health and welfare of the victim is of primary importance. Medicolegal services are important but should be of secondary importance. From service delivery point of view, safety and confidentiality should be one of the vital provision and entire spectrum of therapeutic care must be ethical, objective, humane and compassionate.[6]

General Principles and Ethical Considerations

Ethical principles should be considered while providing services to such clients.
- *Respect for autonomy:* The right of patients to take decision, including giving or refusing consent for any examination or filing a legal suit.
- *Beneficence:* Therapist must act in patient's best interest.
- *Non-maleficence:* Therapist should not cause any harm to patient.
- *Justice or fairness:* Therapist must do the rightful duty displaying sensitivity and compassion.

Sexual assault is a crime against humanity. State has duty to protect women from sexual violence and providing survivors complete care. Rightful entitlement of a victim for certain service delivery provisions is as follows:[6,7]
- *Right to health*: Every survivor has the right to quality reproductive healthcare services including prevention and management of sexually transmitted infections (STIs), HIV/AIDS and pregnancy.
- *Best interest of the child*: This includes the right to protection and to a chance for harmonious development. It refers to not just protecting the child from secondary victimization and hardship while involved in the justice process as victim or witness, but also enhancing the child's capacity to contribute to that process.
- *Right to human dignity*: Victims of sexual violence deserve to be treated with respect and dignity. This means health service providers should take care of privacy, confidentiality, communicating clearly in their native tongue about possible interventions and a safe clinical environment.
- *Right to non-discrimination*: Laws, policies, or health practitioners should not discriminate against a victim of sexual violence on any grounds (including sex, ethnic group, and the like).
- *Right to self-determination*: Survivors of sexual violence should be able to make their own decisions about whether to receive treatment or an examination. It is important that health providers should give victim clear information about her options in order to make an informed decision, including right to refuse examination and treatment.
- *Right to information*: Information about all possible medical, social and legal options should be provided to each victim by the doctors or medical social workers.
- *Right to privacy*: Victims of sexual violence should be afforded complete privacy while giving their statements and undergoing a medical or forensic examination.
- *Right to confidentiality*: All information related to a victim's health status should remain completely confidential.
- *Right to safety and effective assistance.*

How Health Professionals should Conduct themselves

Following strategies and techniques are helpful when dealing with victims of sexual violence:[6,7]
- Introduce yourself to the patient and explain your role.
- Greet the patient by name. Use her preferred name.
- Be respectful, professional and maintain a calm demeanor.
- Be unhurried.

- Give time.
- Maintain eye contact as much as is culturally appropriate.
- Be empathetic and non-judgmental as your patient recounts her experiences.
- Validation of patient's feeling. Body language, gestures and facial expressions all contribute to conveying an atmosphere of believing the patient's account.

Health professionals should display following skills:
- Awareness of the needs and wishes of the patient
- Balance of sensitivity compassion and objectivity
- Knowledge of normal human sexual responses, genital anatomy/physiology and dynamics of sexual violence
- Knowledge of medical and colloquial terms for sexual organs and acts
- Good communication skills
- Understanding of legal issues related to sexual crimes
- Understanding of relevant cultural/religious issues
- Empathy, non-judgmental and sensitivity.

Interdisciplinary Team Approach

For dealing with such cases, its ideal to have a team consisting of following professionals:
- Medical health professionals
- Psychiatrists
- Psychologists
- Psychiatric social workers
- Law enforcement agencies
- Social support agencies
- Non-government organizations (NGOs).

LEGAL RESPONSIBILITIES OF HEALTH PROFESSIONALS

Section 164(A) of the Criminal Procedure Code lays out following legal obligations of the health worker in cases of sexual violence:[8]
- Examination of a case of rape shall be conducted by a registered medical practitioner (RMP) employed in a hospital run by the government or a local authority (not necessarily a gynecologist).
- Examination to be conducted without delay and a reasoned report to be prepared by the RMP.
- Record consent obtained specifically for this examination.
- Exact time of start and close of examination to be recorded.
- RMP to forward report without delay to the Investigating Officer (IO), and in turn, IO to the Magistrate.

MEDICAL EXAMINATION AND REPORTING OF SEXUAL ASSAULT

A client may reach to the health professionals in one of the following ways:
- As voluntary patient for evaluation and or treatment
- Brought by family, victim not in a state to give consent, for evaluation and or treatment
- Brought by police
- Brought via court directives.

In all cases, hospital is bound to provide treatment and police requisition is not essential for same. If client comes without FIR, he/she can be offered for the same. But, if client refuses to lodge FIR and just wants treatment, as per the law, the hospital/examining doctor is required/duty bound to inform the police about the childhood sexual offence.[7,9]

Informed Consent

Consent should be *informed,* i.e. the person giving the consent should be told about the purpose, expected risks, side effects, and benefits of the examination, and the amount of time it will take. This information should be given before the examination is conducted, in a form, language and manner that the child and his parent/guardian can understand.

In all circumstances, it is mandatory to seek an Informed Consent/Refusal for following separately:
- Medical examination
- Medicolegal evidence collection
- Treatment
- Police intimation.

Who can give consent: Doctors shall inform the victim/parent/guardian about the nature and purpose of examination. The consent form must be signed by the victim (>12 years age) or guardian/parent (if victim's age <12 years). The consent form must be signed by the survivor, a witness and the examining doctor.

Waiver of consent: Only in situations, where it is life-threatening, the doctor may initiate treatment without consent as per section 92 of IPC.

Refusal for medicolegal examination: Neither court nor police can force the victim to undergo medical examination. In case, the victim or guardian does not want to pursue a police case, a Medicolegal Case (MLC) must be made and she/he must be informed that she/he has the right to refuse to file FIR. An informed refusal must be documented in such cases. At the time of MLC intimation being sent to the police, a clear note stating "informed refusal for police intimation" should be made. It should not result in denial of treatment for sexual violence.

Refusal for lodging FIR: It is victim's decision whether to lodge an FIR or not.[7]

Overview of Assessment and Examination

Consider arranging same sex examiner preferably: Preferably same sex examiner should do the examination. If the victim is female and examiner is male, a female attendant for the patient should always be present.

CHAPTER 23: Medicolegal Approach for Management of Adult Victims of Sexual Violence

In case of child victim, female victim has to be examined by a female doctor as per section 27 of POCSO Act, in absence of same, it can be carried out in presence of parent or person whom child trusts or a woman nominated by head of medical institute.[9]

All parts of the examination should be explained well in advance; during the examination, patients should be informed when and where touching will occur and should be given ample opportunity to ask questions.

The patient's wishes must be upheld at all times. Patients may refuse all or parts of the physical examination and you must respect the patient's decision. Allowing the patient a degree of control over the physical examination is important to her recovery.

Individuals who have suffered sexual violence, irrespective of the point at which they present within the health sector, should be offered a full medical-forensic examination, the main components of which are as follows:
- An initial assessment, including obtaining informed consent
- A medical history, including a gynecological history
- Account of the alleged incidence
- A "top-to-toe" physical examination
- Mental state assessment
- Appropriate referrals to different departments like gynecology, surgery, medicine as needed
- Mention account of things done in referrals (e.g. detailed genito-anal examination; recording and classification of injuries; collection of indicated medical specimens for diagnostic purposes; collection of forensic specimens; labeling, packaging and transporting of forensic specimens to maintain the chain of custody of the evidence)
- Therapeutic opportunities
- Arranging follow-up care
- Storage of documentation
- Provision of a medicolegal report.

Assess following factors determining psychological impact of sexual assault on victim:
- Whether victim is child or adult
- Prior history of trauma, sexual or otherwise
- Prior mental health issues
- Relationship of the offender to the victim
- Victim's appraisal of the circumstances
- Victim's coping mechanisms
- Positive social support
- *Cultural background:* Perceived and actual response of society to disclosure of sexual violence.

Mental Status Examination of Adult Victims

Besides the usual detailed mental state examination finding, also important to comment on following:
- Current emotional state

- Indicators of self harm behavior, suicidal gestures, plans, ideas, non-fatal deliberate self-harm, presence of potential weapons, sharps, medications or poisonous substance
- Past history of psychiatric illness or self-harm behavior.

Red flag signs warranting need for urgent mental health intervention and admission are:
- Suicidal behavior
- Stuporous state
- Severe depressive disorder
- Presence of psychotic symptoms
- Prolonged adjustment disorder
- Post-traumatic stress disorder (PTSD)
- Comorbid substance dependence/withdrawal
- Client with psychosocial disability
- High level of emotional distress
- High level of disorganization
- Poor social support (for respite care).

Safety Assessment of the Client

- If assessment reveals that victim is unsafe and fears reoccurrence of sexual violence, health professional can offer her alternate arrangements for stay such as temporary admission as respite care in the hospital or referral to shelter services in collaboration with hospital social worker. A safety plan must be made which may include suggestions such as making a police complaint about threats received, building support strategy with family.
- In situations, where a parent is the perpetrator of sexual abuse: Survivor under 18 years is likely to be accompanied by parents/guardians. If a health professional finds out that the perpetrator is the parent, it is critical to involve social worker/counselor from the hospital to discuss safety of the child and informing child welfare committee. As per Protection of Children from Sexual Offences (POCSO) Act 2012, social worker would have to speak with the child to assess whom the child trusts and can be called upon in the hospital itself. Simultaneously, social worker would also have to contact police, who in communication with social worker should assess whether the child is in need of protection and care. Likewise, the child may be admitted to the hospital for a period of 24 hours till a long-term strategy for shelter or child welfare home is made.[9]

TREATMENT GUIDELINES AND PSYCHOSOCIAL SUPPORT

Emergency Medical Care

The Criminal Law Amendment Act, 2013, in Section 357C of CrPC says that both private and public health professionals are obligated to provide free emergency treatment.[10] Denial of treatment of rape survivors is punishable under section 166B IPC with imprisonment for a term, which may extend to one year or with fine or with both.[11]

Interventions for Physical Illnesses and Injuries[7]
- *Sexually transmitted infections (STIs):*
  - If clinical signs are suggestive of STI, collect relevant swabs and start postexposure prophylaxis (PEP). If there are no clinical signs, wait for lab results.
    - For non-pregnant women, the preferred choice is azithromycin 1 g stat or doxycycline 100 mg bd for 7 days, with metronidazole 400 mg for 7 days with antacid.
    - For pregnant women, amoxicillin/azithromycin with metronidazole is preferred. {Metronidazole should NOT to be given in the 1st trimester of pregnancy}.
  - For Hepatitis B: Draw a sample of blood for HBsAg and administer 0.06 mL/kg HB immunoglobulin immediately (any time up to 72 hours after sexual act).
- *Pregnancy prophylaxis (Emergency contraception):*
  - The preferred choice of treatment is 2 tablets of levonorgestrel 750 µg, within 72 hours. If vomiting occurs, repeat within 3 hours OR 2 tablets COCs Mala D—2 tablets stat repeated 12 hours within 72 hours.
  - Although emergency contraception is most efficacious if given within the first 72 hours, it can be given for up to 5 days after the assault.
  - Pregnancy assessment must be done on follow-up and the survivor must be advised to get tested for pregnancy in case she misses her next period.
- *Lacerations:* Clean with antiseptic or soap and water. If the survivor is already immunized with tetanus toxoid (TT) or if no injuries, TT not required. If there are injuries and survivor is not immunized, administer 0.5 mL TT intramuscular (IM). If lacerations require repair and suturing, which is often the case in minor girls, refer to the nearest center offering surgical treatment.
- *Postexposure prophylaxis (PEP):* PEP for HIV should be given if a survivor reports within 72 hours of the assault. Before PEP is prescribed, HIV risk should be assessed.
- *Follow-up:* Please emphasize the importance of follow-up to the survivor. It is ideal to call the survivor for re-examination 2 days after the assault to note the development of bruises and other injuries; thereafter at 3 and 6 weeks. All follow-ups should be documented.
  - Repeat test for gonorrhea if possible
  - Test for pregnancy
  - Repeat after 6 weeks for venereal disease research laboratory (VDRL) test.
  - Assess for psychological sequelae and reiterate need for psychological support.

Psychological Intervention
Most important thing to understand is that it is an experience and not a disorder. Symptomatic clients may be given specific pharmacological treatment depending on the disorder and psychotherapeutic interventions but the difficulty is that one cannot say which specific therapy or combination of therapies will be effective in an individual case as there are paucity of treatment outcome studies. Benzodiazepines may be used in short-term to control acute agitation and excitement. But, to be avoided in outpatient settings and long-term to prevent

potential misuse and dependence. In general, all survivors should be provided the first line of psychosocial support involving expression of feelings about abuse, clarifying misconceptions, teaching prevention skills and diminishing the sense of stigma and isolation in victims. The health professional must provide this support himself/herself or ensure that patient is referred to some trained counselor or social workers of the hospital.[6]

Crisis Intervention

In acute stage, client may need crisis counseling/intervention, which should include the following:
- *Restoring patient's psychological safety:* Ventilatory support with non-judgmental, non-directive, facilitatory attitude and continuous reassurance along with environmental manipulation, if required
- Providing information related to current medical status, addressing fears related to misattributions
- *Restoring and supporting effective coping:* Assistance in preparing for ways in which they can deal with the practical and emotional needs in future using cognitive and problem-solving techniques.

Techniques to Address Immediate Emotional Distress

A victim may be in a heightened state of awareness and emotional turmoil after the assault; he/she may have a range of emotional reactions. Never be judgmental, use words judiciously. Appreciate survivor's strength in help seeking; it can help build therapeutic relationship. Help the client deal with their emotions. Following is the list of common emotional responses seen in such victims and way to deal with them[6,12] **(Table 2)**:

Table 2: Techniques to address immediate emotional distress in victims of sexual assault.

Emotions	Ways to respond
Guilt, self blame	Say, "You are not to blame for what happened to you. The person who assaulted you is responsible for the violence"
Numbness	Say, "This is a common reaction to severe trauma. You will feel again. All in good time"
Hopelessness	"You are a valuable person"
Despair	Focus on the strategies and resourcefulness that the person used to survive
Helplessness	Say, "It sounds as if you were feeling helpless. We are here to help you"
Powerlessness	Say, "You have choices and options today in how to proceed"
Shame	Say, "There is no loss of honor in being assaulted. You are an honorable person."
Anger	A legitimate feeling and avenues can be found for its safe expression. Assist the patient in experiencing those feelings. For example, "You sound very angry."
Fear	Emphasize, "You are safe now." You can say, "That must have been very frightening for you"
Flashback	Say, "These will resolve with the healing process"
Denial	Say, "I am taking what you have told me seriously. I will be here if you need help in the future"
Mood swings, anxiety	Tell the patient that these symptoms will ease with the use of the appropriate stress management techniques and offer to explain these techniques

Other Specific Therapies of Utility as per Need
For adults:
- Cognitive behavioral therapy
- Group therapies including stress inoculation; assertion training; feminist therapy
- Supportive psychotherapy;
- Eye movement desensitization reprocessing.

For children:
Art therapy, play therapy, and supportive psychotherapy. Trauma focused debriefing is not advised anymore.

DOCUMENTATION
How to document:
- Document all pertinent information accurately and legibly during the consultation.
- Notes and injury chart should be created during the consultation, not by memory.
- Notes should not be altered unless this is clearly identified as a *later* addition or alteration.
- Deletions should be scored through once and signed, and not erased completely.
- Record the extent of the physical examination conducted and all "normal" or relevant negative findings.
- Record verbatim any statements made by the victim regarding the assault. This is preferable to writing down your own interpretation of the statements made.

What to document: In sexual assault cases, documentation should include the following:
- Demographic information (i.e. name, age, sex);
- Consents obtained;
- History (i.e. general medical and gynecological history);
- An account of the assault;
- Results of the physical examination;
- Tests and their results;
- Treatment plan;
- Medications given or prescribed;
- Patient education;
- Referrals given.

Confidentiality of records: Patient records and information are strictly confidential. All healthcare providers have a professional, legal and ethical duty to maintain and respect patient confidentiality and autonomy. Records and information should not be disclosed to anyone except those directly involved in the case or as required by local, state and national statutes.

PATIENT INFORMATION
On completion of the assessment and medical examination, it is important to discuss any findings, and what the findings may mean, with the patient. In particular:
- Give the patient ample opportunity to voice questions and concerns.

- Reassure the patient that he/she did not deserve to be sexually assaulted and that the assault was not his/her fault.
- Teach patients how to properly care for any injuries they have sustained.
- Explain how injuries heal and describe the signs and symptoms of wound infection.
- Teach proper hygiene techniques and explain the importance of good hygiene.
- Discuss the signs and symptoms of STIs, including HIV and the need to return for treatment if any signs and symptoms should occur. Stress the need to use a condom during sexual intercourse until STI/HIV status has been determined.
- Explain the importance of completing the course of any medications given.
- Discuss the side effects of any medications given.
- Explain the need to refrain from sexual intercourse until all treatments or prophylaxis for STIs have been completed and until their sexual partner has been treated for STIs, if necessary.
- Explain rape trauma syndrome (RTS) and the range of normal physical, psychological and behavioral responses that the patient can expect to experience to both the patient and (with the patient's permission) family members and/or significant others. Encourage the patient to confide in and seek emotional support from a trusted friend or family member.
- Inform patients of their legal rights and how can they exercise those rights. Also inform the client about free legal aid from state legal service authority.
- Give patients written documentation regarding:
  - Any treatments received;
  - Tests performed;
  - Date and time to call for test results;
  - Meaning of test results;
  - Date and time of follow-up appointments;
  - Information regarding the legal process.
- Stress the importance of follow-up examinations at 2 weeks and 3 and 6 months.
- Tell the patient that he/she can come to the healthcare facility at any time if he/she has any querries, complications related to the assault, or other medical problems.

ROLE OF FAMILY, FRIENDS AND COMMUNITY

Recovery from sexual violence is dependent on the extent of support received from family, friends and community. Health professionals are best suited to engage with family and discuss ways of promoting survivors' well-being. It must be discussed with all caregivers that survivor should not be held responsible for the assault. Judgmental statements from family members such as; "she should have been careful", "she should have resisted" make the survivors journey to recovery more difficult, so, should be avoided.

INTERFACE WITH LEGAL AGENCIES

Health professionals have to interface with other agencies such as the police, public prosecutors, judiciary and child welfare committees to ensure comprehensive care to survivors of sexual violence.

Interface of Health Systems and the Police

- Whenever a survivor reports to the police, the police must take her/him to the nearest health facility for medical examination, treatment and care. Delays related to the medical examination and treatment can jeopardize the health of the survivor.
- Health professionals should also ask survivors whether they were examined elsewhere before reaching the current health set-up and if survivors are carrying documentation of the same. If this is the case, health professionals must refrain from carrying out an examination just because the police have brought a requisition and also explain the same to them unless court directives for re-examination present.
- The health sector has a therapeutic role and confidentiality of information must be ensured. The police should not be allowed to be present while details of the incident of sexual violence, examination, evidence collection and treatment are being sought from the survivor.
- The police cannot interfere with the duties of a health professional. They cannot take away the survivor immediately after evidence collection but must wait until treatment and care is provided.
- In the case of unaccompanied survivors brought by the police for sexual violence examination, police should not be asked to sign as witness in the medicolegal form. In such situations, a senior medical officer or any health professional should sign as witness in the best interest of the survivor.
- Doctors may also be asked to opine regarding client's fitness for statement under section 164A of CrPC.

Interface of Health Systems and the Judiciary

Doctors are termed as "expert witness" by Law. As per Section 164A, CrPC, an examining doctor has to prepare a reasoned medical opinion without delay.[10] A medical opinion has to be provided on the following aspects:

- Was victim administered drugs/psychotropic substance/alcohol, etc.
- Evidence that the victim has an intellectual, or mental disability
- Evidence of physical health consequences such as bruises, contusions, contused lacerated; wounds, tenderness, swelling, pain in micturition, pain in defecation, pregnancy, etc.
- Age of the victim if in doubt
- Client's fitness for giving statement or fitness to stand trial or fitness to testify as witness.

The examining doctor should clarify in the court that normal examination findings neither refute nor confirm whether the sexual offence occurred or not. They must ensure that a medical opinion cannot be given on whether 'rape' occurred because 'rape' is a legal term.

Capacity Assessment as Asked by Court Regarding Victims of Sexual Violence

The legal test of capacity for persons with mental health issues can be seen in 2 parts:
Part 1: Presence of a mental disorder.

Part 2: "Impairment of Capacity"—The person must be unable to do any one of the following:
- Understand the information relevant to the decision
- Remember the information relevant to the decision
- Weigh up the information—consider the advantages and disadvantages, risks and benefits of saying "yes" or "no"
- Be able to communicate their decision (by whatever means they are able to use to communicate.

Two types of capacity assessments for victims of sexual assault with mental health issues is often asked by court of law:
1. Assessing the capacity of victims to give evidence or statement in court (competence to give evidence)
2. Assessing capacity of victim to consent to a sexual relationship.

Competence to Give Evidence

"The law states that all people are competent to give evidence. Competent in this context means 'lawfully able to give evidence'. This is the starting point from which all witnesses should be assessed when prosecutors are considering their evidence. A witness is not competent to give evidence if he/she:
- Is not able to understand questions put to him/her as a witness
- And give answers to those questions which can be understood.

(Indian Evidence Act section 118 states that "All persons shall be competent to testify unless the Court considers that they are prevented from understanding the questions put to them, or from giving rational answers to those questions, by tender years, extreme old age, disease, whether of body or mind, or any other cause of the same kind. (Explanation. -- A lunatic is not incompetent to testify, unless he is prevented by his lunacy from understanding the questions put to him and giving rational answers to them.)[13]

Mental health assessment for fitness to give statement should focus on:
- How might the nature or extent of the witness's mental health condition affect his/her ability to give evidence: Could the nature or extent of the witness's mental health condition affect his/her:
  – Understanding
  – Perception or
  – Recollection of an incident? as assessed by following:
    * Ability to recall and accurately interpret events;
    * Ability to consistently tell the events;
    * Quality of short- and long-term memory.[14]
- How might the nature or extent of the witness's mental health condition affect his/her ability to withstand cross-examination, particularly with reference to:
  – Response to questioning and cross-examination;
  – Concentration and attention;
  – Ability to communicate; and
  – Interaction with other people.[14]

Additional assessment of supportive measures to address impact of evidence giving on person's mental health:

Special measures: Mental health professional must also communicate to court the likelihood of impact of evidence giving on person's mental health and need of any support measures required to decrease this likelihood like:
- Giving evidence in private—particularly where sensitive personal or medical information is being disclosed;
- Removal of wigs and gowns—which may reduce the risk of a witness becoming anxious, distressed or experiencing feelings of paranoia or panic;
- Use of intermediaries as support persons—to assist with interpreting questions and answers appropriately.
- Asking the Judge or Magistrates to allow witnesses to take regular comfort breaks;[14]

- *Mental health assessment for assessing capacity to consent to a sexual relationship:* At times, mental health professionals are also asked for retrospective assessment like to assess whether the victim with mental health issues had capacity to give consent for sexual relationship, when alleged perpetrator takes the plea of consensual relationship not sexual assault and judiciary or family of victim has reason to believe that alleged victim's capacity for giving consent for same was impaired, e.g. In case with intellectual disability.
  - In order to have capacity to consent to a sexual relationship the person need to know the following:
    - The mechanics of the act (that is, what people actually do when they have sex)
    - That there are health risks involved, particularly the acquisition of sexually transmitted and sexually transmissible infections (HIV, syphilis, etc.)
    - That sex between a man and a woman may result in the woman becoming pregnant or the concept of same sex relationships
    - They also needed to be able to "exercise their capacity". In other words, the mental disorder should not make someone be unable to refuse.[14]

INTERFACE WITH SOCIAL WELFARE AGENCIES

Clients in need can also be referred to self-help groups/non-governmental organizations (NGOs)/rape crisis cells. They should be informed regarding women in distress helpline (1099), provisions of contacting protection officers in case of domestic violence and various social welfare schemes under department of women and child welfare. Help from a social worker should be taken for formulating a comprehensive rehabilitation plan for the client.

CONCLUSION

Sexual assault is a crime against humanity. Victims are facing the pain of trauma, societal discrimination and associated medical morbidities. A comprehensive medical care can be instrumental in recovery. Health professionals should provide an impartial, non-judgmental, empathetic care and help in collecting evidence neutrally. Client should not only receive medical care, but a complete package of access to legal and social welfare aids.

REFERENCES

1. Sexual violence. WHO publication. Available at: http://www.who.int/violence_injury prevention/violence/global campaign/en/chap6.pdf. Last accessed on 7 February 2018
2. Sarah B, Morrison A, Ellsberg M. Preventing and responding to gender-based violence in middle and low-income countries: a global review and analysis. World Bank Policy Research Working Paper no. 3618, 2005: 27
3. Crime in India Crime 2015 statistics. National Crime Record Bureau, Ministry of Home Affairs, Government of India. 2015. Available at: http://ncrb.gov.in/StatPublications/CII/CII2015/FILES/CrimeInIndia2015.pdf. Last accessed on 7 February 2018
4. Crime in India 2015 Compendium. National Crime Record Bureau. Ministry of Home Affairs, Government of India. Available at: http://ncrb.gov.in/StatPublications/CII/CII2015/FILES/Compendium-15.11.16.pdf. Last accessed on 7 February 2018
5. Campbell R, Raja S. Secondary victimization of rape victims: insights from mental health professionals who treat survivors of violence and victims. Vol. 14 (3), 1999. [Cited 2016 Feb 13]. Available at: https://mainweb-v.musc.edu/vawprevention/research/victim rape.shtml. Last accessed on 7 February 2018
6. Kukreti P, Kishore J, Tanwar R. Psychological and medico legal aspects of management of sexual assault: Indian perspective International Journal of Health Sciences & Research. 2016;6(4):507-15.
7. Guidelines and protocols of Medico-legal care for survivors/victims of sexual violence Ministry of Health and Family Welfare. Government of India. November 2014
8. The Code of Criminal Procedure, 1973. Current Publications, 2015.
9. Model Guidelines of the Protection of Children from Sexual Offences Act, 2012. Guidelines for the Use of Professionals and Experts under the POCSO Act, 2012. Ministry of women and child development. Government of India. September 2013.
10. The Criminal Law (Amendment) Act 2013, No.13 of 2013. Gazette of Govt. of India Extraordinary. Ministry of Law & Justice (Legislative Division) 2013.
11. Gandhi BM. Indian Penal Code, EBC, 1–796. Current Publications, 2015.
12. Responding to intimate partner violence and sexual violence against women, WHO clinical and policy guidelines, 2013. [Cited 2016 Feb 13]. Available at: http://www.who.int/ reproductive health/publications/violence/9789241548595/en.
13. The Indian Evidence Act 1872, Act No. 1 of 1872.Available at: ncw.nic.in/Acts/The Indian Evidence Act 1872.pdf. Last accessed on 7 February 2018
14. Joyce T. Assessing capacity to consent and to give evidence. Estia Centre; South London & Maudsley NHS Trust, London, UK. Available at: www.nomasabuso.com/wp-content/uploads/2012/06/theresa_joyce_1Ponencia8.pdf. Last accessed on 7 February 2018.

CHAPTER 24

Medicolegal Approach for Management of Victims of Child Sexual Abuse

LEARNING OBJECTIVES
- Psychological effects of CSA
- Legal provisions of POCSO Act
- Perpetrator-victim dynamics: Understanding CSA
- Effects of child sexual abuse
- Medicolegal approach to case of child sexual abuse
- Handling disclosure
- Mandatory reporting
- Forensic interviewing: Liaisoning with legal agencies as child development expert
- Capacity assessment for courts

INTRODUCTION

Child sexual abuse (CSA) is a major problem across the globe.[1] The World Health Organization (WHO) defines CSA as "the involvement of a child in sexual activity that he or she does not fully comprehend and is unable to give informed consent to, or for which the child is not mentally prepared, or else that violate the laws or social taboos of society".[2] The term CSA includes a range of activities like "intercourse, attempted intercourse, oral-genital contact, fondling of genitals directly or through clothing, exhibitionism or exposing children to adult sexual activity or pornography, and the use of the child for prostitution or pornography".[2]

EPIDEMIOLOGY

The prevalence of CSA is high globally, in a study conducted by WHO in 2002, 73 million minor boys and 150 million minor girls reported having experienced different forms of sexual violence and largest number of cases were from India.[1] A statistical analysis of reported cases reveals, a child less than 16 years being raped every 155th minute, a child less than 10 years, being raped every 13th hour, and nearly one in 10 children report having sexually abused at some point of time in childhood.[2] Another Indian survey conducted by United Nations International Children Education Fund (UNICEF) from 2005 to 2013 revealed that 10% of girls reported having experienced sexual violence during 10–14 years of age and 30% during 15–19 years of age.[3] A study was conducted in 2007 by Ministry of Women and Child Development in India covering 13 states. The study reported that about 21% of the participants were exposed to extreme forms of sexual abuse. Among the participants who reported being abused, 57.3%

were boys and 42.7% were girls, about 40% were 5–12 years of age. About half of the participants were exposed to other forms of sexual abuse.[4]

PSYCHOLOGICAL EFFECTS OF CHILD SEXUAL ABUSE

Child sexual abuse (CSA) is associated with range of psychological problems like low self-esteem, guilt, anger, hopelessness and suicide attempts. High prevalence of post-traumatic stress disorder, depression, anxiety disorders, body image concerns, eating disorders and substance use disorders have been reported in this population. Later on, these children also show behavioral problems like violation of law, social misconduct, violent behavior, lower academic performance, absenteeism and abnormal sexual behaviors. Act of sexual abuse can adversely affect cognitive and emotional development of the child.[5]

Role of Mental Health Professionals

Child sexual abuse is a hidden epidemic; most of the cases are not disclosed due to poor understanding of child itself or inability of health professionals to pick up hidden indicators. Most cases report to emergency or pediatricians or gynecologists, sometimes, presentation can be first to a mental health professional due to altered behavior or immediate psychological impact of CSA. Also, in many cases of CSA, physical signs of sexual assault are not apparent due to grooming technique used by perpetrators for long time, in such cases, only good history taken in a sensitive and developmentally appropriate way can be the only way to achieve justice. Thus, mental health professionals can play a great role in these cases being apt for the dual role of therapists as well as child mental health experts to facilitate forensic interviewing for law enforcement agencies. Besides this, they can also play an important role of sensitizing other medical professionals and law enforcement officials in skills of dealing with such cases to prevent secondary victimization of child. Hence, having clear knowledge of clinical, legal, ethical issues concerning such cases can enable mental health professionals to deal with such cases in a better way.

UNDERSTANDING CHILDHOOD SEXUAL OFFENCES THROUGH LEGAL PERSPECTIVE IN INDIA

List of offences under the Protection of Children from Sexual Offences (POCSO) Act, 2012 and the punishment for the offence:

To deal with child sexual abuse cases, the Government has brought in a special law, namely, POCSO Act, 2012.

Who is a Child: The said Act defines a child as any person below 18 years of age.[6]

Mandate of Act: The POCSO Act, 2012 is a comprehensive law to provide for the protection of children from the offences of sexual assault, sexual harassment and pornography, while safeguarding the interests of the child at every stage of the judicial process by incorporating child-friendly mechanisms for reporting, recording of evidence, investigation and speedy trial of offences through designated Special Courts.[6]

Aggravated offences: Any of the following listed sexual assault is said to be "aggravated" under certain circumstances, such as when the abused child is mentally ill or when the abuse is committed by a person in a position of trust or authority *vis-à-vis* the child, like a family member, police officer, teacher, or doctor **(Table 1)**.[6]

Table 1: Offences and punishment under the Protection of Children from Sexual Offences Act, 2012.

S.No.	Offences description	Punishment
1.	Section 3: Penetrative Sexual Assault is defined as— • Penetration of the penis to any extent into any vagina, urethra, or anus of a child's body, • Insertion of an object to any extent into the vagina, urethra, or anus of a child, • Manipulating the body of a child so as to cause penetration into the vagina, urethra or anus, and applying the mouth to the vagina, penis, anus or urethra of a child or making a child do any of the above with him or any other person.	Section 4: Not less than 7 years of imprisonment which may extend to imprisonment for life, and liable to be fined
2.	Section 7: Sexual Assault includes—Touching the vagina, penis, anus or breast of the child with sexual intent or making the child touch the vagina, penis, anus or breast of such person or any other person, Any other act with sexual intent which involves physical contact without penetration.	Section 8: Not less than 3 years of imprisonment which may extend to 5 years, and liable to fine
3.	Section 11: Sexual Harassment of the Child with Sexual Intent: Utters any word or makes any sound, or makes any gesture or exhibits any object or part of body with the intention that such word or sound shall be heard, or such gesture or object or part of body shall be seen by the child; or makes a child exhibit his body or any part of his body so as it is seen by such person or any other person; or shows any object to a child in any form or media for pornographic purposes; or repeatedly or constantly follows or watches or contacts a child either directly or through electronic, digital or any other means; or threatens to use, in any form of media, a real or fabricated depiction through electronic, film or digital or any other mode, of any part of the body of the child or the involvement of the child in a sexual act; or entices a child for pornographic purposes or gives gratification therefore.	Section 12: Up to 3 years of imprisonment and liable to fine

Contd...

Contd...

S.No.	Offences description	Punishment
4.	*Section 13:* Use of Child for Pornographic Purposes: Use of child in any form of media (including program or advertisement telecast by television, internet or electronic or printed form, whether or not such program or advertisement is intended for personal use or for distribution), for the purpose of sexual gratification which includes representation of the sexual organs of the child, usage of a child engaged in real or simulated sexual acts (with or without penetration), indecent or obscene representation of a child	*Section 14 (1):* Imprisonment up to 5 years and fine and in the event of subsequent conviction, up to 7 years and fine
5.	*Section 15:* Storage of pornographic material in any form, involving a child for commercial purposes	*Section 15:* Three years of imprisonment and/or fine
6.	*Section 16:* Abetment of an offence: A person abets an offence if he • Instigates any person to do that offence • Engages with one or more other person/s in any conspiracy for the doing of that offence, if an act or illegal omission takes place in pursuance of that conspiracy, and in order to the doing of that offence Intentionally aids, by any act or illegal omission, the doing of that offence	*Section 17:* If the act abetted is committed in consequence of the abetment, the person shall be punished with punishment provided for that offence
7.	*Section 18:* Attempt to commit an offence	*Section 18:* Imprisonment of any description provided for the offence for a term which may extend to one half of the imprisonment for life, or one half of the longest term of imprisonment provided for that offence and/or with fine
8.	*Section 21:* Punishment for failure to report or record a case by (i) Any person; (ii) Any person, being in charge of any company or an institution. (This offence does not apply to a child)	*Section 21* (i) Imprisonment of either description which may extend to 6 months or with fine or with both, (ii) Any person, being in charge of any company or an institution (by whatever name called) who fails to report the commission of an offence under sub-section (1) of section 19 in respect of a subordinate under his control shall be punished with imprisonment for a term which may extend to 1 year and with fine
9.	*Section 22:* (1) Punishment for false complaint or false information in respect of an offence committed under sections 3, 5, 7 and 9 solely with the intention to humiliate, extort or threaten or defame him. (3) False complaint or providing false information against a child knowing it to be false, thereby victimizing such child in any of the offences under this Act. (This offence does not apply to a child)	*Section 22:* (1) Imprisonment for a term which may extend to 6 months or with fine or with both. (3) Imprisonment which may extend to 1 year or with fine or with both

VICTIM PERPETRATOR DYNAMICS: UNDERSTANDING CSA THROUGH PSYCHOLOGICAL PERSPECTIVE

Finkelhor and Browne reviewed the literature on the effects of sexual abuse and postulated traumagenic dynamics (TD) framework. This framework tells how CSA alters children's cognitive and emotional orientation to the world, and creates trauma focused orientation by distorting children's self-concept, world view, and affective capacities.[7-9] According to the TD framework, CSA may lead to four consequences:

- *Betrayal and lack of trust:* Child feels betrayed by the abuser and reaction of others to disclosure or by failure of others to recognize and stop the abuse;
- *Stigmatization:* Child feels stigmatized and sexually different because of abuse and feels shame and guilt;
- *Powerlessness:* Child feels unable to control the sexual aspects of relationships
- *Traumatic sexualization:* If the child was being rewarded for involvement in sexual activity by the abuser, child develops maladaptive attitude towards sexual behavior.[8,9] It can happen in following way:
    - If molester "grooms" the child, i.e. gives undue affection, attention or special privileges and gifts to a child in exchange of certain sexual behavior, then there is high possibility that this child learns to use sexual behavior as a strategy for manipulating others to satisfy a variety of his or her needs.[8]
    - If certain anatomical sexual organs of child are fetishized and offender gives it distorted importance and meaning, it creates misconceptions and confusions about sexual behavior and sexual morality in the child and becomes associated with frightening memories and events in the child's mind with sexual activity.[8]
    - Characteristics of sexual abuse experiences are very important in determining the amount and kind of traumatic sexualization like whether the molester made the child active or passive during sexual experience or brute force was used by the molester or not. Experiences in which the offender makes an effort to evoke the child's sexual response, for example, are probably more sexualizing than those in which an offender simply uses a passive child to masturbate with.[8]
    - The degree of a child's understanding about sex and related behavior may also affect the degree of sexualization. In a child who has less awareness of sexual and related issues, because of early age or developmental level, the sexual experience may be less sexualizing than that involving a child with greater awareness.[8]

Children who have been traumatically sexualized emerge from their experiences with inappropriate repertoires of sexual behavior, with confusions and misconceptions about their sexual self-concepts, and with unusual emotional associations to sexual activities.[8]

EFFECTS OF CHILD SEXUAL ABUSE

Short-term effects of child sexual abuse are as follows:[10]
- Feeling of powerlessness
- Anger
- Anxiety
- Fear

- Phobias
- Nightmares
- Difficulty concentrating
- Flashbacks of the events
- Fear of confronting the offender
- Loss of self-esteem and confidence
- Feelings of guilt.

If childhood sexual abuse is not treated, long-term symptoms can go on through adulthood. These may include:[9]

- Post-traumatic stress disorder (PTSD) and anxiety
- Depression and thoughts of suicide
- Sexual anxiety and disorders, including having too many or unsafe sexual partners
- Difficulty setting safe limits with others (e.g. saying no to people) and relationship problems
- Poor body image and low self-esteem
- Unhealthy behaviors, such as alcohol, drugs, self-harm, or eating problems. These behaviors are often used to try to hide painful emotions related to the abuse
- Issues in maintaining relationships.

MEDICOLEGAL APPROACH TO A CASE OF CSA (BASED ON GUIDELINES ISSUED BY MINISTRY OF WOMEN AND CHILD WELFARE)

Health professionals have to play the simultaneous role of treating and facilitating evidence collection for justice. But, health and welfare of the victim is of primary importance. Medicolegal services are important but should be of secondary importance. From service delivery point of view, safety and confidentiality should be one of the vital provision and entire spectrum of therapeutic care must be ethical, objective, humane and compassionate.[6]

General Principles and Ethical Considerations

Ethical principles should be considered while providing services to such clients.
- *Respect for autonomy*. The right of patients to take decision, including giving or refusing consent for any examination or filing a legal suit.
- *Beneficence*. Therapist must act in patient's best interest.
- *Non-maleficence*. Therapist should not cause any harm to patient.
- *Justice or fairness*. Therapist must do the rightful duty displaying sensitivity and compassion.

Ways in which CSA Cases can Present to Mental Health Professionals

Presentation of childhood sexual abuses can be in following ways:

Adulthood presentation: Retrospective revelation of CSA as an accidental disclosure when adults may present to mental health professionals for one of the following mental health issues developed as a result of traumatic sexualization:

- Relationship problems
- Distorted views about sexuality
- Sexual dysfunctions
- Personality changes
- Substance use disorder.

Childhood presentation: It can happen in following ways:

Spontaneous disclosure
- Self referral/brought by parent after the incidence for treatment
- Brought by police for examination
- Came with court's directive.

Accidental disclosure
Child presenting with any of the behavioral problems and on exploring the history or during examination, history of CSA is divulged accidentally.

Consent of the Victim

According to the medical protocol, where the child is over 12 years old, consent for the medical examination should be sought from the child himself or herself. Where he/she is below the age of 12, a parent or the guardian may be asked for such consent.

Consent should be taken for the following purposes separately:
- Medical examination for therapeutic purpose,
- Sample collection for clinical and forensic examination,
- Medical treatment and
- Police intimation.

Informed Consent

Consent should be *informed,* i.e. the person giving the consent should be told about the purpose, expected risks, side effects, and benefits of the examination, and the amount of time it will take. This information should be given before the examination is conducted, in a form, language and manner that the child and his parent/guardian can understand.

A child victim and family may approach a health facility under three circumstances, and informed consent must be taken in all:[11]
a. On his/her own only for treatment for effects of assault;
b. With a police requisition after police complaint; or
c. With a court directive.
   - If a person has come directly to the hospital without the police requisition, the hospital is bound to provide treatment and conduct a medical examination with consent of the survivor/parent/guardian (depending on age).
   Note: Even if the child or parent does not give consent for medical examination you can still provide them with medical treatment.

- If a person has come on his/her own without FIR, she/he may or may not want to lodge a complaint but may require a medical examination and treatment, even in such cases the doctor is bound to inform the police as per POCSO Act.
- However, neither court nor police can force the child to undergo medical examination. In case the child or the parent/guardian does not want to pursue a police case, a Medicolegal Case (MLC) must be made and she/he must be informed that she/he has the right to refuse to file FIR. An informed refusal must be documented in such cases.
- If the person has come with a police requisition or wishes to lodge a complaint later, the information about Medicolegal Case (MLC) number and police station should be recorded.
- Police personnel should not be present during any part of the examination.[11]

Medical Examination for Legal Purposes

After taking the consent, the examination needs to be conducted in the presence of a person trusted by the child (e.g. parent/relative/social worker), in the absence of which, a woman nominated by the hospital, needs to be present during examination.[11]

Physical Treatment

Emergency medical care: Under Rule 5 of the POCSO Act, 2012 emergency medical care is to be provided by any medical facility, private or public; and no magisterial requisition or other document is to be demanded as a precondition to providing emergency medical care. Such care includes treatment for cuts, bruises, and other injuries including genital injuries, if any. Inpatient care is recommended if the child's safety is in jeopardy or if the child has an acute traumatic injury requiring inpatient treatment.[11]

Reproductive health care: Pregnancy and STDs in sexually abused children:
- Pregnancy test should be done on girls 11 years and older and on any girl who has either had any menstrual periods, or who has breast development or pubic hair.
- Urine test is as sensitive and accurate as blood test, and easier for patient.
- The doctor must provide information about emergency contraception, and, unless medically contraindicated, offer emergency contraception.
- Legally, the child can provide consent and must be given an assurance of confidentiality for reproductive health care. The patient must provide informed consent.
- If the patient is not able to give informed consent, consent must be obtained from parents, guardian, or surrogate decision-maker.[11]

Psychological Assessment of CSA Case

There is high prevalence of history of sexual abuse in all diagnostic categories and the disclosure rates are low, because of following reasons, children are not comfortable in sharing the history:
- Sense of embarrassment
- Inability to understand they are being abused

- Poor cognitive or verbal ability to convey
- The abuser is a known person and the child does not want to get them in trouble
- The abuser told the child to keep it a secret
- Fear of not being believed
- The abuser bribes or threatens the child
- He/she thinks you already know.

Thus, it is essential to ask all patients about abuse history in a sensitive manner and appropriate response should be provided. It is prudent to thus, ask routinely in personal history, and better to approach by moving from general (less threatening/more neutral) to specific questions:[12]

- Can you tell me about your daily routine?
- Can you tell me about your best memory and the worst?
- Who are your favorite people? Tell me what you like about them and activities you enjoy with them.
- Who are the people you do not like? What are reasons you dislike them or why do they make you feel uncomfortable/upset?
- Have you ever been upset or bothered by someone's behavior towards you?
- Has anyone touched you in ways that you do not like?
- Has anyone touched your private parts and made you feel uncomfortable?

Also it is important to be aware about other indicators of CSA:[11]

Behavioral indicators:
- Abrupt changes in behavior such as self-harm, talks of suicide or attempt to suicide, poor impulse control, etc.
- Reluctance to go home.
- Sexualized behavior or acting out sexually.
- Low self-esteem.
- Wearing many layers of clothing regardless of the weather.
- Recurrent nightmares or disturbed sleep patterns and fear of the dark.
- Regression to more infantile behavior like bed-wetting, thumb-sucking or excessive crying.
- Poor peer relationships.
- Eating disturbances.
- Negative coping skills, such as substance abuse and/or self-harm.
- An increase in irritability or temper tantrums.
- Fears of a particular person or object.
- Aggression towards others.
- Poor school performance.
- Knowing more about sexual behavior than is expected of a child of that age:
    a. Child may hate own genitals or demand privacy in an aggressive manner.
    b. Child may think of all relationships in a sexual manner.
    c. Child may dislike being his/her own gender.
    d. Child may use inappropriate language continuously in his or her vocabulary or may use socially unacceptable slang.

e. Child may carry out sexualized play (simulating sex with other children).
f. Unwarranted curiosity towards sexual act like visiting adult sites or watching adult images or content.

Physical indicators[11]
- Sexually transmitted diseases,
- Pregnancy,
- Complaints of pain or itching in the genital area,
- Difficulty in walking or sitting,
- Repeated unusual injuries,
- Pain during elimination, and
- Frequent yeast infections.

Technique for Interviewing the Child[11]

- The first step is to establish a trusting relationship with the child, so that the child can communicate freely. Try to speak to the child in its own language, taking into account his or her age, maturity and emotional state.
- It is important to explain the purpose of interview and to explain that it will include discussion about the abuse suffered by the child. This will help the child to be prepared for the discussion, and prevent him or her from withdrawing when an uncomfortable topic comes up.
- Allow for free flow of talk without too many intensive questions. Do not begin questioning the child immediately about his/her problem.
- Try not to be intimidating authoritarian or too patronizing. Do not control the child's conversation – follow the child's lead.
- Children often lack the vocabulary to discuss sexual acts, and it is important for the counselor to be aware of the child's sensitivities and difficulties before talking about sexual issues with him or her.

Handling Disclosure of Abuse by Child[11,12]

- Believe him or her. The most important thing is to believe the child. Children rarely lie about abuse; what is more common is a child denying that abuse happened when it did. Tell the child you believe him/her.
- Do not be emotionally overwhelmed and try to remain composed while talking to the child.
- Do not interrogate the child. It can be traumatic for the child to repeat his/her story numerous times. Leave the questioning to the legal and police personnel.
- Reassure the child that the abuse is not their fault. Acknowledge that it is difficult to talk about, regard it as a positive step. The child's greatest fear is that he or she is responsible for the abuse. Be sure to make it clear that what happened is not a result of anything he/she did or did not do. This is particularly important when the accused person is a member of the child's family, such as his or her father, and the child feels guilty at having put that person to trouble. Reassure them that prompt and adequate steps will be taken to stop the abuse.

- Do not make promises you cannot keep. Do not make promises such as the child will never have to see the abuser again, that nothing will change, or other such promises like it will be confidential between you and me.
- Believing and supporting the child are two of the best actions to start the healing process. Appropriate and helpful responses to disclosures are as follows:
  a. "I am glad you told me, thank you for trusting me."
  b. "You are very brave and did the right thing."
  c. "It was not your fault."
- Ask the child if he/she has told about it to someone else and what the response were.
- Must ascertain for ongoing abuse and address safety concerns of child.
- Psychological education on safe/unsafe touches, feelings, thoughts and behavior, safer coping techniques can be done at some stage, considering child's emotional state.
- Explain about limitations of confidentiality: The next appropriate step would be to inform the parents and then the concerned authorities. Clinician must inform the child in the initial session that most of what is spoken is confidential but that there may be scenarios in which the clinician may need to set aside confidentiality, and inform the parents, such as in situations of personal neglect, imminent harm to self or others and high-risk behavior, ongoing physical/sexual abuse, all of which may harm or hurt the child.

How to Handle Child's Refusal for Informing Significant Others?

It can be a dilemma between rights to confidentiality of child versus beneficence of child versus therapist's legal duty to inform. In such cases, it is good to explore the reasons or reservations child has. The clinician must also assure the child that as far as possible the nature of this disclosure to the parents will be discussed and agreed upon with the child and done in ways most comfortable to his/her. Such an approach that balances confidentiality and the child's well-being, presented from a perspective of genuine concern that the clinician has for the child safety and is likely to help the child move towards making decisions about disclosure. Upon consent from the child, best to disclose parents in the presence of the child so that she is convinced that the disclosure process was conducted as per her permission and discussions with the clinician.

However, in cases where the child refuses to give consent for disclosure, the clinician might need to override confidentiality for child's safety concern and should inform the child about his/her duty to inform.[12]

Handling Parent's Response on Disclosure

When parents first find out about their children being sexually abused, they will experience a wide range of feelings. They may experience denial, anger, betrayal, confusion and disbelief. Parents often tend to blame themselves for not paying attention to their child's behaviors or complaints earlier on. They may feel that they have failed as parents and they did not protect their children. For some parents, they may wonder why their children did not disclose to them directly but to others. Some parents also become angry at themselves or at their spouses for not supporting the family. In addition to a wide range of emotional experiences, parents may also experience insomnia, change of appetite or other physical complaints.

Some parents also feel conflicting emotions, especially if the accused perpetrator is someone they have trusted, a close friend or a family member. There may be feelings of loyalty and love towards the offending person as well as towards the victim. Family members may choose sides with some believing it happened and others refusing to believe it could have. Parents may disagree about how to handle the situation. If the offender is the spouse or partner of the parent, what the relationship is like can strongly influence the parent's actions once he/she learns of the abuse. If feelings toward the offending spouse/partner are positive or mixed, decisions about staying together, or to divorce or separate will be more difficult to sort through. Parents may be faced with making decisions about whether to continue the relationship with the offender, how to deal with contact between the offender and the child, and re-establishing trust and communication in the family.

The feelings a parent has toward the offender may affect a parents' ability to believe in and support the child. When offenders deny or minimize the abuse or blame the child, the situation gets very complicated. If a parent does not believe a child who has been abused and supports the offender, there can be severe damage to the child. The child will feel betrayed by the parent as well as the offender. What every child victim needs is to be believed and to know that he or she is not at fault. When the parent is able to support and stand up for the child, the child has an excellent chance of recovering from the effects of sexual abuse. It is very important to get help and support for their feelings because parents' reactions make a big difference in children's recovery. Families are children's most important resource for recovery.[11]

Mandatory Reporting

Legal provision: Section 21(1) of the POCSO Act, 2012 requires mandatory reporting of cases of child sexual abuse to the law enforcement authorities, and applies to all individuals who has awareness about the possibility of act including doctors.

Why report?: The purpose of reporting is to identify children suspected to be victims of sexual abuse and to prevent further harm.

Whom to report: Special Protection Juvenile Unit (SPJU), concerned local police station, concerned child welfare committee, child helpline number (1098).

Obligation to inform the child: The POCSO Act does not lay down that a mandatory reporter has the obligation to inform the child and/or his/her parents or guardian about his/her duty to report. However, it is good practice to let them know that this will need to be done. This will help establish an open relationship and minimize the child's feelings of betrayal if a report needs to be made. When possible, discuss the need to make a child abuse report with the family. However, be aware that there are certain situations where if the family is warned about the assessment process, the child may be at risk for further abuse, or the family may leave with the child.

What to report?: Explain, as well as you can, what happened or is happening to the child. Describe the nature of the abuse or neglect and the involved parties.

The reporter is not expected to investigate the matter, know the legal definitions of child abuse and neglect, or even know the name of the perpetrator. This should be left to the police and other investigative agencies.

A report of sexual abuse should contain the following information, if it is known:
- The names and home address of the child and the child's parents or other persons believed to be responsible for the child's care.
- The child's present whereabouts.
- The child's age.
- The nature and extent of the child's injuries, including any evidence of previous injuries.
- The name, age, and condition of other children in the same household.
- Any other information that you believe may be helpful in establishing the cause of the abuse to the child.
- The identity of the person or persons responsible for the abuse or neglect to the child, if known.
- Your name and address.

Legal Sanctions of not Reporting or Falsely Reporting

Failure to Report Child Abuse: The POCSO Act, 2012 provides under Section 21(1) that any person, who fails to report the commission of an offence or who fails to record such offence shall be punished with imprisonment of either description which may extend to 6 months or with fine or with both.

Reporting False Information: The POCSO Act, 2012 makes it an offence to report false information, when such report is made other than in good faith. It states that any person, who makes false complaint or provides false information against any person, solely with the intention to humiliate, extort or threaten or defame him, shall be punished with imprisonment for a term which may extend to 6 months or with fine or with both.[11]

Ethical Dilemma of Reporting

Family's concerns: Families have concern about reporting, being subjected to social humiliation and facing ordeal of long judicial process. Sometimes they may not bring the patient back for treatment also from fear of reporting. Such dilemmas are more when perpetrator is within family or in some cases the sole breadwinner for the family. Clinician can make an attempt of informing family about child-friendly measures of new law, POCSO and the immediate welfare mechanisms inherited in it to help victims and family.

Health professionals concerns: Ethical concern of overriding confidentiality can be there. Also, there is a concern that many adolescents with consensual sexual activity who report for a subsequent psychological distress or for medical termination to hospitals, now may not seek help or may resort to seeking treatment from quacks for fear of reporting.

The answer from legal stand point of view is clear but ethical dilemma will needs fine balancing. But, as per the current law of the land not reporting is a punishable offense.

Inform Family about Child-friendly Provisions of POCSO

- *Burden of proof on the accused:* What makes POCSO special is that it asks us to trust our children. If a child complains of sexual abuse, the law ensures that the pressure is not on the child to prove that the crime took place. Rather, it places the onus squarely on the accused to prove that he/she is innocent. The Court presumes "culpable mental state" (intention, motive, etc.) of the accused.
- *Child-friendly measures for recording statement:* Child need not be taken to police station, rather police personnel, preferable a women not in uniform) has to reach out at a place of child's comfort and convenience for recording the statement to be appointed as "*support person*".
- *Support to the child and family:* POCSO takes into account that handling a sexual offence is not easy for the child and family. So, it makes provisions for experienced and professional individuals who can provide support and guidance in the case.
- *Confidentiality of the child and the family:* The law puts in place measures to secure the confidentiality of the child and family. Disclosing or publishing the identity of the child by mentioning name, address, neighborhood, school name and other particulars is punishable under POCSO. It also covers making of negative reports that cause harm to the child's reputation.
- *Speedy procedures:* Act requires that the evidence of the child is recorded by the Special Court within 30 days of taking cognizance of the offence. Any delay must be explained in writing. As far as possible, the trial should be completed in a year's time.
- *Compensation:* A child victim may receive interim compensation for immediate need for relief or rehabilitation and final compensation for the loss or injury caused to him or her. Compensation is given irrespective of whether the accused is found guilty or not.
- *Free legal aid:* Under Section 12(c) of the Legal Services Authorities Act, 1987, every child who has to file or defend a case shall be entitled to legal services under this Act. The POCSO Act, 2012 confirms the right to free legal aid under section 40, providing that the child or his/her family shall be entitled to a legal counsel of their choice, and that where they are unable to afford such counsel, they shall be entitled to receive one from the Legal Services Authority. In every District, a District Legal Services Authority has been constituted to implement the Legal Services Programs in the District. The District Legal Services Authority is usually situated in the District Courts Complex in every District and chaired by the District Judge of the respective district.[11]

Forensic Interviewing: Liasioning with Legal Agencies as Child Development Expert[11]

- If possible, a primary case worker from hospital should accompany the child in all referrals, procedures and enquiries and be a familiar, consistent figure in the process to avoid re-victimization at different point of time. However, due to manpower constrain it may not be possible in all situations.

CHAPTER 24: Medicolegal Approach for Management of Victims of Child Sexual Abuse

- Clinician may aid police in conducting forensic interview in order to prevent re-traumatization and this interview can be embedded in the therapeutic process.
- Liasion between clinical team, police and CWC can be ideal situation, though difficult to achieve in individual clinic based systems.

Clinicians Assisting Forensic Interviewing

- *What it is:* It is a non-therapeutic interview done by law officials or forensic psychiatrist who is not the therapist with goal of obtaining statement from child in a developmentally-sensitive, unbiased and truth-seeking manner to support fair decision-making.
- *Role of mental health professional*: Absence of sufficient trained manpower in India and sometimes due to clinical urgencies, treating clinician may consider doing forensic interview to reduce further trauma through multiple or unskilled interviewing. Also for cases with "special needs" including mental disability, following provisions exist in POCSO:
    - Court can order "child development expert" to assist in forensic interviewing. As per the POCSO Act, 2012, Rule 2(c) states: *"Expert" means a person trained in mental health, medicine, child development or other related discipline, who may be required to facilitate communication with a child whose ability to communicate has been affected by trauma, disability or any other vulnerability.*
    - Section 26(3) states, *"the Magistrate or the police officer, as the case may be, may, in the case of a child having a mental or physical disability, seek the assistance of a special educator or any person familiar with the manner of communication of the child or an expert in that field, having such qualifications, experience and on payment of such fees as may be prescribed, to record the statement of the child.*
    - Section 38(2) states, *"if a child has a mental or physical disability, the Special Court may take the assistance of a special educator or any person familiar with the manner of communication of the child or an expert in that field, having such qualifications, experience and on payment of such fees as may be prescribed to record the evidence of the child".* Thus, the Act envisages a role for child development experts (like a child psychiatrist or concerned treating mental health professional) at the stage of taking evidence from the child and recording his/her statement for the purpose of investigation and trial under the Act. The role of this expert is to facilitate communication between the child and the authority concerned.
- No uniform forensic interview protocol is approved in India, The Cornerhouse Forensic Interview Protocol or National Institute of Child Health and Human Development Protocol may be adopted.
- Consider using dolls or human body diagrams to aid interview for younger children. Use of videos and storybook should be avoided, it can increase suggestibility.

Ethical dilemma in forensic interviewing: Clinician is surrounded by dilemma of re-traumatizing the child in such interviews versus bringing legal justice. In such instances, the clinician may need to follow the principle of "Primum non nocere"– First, do no harm. The most important goal cannot be to obtain the all or accurate the details of the abuse but to understand the effects on the child and help in management of the consequences. Thus, even when the clinician does take on an investigator's role, in circumstances where the child responds to the investigation with extreme distress, the decision to continue with questioning should be guided by the child's best interests in terms of his/her psychosocial and mental health.

CAPACITY ASSESSMENT AS ASKED BY COURT REGARDING VICTIMS OF SEXUAL VIOLENCE

The legal test of capacity for persons with mental health issues can be seen in 2 parts:
Part 1: Presence of a mental disorder
Part 2: "Impairment of Capacity": the person must be unable to do any one of the following:
- Understand the information relevant to the decision
- Remember the information relevant to the decision
- Weigh up the information - consider the advantages and disadvantages, risks and benefits of saying "yes" or "no"
- Be able to communicate their decision (by whatever means they are able to use to communicate.[13]

Usually Assessment regarding capacity of victims to give evidence or statement in court (competence to give evidence) is asked by court of law:

"The law states that all people are competent to give evidence. Competent in this context means 'lawfully able to give evidence'. This is the starting point from which all witnesses should be assessed when prosecutors are considering their evidence.

A witness is not competent to give evidence if he/she:
- Is not able to understand questions put to him/her as a witness
- And give answers to those questions which can be understood."

(Indian Evidence Act section 118 states that "All persons shall be competent to testify unless the Court considers that they are prevented from understanding the questions put to them, or from giving rational answers to those questions, by tender years, extreme old age, disease, whether of body or mind, or any other cause of the same kind. (Explanation. -- A lunatic is not incompetent to testify, unless he is prevented by his lunacy from understanding the questions put to him and giving rational answers to them)"[14]

- Mental health assessment for fitness to give statement should focus on:
  – How might the nature or extent of the witness's mental health condition affect his/her ability to give evidence: Could the nature or extent of the witness's mental health condition affect his/her:
    • Understanding
    • Perception or
    • Recollection of an incident? as assessed by following:
      - Ability to recall and accurately interpret events;
      - Ability to consistently tell the events;
      - Quality of short- and long-term memory;[13]

CHAPTER 24: Medicolegal Approach for Management of Victims of Child Sexual Abuse

- How might the nature or extent of the witness's mental health condition affect his/her ability to withstand cross-examination, particularly with reference to:
  - Response to questioning and cross examination;
  - Concentration and attention;
  - Ability to communicate; and
  - Interaction with other people.[13]
    - Additional assessment of supportive measures to address impact of evidence giving on person's mental health:

Special measures: Likelihood of impact of evidence giving on person's mental health and need of any support measures to decrease this likelihood that needed to be communicated to judiciary accordingly like:

- Giving evidence in private—particularly where sensitive personal or medical information is being disclosed;
- Removal of wigs and gowns—which may reduce the risk of a witness becoming anxious, distressed or experiencing feelings of paranoia or panic;
- Use of intermediaries as support persons—to assist with interpreting questions and answers appropriately.
- Asking the Judge or Magistrates to allow witnesses to take regular comfort breaks.[14]

MANAGEMENT

Child sexual abuse (CSA) is an experience not a disorder, so, there cannot be a one shoe fit all approach for treatment. Response to CSA is highly variable and depends on several factors enlisted above. Which specific therapy will be effective and is there any role of preventive therapy, is difficult to answer. In general encouraging expression of feelings about abuse, clarifying misconceptions, teaching prevention skills and diminishing the sense of stigma and isolation in victims should be targeted.[15]

CONCLUSION

Child sexual abuse is a complex phenomenon with long-lasting impact. Some of the aspects of management are challenging and ethically thought provoking. Mental health professional must take child's best interest as central view and then should try to balance expectations of legal, medical, familial and social interests.

REFERENCES

1. Geneva: World Health Organisation (WHO); child maltreatment. Available from: http://www.who.int/topics/child_abuse/en/ [Last accessed on 04-03-2018].
2. Childline organisation. Childline 1098 service. Available from: http://www.childlineindia.org.in/1098/1098.htm [Last accessed on 04-05-2015].
3. 42% of Indian girls are sexually abused before 19: UNICEF. The Times of India. 2014. Sep 12, Available from: http://timesofindia.indiatimes.com/india/42-of- Indian-girls-are-sexually-abused-before-19-Unicef/ article show/42306348.cms? [Last accessed on 04-03-2018].

4. Study on Child Abuse: India 2007. India, Ministry of Women and Child development Government of India. 2007. Available from: wcd.nic.in/childabuse.pdf. [Last accessed on 04-03-2018].
5. Singh MM, Parsekar SS, Nair NS. An epidemiological overview of child sexual abuse. Journal of Family Medicine and Primary Care. 2014;3(4):430-5.
6. Guidelines & protocols for medico-legal care for survivors/victims of sexual violence. Ministry of Health and Family Welfare, Government of India. Available at: http://www.mohfw.nic.in/showfile.php?lid=2737. [Last accessed on 04-03-2018].
7. Yaduvanshi R, Agarwal A, Mohapatra S. Child sexual abuse and traumatic sexualization. In: Kar SK, Mishra SR (Eds). Sexual Assault and Life Beyond. Indian Institute of Sexology, Midyear Publication June 2015.
8. Finkelhor D, Browne A. The traumatic impact of child sexual abuse: a conceptualization. Am J Orthopsychiatry. 1985;55(4):530-41.
9. Senn TE, Carey MP, Coury-Doniger P. Mediators of the relation between childhood sexual abuse and women's sexual risk behavior: a comparison of two theoretical frameworks: Arch Sex Behav. 2012;41(6):1363-77.
10. Kukreti P, Kishore J, Tanwar R. Psychological and medicolegal aspects of management of sexual assault: Indian perspective. International Journal of Health Sciences & Research. 2016;6(4):507-15.
11. Model Guidelines under Section 39 of The Protection of Children from Sexual Offences Act, 2012. Guidelines for the Use of Professionals and Experts under the POCSO Act, 2012. Ministry of women and child development. Government of India. September 2013.
12. Bhaskaran S, Sheshadri SP. Child sexual abuse- clinical challenges and practical recommendations. J Indian Assoc Child Adolesc. Ment. Health 2016;12(2):143-61.
13. Joyce T. Assessing capacity to consent and to give evidence. Estia Centre; South London & Maudsley NHS Trust, London, UK. Available at: www.nomasabuso.com/wp-content/uploads/2012/06/theresa_joyce_1Ponencia8.pdf. Last accessed on 7 February 2018.
14. The Indian Evidence Act 1872, Act No. 1 of 1872. Available at: ncw.nic.in/Acts/The Indian Evidence Act 1872.pdf. Last accessed on 7 February 2018.
15. Finkelhor D, Berliner L. Research on the treatment of sexually abused children: a review and recommendations. J Am Acad Child Adolesc Psychiatry [Internet]. 1995 Nov [cited 2014;34(11):1408-23. Available from: http://www.ncbi.nlm.nih.gov/pubmed/8543508.

SECTION VII
Legal Statutes of Relevance to Mental Health

CHAPTER 25

Mental Healthcare Act, 2017

> **LEARNING OBJECTIVES**
> - Indian Lunacy Act (ILA), 1912
> - Mental Health Act (MHA), 1987
> - UN Convention on Rights of Persons with Disabilities
> - Salient features of Mental Healthcare Act, 2017
> - New concepts in Health Care Act
> - Advance directive
> - Nominated representative
> - Regulatory agencies: Authorities and Board
> - Specifics of registering and running mental health establishment
> - Rights of persons with mental illness
> - Basic medical record and right to access records
> - Admission treatment discharge procedures
> - Implications for research on persons with mental illness

NEED FOR LEGISLATION IN MENTAL HEALTH: CHALLENGES AND SPECIAL ISSUES CONCERNING MENTALLY ILL[1]

Mentally ill people are often victims of abuse, cruelty and neglect with their legitimate rights violated. Legislation therefore comes to their rescue and provides a safeguard against such atrocities. However, legislation if not in accordance with the riding principles of equal rights and dignity can worsen the stigma associated with such illnesses giving them a judicial fervor than a medical one.

The need for mental health legislation also arises with a better understanding of the heavy burden of mental illness on peoples' personal, social, and economic lives. Mental disorders account for a high proportion of all disability adjusted life years lost, and this burden is predicted to grow significantly, in the future. In addition, the hidden burden of stigma and discrimination further leads to deterioration in their condition. Therefore, legislation plays an important role in providing a legal framework for addressing critical issues such as:

1. Community integration of persons with mental disorders
2. Provision of high quality care, improvement of access to care
3. Protection of civil rights, promotion of rights to housing, education and employment.

History of Mental Health Laws in India

India's first Lunacy Act (Act 36) drafted in 1858 came with the guidelines to establish mental asylums and procedures to admit patients, which was replaced by the Indian Lunacy Act (ILA) (Act 4) 1912. The period postindependence saw tremendous growth in health services and a paradigm shift in the management of mentally ill, moving from captivity to community integration. The main focus of concern remained the lack of infrastructure and manpower. In view of limited resources, integration of mental health with primary health care services was considered the solution to the growing problems of mental illness and substance abuse.

The dawn of the new era was brought by the replacement of the ILA 1912 with MHA 1987 and the enactment of the Persons with Disabilities Act, 1995 which brought forward the concept of equal opportunities, rights and full participation of disabled persons and included mental illness under the broader ambit of disability. Another key development that has affected the growth of legislation in psychiatry has been the development of private psychiatry in a big way and problems associated with the regulation of provision of services.

It is of crucial interest to understand the salient features of the previous legislations and their limitations for understanding led to the culmination of the Mental Healthcare Act, 2017.

1. *Indian Lunacy Act (ILA), 1912*: The purpose of this Act was to ensure custodial care and to prevent harm to the society, which reflected the general perception of mental illness at that time. There was no provision of treatment, protection of rights or provision of welfare, and there was no time limit specified for involuntary admissions. The draconian law prevailed for more than seventy five-years and could not keep pace with the fast occurring developments in the field of psychiatry.[2]
2. *The Mental Health Act (MHA), 1987*: MHA 1987 spread in 10 chapters and 98 sections came as a result of mammoth efforts of India's mental health professionals. It was a step towards the treatment centric paradigm of psychiatry and renamed mental hospitals as psychiatric hospitals/nursing home attempting to bring mental illnesses at par with physical illnesses.[3]

Creation of Mental Health Authorities, provision of judicial safeguard for human rights and property, were the important aspects of the Act. However, it did not promote community mental health care or integration with primary health care and neither made provisions of rehabilitation or choice and consent for treatment.

Mental Healthcare Act (MHCA), 2017[4]

Mental Healthcare Act provides for mental healthcare and services for persons with mental illness and to protect, promote and fulfill the rights of such persons during delivery of mental healthcare and services and for matters connected. It is divided into 16 chapters and 126 sections **(Table 1)**.

Table 1: Provisions of Mental Healthcare Act.

Chapter number	Heading	Salient features
I	Preliminary	Definitions of various terminologies used in the Act
II	Mental illness and capacity to make mental healthcare and treatment decisions	Directions regarding the diagnosis of mental illness; capacity to make decisions
III	Advance directive	Description of advance directive, its making, and provision of online register for recordkeeping
IV	Nominated representative	Description of the appointment, revocation and duties of the nominated representative
V	Rights of persons with mental illness	Enlist the basic rights of persons with mental illness and directs the government to make provisions regarding their fulfillment
VI	Duties of appropriate government	Entails the duties of the appropriate government
VII	Central mental health authority	Describes the composition and functions of the central mental health authority
VIII	State mental health authority	Describes the composition and functions of the state mental health authority
IX	Finance, accounts and audit	Describes the grants by the central government and use of funds by the central authority
X	Mental health establishments	Procedure for Registration of mental health establishments, inspection and inquiry and provisions of their adequate functioning
XI	Mental health review boards	Composition and functions of the mental health review board and judiciary powers
XII	Admission, treatment and discharge	Describes the admission procedures, emergency and prohibitory treatment modalities.
XIII	Responsibilities of other agencies	Outlines the duties of police officers in regards to the wandering persons with mental illness and suspected neglect of such persons; prisoners with mental illness
XIV	Restriction to discharge functions by professionals not covered by profession	Limitations of the professionals to work under the act and principles of ethical evidence based treatments.
XV	Offences and penalties	Describes the offences and penalties in contravention to the act
XVI	Miscellaneous	Deals with locus of power, special provision for neglected areas, decriminalizing suicide and laying of rules and regulations

IMPLICATIONS OF MENTAL HEALTHCARE ACT (MHCA), 2017 IN CLINICAL PRACTICE

Need of New Act

United Nations adopted Convention on Rights of Persons with Disabilities (CRPD) and its Optional Protocol on 13th December, 2006 and it came into force on the 3rd May, 2008.

India signed and ratified the said Convention on the 1st day of October, 2007; and it was needed to harmonize existing laws in synchrony with it.

Aim of the Act: An Act to provide following during delivery of mental healthcare and services and for matters connected therewith or incidental thereto:
- Mental healthcare and services for persons with mental illness and
- To protect, promote and fulfill the rights of such persons.

Official Enactment

- Received the assent of the President on 7th April, 2017
- It came into force on 29 May, 2018

Scope: It extends to whole of India.

Basic Definitions

I. What is mental health care and mental illness?
   - **"Mental healthcare (MHC)"** refers to any of the following being done for any person's **mental illness** or **suspected mental illness:**
     - Analysis and **diagnosis** of a person's mental condition and
     - **Treatment** as well as
     - **Care** and
     - **Rehabilitation** of (Chapter I, Section 2)
   - **"Mental illness"** means a **substantial disorder** of thinking, mood, perception, orientation or memory that **grossly impairs judgment, behavior, capacity to recognize reality or ability to meet the ordinary demands of life**. It **includes** mental conditions associated with the **abuse of alcohol and drugs**, but **excludes mental retardation (Chapter I, Section 2).**

II. MHCA is applicable on whom all?
   - It is applicable on all mental health establishments as detailed below:
     - **"Mental health establishment (MHE)"** refers to: (Chapter I, Section 2)
       - Any health establishment, **including Ayurveda, Yoga and Naturopathy, Unani, Sidha and Homoeopathy (AYUSH)** establishment,
       - Where persons with mental illness are **admitted and reside at/kept in**,
       - For **care, treatment, convalescence and rehabilitation**,
       - **Either temporarily or otherwise**;
       - Includes any general hospital or general nursing home
       - Whether private or public

(But does not include a family residential place where a person with mental illness resides with his relatives or friends)
- (Chapter X, Section 65) State mental health authority (SMHA) will classify MHEs into different category as specified in Central Authority regulations.

III. Who all as professionals can be involved in mental health care service delivery?
- **"Mental health professionals (MHP)"** (Chapter I section 2)
  - *Psychiatrist:* **Postgraduate degree** (MD/DPM/DNB) in Psychiatry from **any of the AYUSH** disciplines from recognized universities (approved by UGC, NBE, MCI), **registered** in state council
  - *Clinical Psychologist:* **Postgraduate degree** in Psychology/Clinical Psychology/Applied Psychology **or MPhil** in Clinical Psychology/Medical psychology/Social Psychology following a **full time** 2-year **course** including Clinical training; **recognized** and approved by **UGC** Act, 1956 and **RCI** Act,1992
  - *Psychiatric Social Worker:* **Postgraduate degree** in Social work or MPhil in PSW following a **full time** 2-year **course** including Clinical training; **recognized** and approved by **UGC** Act, 1956
  - *Mental Health Nurse:* **Diploma or degree** in **General nursing/ Psychiatric nursing** recognized by the **NCI** and **registered** with the relevant State nursing council
- **"Other medical professionals"** (Chapter VI, Section 31): The appropriate Government shall, at the minimum, train all medical officers in public healthcare establishments and in prisons to provide basic and emergency mental healthcare.
- **Duty of above mentioned professionals to adhere to functions authorized by the Act**
  - **Restriction to discharge functions by professionals not covered by profession** (Chapter XIV, Section 106) "No mental health professional or medical practitioner shall discharge any duty or perform any function not authorized by this Act or specify or recommend any medicine or treatment not authorized by the field of his profession."

CERTAIN NEW CONCEPTS OF CLINICAL RELEVANCE IN MHCA

Capacity Assessment (Chapter II, Section 4)

Assessment of Capacity to Make Mental Health Care and Treatment Related Decision

Capacity to make decisions regarding his mental healthcare or treatment refers to **ability to:**
a. **Understand the information** that is relevant to take a decision on the treatment or admission or personal assistance; or
b. **Appreciate** any reasonably **foreseeable consequence of a decision or lack of decision** on the treatment or admission or personal assistance; or
c. **Communicate the decision** under sub-clause (a) by means of speech, expression, gesture or any other means.

Central mental health authority (CMHA) expert committee will bring guideline on its operationalization.

Advance Directive (AD)

What it is: A document expressing the way one wishes to receive or not receive mental health care or treatment and the individuals one wants to appoint as Nominated representative (NR) in order of precedence (Chapter III, Section 5).

Who Can Make Advance Directive?

- Any major who has capacity to make mental health care and treatment related decision can make Advance directive (Chapter III, Section 5)
- The legal guardian shall have right to make an advance directive in writing in respect of a minor and all the provisions relating to advance directive, mutatis mutandis, shall apply to such minor till such time he attains majority. (Chapter III, Section 11 (4)).

Procedure of making/revoking AD: Operationalization and validity shall be notified by CMHA rules.

When it comes into action or is evoked: Once person ceases to have capacity to make mental health care and treatment related decision

Remain effective only till: Person regains capacity

Can it be changed: Can be changed any number of times

AB initio void: If made contrary to any existing law.

How Can a MHP/MHE Access Advance Directive?

- The **person writing the advance directive** and his **nominated representative** shall have a duty to ensure that the Medical officer in charge of MHE, Medical practitioner or MHP, has access to AD when required (Chapter III, Section 11(3)).
- Section 91, every **Board** shall maintain **online register** of all ADs registered with it and make them available to concerned MHP as required.

What is Liability of MHP/MHE in Relation to Advance Directive?

- Chapter III Section 10 states that it shall be the duty of every medical officer in charge of a mental health establishment and the psychiatrist in charge of a person's treatment to propose or give treatment to a person with mental illness, in accordance with his valid advance directive
- A mental health professional or a relative or a caregiver of a person, if do not wish to follow AD, they can apply to Mental Health Review Board (MHRB), then possibility of following situations is explored regarding AD
    a. Whether the advance directive was made by the person out of his own free will and free from force, undue influence or coercion; or
    b. Whether the person intended the advance directive to apply to the present circumstances, which may be different from those anticipated; or

c. Whether the person was sufficiently well informed to make the decision; or
  d. Whether the person had capacity to make decisions relating to his mental healthcare or treatment when such advanced directive was made; or
  e. Whether the content of the advance directive is contrary to other laws or constitutional provisions.

What is Liability of MHP in Relation to AD?

- Duty bound to follow AD (Chapter III Section 10)
- A medical practitioner or a mental health professional shall not be held liable for any unforeseen consequences on following a valid advance directive Chapter III section 13(1).
- The medical practitioner or mental health professional shall not be held liable for not following a valid advance directive, if he has not been given a copy of the valid advance directive [Chapter III, Section 13 (2)].

Nominated Representative (NR)

Who can appoint NR?: Any major person (Chapter IV, Section 14)

Who can be appointed as NR?:

- Any major person as per wish of persons making NR (Chapter IV, Section 14)
- Who is competent to discharge the duties or perform the functions assigned to him under this Act, (Chapter IV, Section 14)?
- Who gives his consent in writing to the mental health professional to discharge his duties under this Act. (Chapter IV, Section 14)?
- Guardians are NR for minors unless the board decides otherwise (Chapter IV, Section 15)
- Any appointed NR may revoke or alter such appointment at any time (Chapter IV, Section 15).

How can NR be made?: Nomination shall be made in writing on plain paper with the person's signature or thumb impression of the person referred (Chapter IV Section 14).

What to do Where no NR has been Appointed?

The following persons for the purposes of this Act in the order of precedence shall be deemed to be NR:
a. A relative
b. A caregiver,
c. A suitable person appointed as such by the concerned Board; or
d. If no such person is available, the Board shall appoint the Director, Department of Social Welfare, or his designated representative, as NR.

Pending such appointment by a board, MHP can engage temporarily any person from a registered society working for persons with mental illness and willing to volunteer their inclination in written (Chapter IV, Section 14).

Can NR be Revoked?

The Board, on an application made to it by the person with mental illness, or by a relative of such person, or by the psychiatrist responsible for the care of such person, or by the medical officer in-charge of the mental health establishment where the individual is admitted or proposed to be admitted, may revoke, alter or modify if it feels NR is not acting in best interest of person or is not fit to discharge duties or is not willing (Chapter IV Section 16).

Duties of NR

a. Consider the current and past wishes, the life history, values, cultural background and the best interests of the person with mental illness;
b. Give particular credence to the views of the person with mental illness to the extent that the person understands the nature of the decisions under consideration;
c. Provide support to the person with mental illness in making treatment decisions in high support admissions;
d. Have right to seek information on diagnosis and treatment to provide adequate support to the person with mental illness;
e. Have access to the family or home based rehabilitation services on behalf of and for the benefit of the person with mental illness;
f. Be involved in discharge planning
g. Apply to the mental health establishment for admission;
h. Apply to the concerned Board on behalf of the person with mental illness for discharge;
i. Apply to the concerned Board against violation of rights of the person with mental illness in a mental health establishment;
j. Appoint a suitable attendant
k. Have the right to give or withhold consent for research.

MONITORING AND REGULATORY AGENCIES IN MHCA

Central Mental Health Authority (CMHA) and its Functions

Chapter VII, Section 43. The Central Authority shall:
a. Register all mental health establishments under the control of the Central Government and maintain a register of all mental health establishments in the country based on information provided by all State Mental Health Authorities of registered establishments and compile update and publish (including online on the internet) a register of such establishments;
b. Develop quality and service provision norms for different types of mental health establishments under the Central Government;
c. Supervise all mental health establishments under the Central Government and receive complaints about deficiencies in provision of services;
d. Maintain a national register of clinical psychologists, mental health nurses and psychiatric social workers based on information provided by all State Authorities of persons registered to work as mental health professionals for the purpose of this Act and publish the list (including online on the internet) of such registered mental health professionals;

e. Train all persons including law enforcement officials, mental health professionals and other health professionals about the provisions and implementation of this Act;
f. Advise the Central Government on all matters relating to mental healthcare and services;
g. Discharge such other functions with respect to matters relating to mental health as the Central Government may decide.

State Mental Health Authority (SMHA) and its Functions

Chapter VIII, Section 55. The State Authority shall:
a. Register all mental health establishments in the State except those referred above and maintain and publish (including online on the internet) a register of such establishments;
b. Develop quality and service provision norms for different types of mental health establishments in the State;
c. Supervise all mental health establishments in the State and receive complaints about deficiencies in provision of services;
d. Register clinical psychologists, mental health nurses and psychiatric social workers in the State to work as mental health professionals, and publish the list of such registered mental health professionals in such manner as may be specified by regulations by the State Authority;
e. Train all relevant persons including law enforcement officials, mental health professionals and other health professionals about the provisions and implementation of this Act;
f. Discharge such other functions with respect to matters relating to mental health as the State Government may decide:

Mental Health Review Board (MHRB)

Chapter XI, Section 73/74 states: Mental health review board will be a quasi judicial board appointed by SMHA.

Power and Functions of MHRB

a. To register, review, alter, modify or cancel an advance directive;
b. To appoint a nominated representative;
c. To receive and decide application from a person with mental illness or his nominated representative or any other interested person against the decision of medical officer or mental health professional in-charge of mental health establishment or mental health establishment under Section 87 or Section 89 or Section 90;
d. To receive and decide applications in respect non-disclosure of information
e. To adjudicate complaints regarding deficiencies in care and services
f. To visit and inspect prison or jails and seek clarifications from the medical officer in-charge of health services in such prison or jail.

Constitution of MHRB

a. A District Judge/officer of the State judicial services/retired District Judge (chairperson)
b. Representative of District Collector/Magistrate/Deputy Commissioner

c. Two members of whom **1 psychiatrist** and the other a medical practitioner.
d. Two members PMI/Caregivers/member of organizations of PMI or Caregivers or NGOs working in this field.

There can be 1 review board for many districts or vice versa as per need of district

CMHA Rules 2018, Chapter V, Section 17 states that at least one Board shall be constituted for a district and where it is not feasible, one Board for a group of two or more districts, not exceeding three districts, in the State.[5]

SPECIFICS OF ESTABLISHING OR MAINTAINING A MENTAL HEALTH ESTABLISHMENT

- *Minimum standards for different categories of mental health establishments:* Chapter X, Section 65) State mental health authority (SMHA) will classify MHEs into different category as specified in Central Authority regulations and within eighteen months from the commencement of this Act will specify minimum standards for different categories of mental health establishments
- Qualifications of mental health professionals to be in accordance with Act
- *Registration of mental health establishment:* (Chapter X, Section 65). Every person or organization who proposes to establish/run a MHE shall register with Central mental health authority, i.e. CMHA (central government MHE)/State mental health authority i.e. SMHA (all state government MHE and other MHEs in state)
  – (Exception: Central Government, may, by notification, exempt any category or class of existing mental health establishments from the requirement of registration)
- Penalty on running unregistered MHE or working in it **(Table 2)**.

Table 2: Penalty for running or working in unregistered MHE.

Chapter XV, Section 107	1st Contravention	2nd Contravention	Every subsequent contravention
Running MHE without registration	₹ 5–50,000	₹ 50,000–2 Lac	₹ 2–5 Lac
Knowingly working in a mental health professional in unregistered MHE: ₹ 25,000			

  – Registration: Whom to apply, When to apply, What to expect

Whom to apply
- All central government MHE to apply to Central mental health authority i.e. CMHA in form B of CMHA Rules with demand draft of ₹ 20,000 drawn in favor of the Chairperson, Central Mental Health Authority payable at New Delhi ("The Mental Healthcare (Central Mental Health Authority and Mental Health Review Boards) Rules, 2018" Chapter III, Section 11)[5]
- All state government MHE and any other non-governmental MHEs of the state to apply to State mental health authority i.e. SMHA in form B of SMHA Rules with demand draft of ₹ 20,000 drawn in favor of the Chairperson, State Mental Health Authority payable at the place where the State Authority is situated ("The Mental Healthcare (State Mental Health Authority) Rules, 2018", Chapter III, Section 11).[6]

When to apply (Chapter X, Section 66)
- Every MHE existing on date of commencement of Act, shall apply for **provisional registration** within 6 months of constitution of Authority.

What to expect (Chapter X, Section 66)
Provisional registration
- Within 10 days, SMHA will issue Provisional registration without any inspection.
- Within 45 days, name and details of MHE on SMHA website
- Provisional registration is valid for 12 months
- Till rules are laid by SMHA for requirement of minimum standards for different categories of MHEs, provisional registration renewal has to be done within 30 days of expiry of previous provisional registration
- In case of delay, MHE shall be liable to pay the renewal fee of ₹ 20,000 to respective mental health authority (MHA) (CMHA Rules 2018 Chapter III, Section 11 and SMHA Rules 2018 Chapter III, Section 11).[5,6]

Permanent registration: Once rules are laid for requirement of minimum standards for different categories of MHEs, one can apply for permanent registration to respective authorities with evidence of MHE fulfilling those standards.
- If MHA on enquiry agrees, permanent registration given, valid for 3 years
- If files objection to application—It shall give public notice and display the same on its website for a period of thirty days for filing objections
- MHE has to submit compliance
- After receiving compliance, MHA has to give decision within 45 days of either granting permanent registration or rejection
- If compliance is found unacceptable by MHA—6 months given to MHE for rectification.

In case of change of ownership of MHE
- Registration remains valid for that MHE—Informed MHA within 1 month about change.

In case of change of category of MHE
- In case of change of category—Fresh registration has to be applied for.

Audit and Inquiry/Inspection of MHES: Continuous Duty to Maintain Standards

Audit and Process of Inquiry
1. *Audit in routine course:* Every 3 year to ensure standards of registration are met with
- Audit Fee: ₹ 10,000 to be paid to respective MHA
- Audit team will comprise of one or more of following:
    a. A representative of the District Collector or District Commissioner of the district where the mental health establishment is situated;
    b. A representative of the State Human Rights Commission of the State where the mental health establishment is situated;

c. A Psychiatrist who is in Government service;
  d. A Psychiatrist who is in private practice;
  e. A mental health professional who is not a psychiatrist;
  f. A representative of a non-governmental organization working in the area of mental health;
  g. Representatives of the caregivers of persons with mental illness or organizations representing caregivers; and
  h. Representatives of the persons who have or have had mental illness.
2. **Inspection and inquiry of MHE after show cause notice or as suo moto action**:
   - If MHE fails to maintain minimum standards
   - Management official of MHE convicted of any offence under MHCA
   - Violation of rights of persons with mental illness happening in MHE.

   Inspection team: It will be conducted by committee of one or more of following:
   a. A Psychiatrist in Government service;
   b. A Psychiatrist in private practice;
   c. A mental health professional who is not a psychiatrist; ,
   d. A representative of non-governmental organization working in the area of mental health;
   e. A police officer in-charge of the police station under whose jurisdiction, the mental health establishment is situated;
   f. A representative of the District Collector or District Commissioner of the district where the mental health establishment is situated.

Reporting of Audit/Inquiry

- Within two days of Audit/Inquiry, report is submitted to Chairperson of respective MHA and chairperson can take suitable action against MHE as per norms of Act
- The Authority shall communicate to the mental health establishment the results of audit and after ascertaining the opinion of MHE may suggest suitable changes—If MHE fails to follow it, may lead to cancellation of registration.

Right to Appeal to High Court

Any MHE aggrieved by any order of MHA refusing to grant registration or renewal of registration or cancellation of registration, may appeal to respective High Court within 30 days of such order.

RIGHTS OF PERSONS WITH MENTAL ILLNESS THAT MENTAL HEALTH ESTABLISHMENTS MUST SAFEGUARD[7]

Right to Access to Health

- As per Chapter V, Section 18 every individual has right to access to mental healthcare in every district. If there is no public MHE in a district where a person with mental illness resides, government will bear the costs of treatment at such establishments in that district

- The Mental Healthcare (Rights of Persons with Mental Illness) Rules, 2018 Chapter II Section 5 states that person can apply to Chief Medical Officer (CMO) of such District for reimbursement of costs of treatment. CMO shall examine the application and issue an order to reimburse such costs by the officer in-charge of the Directorate of Health Services of that State Government.[7]

Right to Protection from Cruel, Inhuman and Degrading Treatment (Chapter V, Section 20)

Ensure infrastructure of organization is conducive to safeguard following rights of person with mental illness:
a. Right to live in safe and hygienic environment;
b. To have adequate sanitary conditions;
c. To have reasonable facilities for leisure, recreation, education and religious practices;
d. To privacy
e. For proper clothing so as to protect such person from exposure of his body to maintain his dignity;
f. To not be forced to undertake work in a mental health establishment and to receive appropriate remuneration for work when undertaken;
g. To have adequate provision for preparing for living in the community;
h. To have adequate provision for wholesome food, sanitation, space and access to articles of personal hygiene, in particular, women's personal hygiene be adequately addressed by providing access to items that may be required during menstruation;
i. To not be subject to compulsory tonsuring (shaving of head hair);
j. To wear own personal clothes if so wished and to not be forced to wear uniforms provided by the establishment; and
k. To be protected from all forms of physical, verbal, emotional and sexual abuse.

Right to Equality and Non-discrimination

Ensure no discrimination happens in MHE on basis of gender, sex, sexual orientation, religion, culture, caste, social or political beliefs, or disability.

Ensure within MHE, every person with mental illness shall be treated as equal to persons with physical illness in terms of following healthcare service delivery provision:
a. Quality and availability of emergency facilities and emergency services
b. Extent and quality of use of ambulance services
c. Manner and extent of living conditions in health establishments and
d. Manner, extent and quality of any other health services provided (Chapter V, Section 21).

Right to Information

At time of admission, MHP is duty bound to inform person with mental illness/ NR about:
- Diagnosis, nature of illness, section of admission
- Proposed treatment plan, anticipated side effects

- Right about appealing against admission to Board with contact details of board members and forms
- Right to complaint about any deficiency in services to in-charge MHE/SMHA/Board If any information when withheld → MHE. MHP must inform Board citing reasons (Chapter V, Section 22).

Right to Confidentiality

All health professionals shall have a duty to keep all such information confidential which has been obtained during care or treatment with the following exceptions, namely:
a. Release of information to the nominated representative to enable him to fulfill his duties under this Act;
b. Release of information to other mental health professionals and other health professionals for care and treatment;
c. Release of information if it is necessary to protect any other person from harm or violence;
d. Only such information that is necessary to protect against the harm identified shall be released;
e. Release only such information as is necessary to prevent threat to life;
f. Release of information upon an order by concerned Board or the Central Authority or High Court or Supreme Court or any other statutory authority competent
g. Release of information in the interests of public safety and security. (Chapter V, Section 23).

Right to Restriction on Release of Information in Respect of Mental Illness

(1) No photograph or any other information relating to a person with mental illness undergoing treatment at a mental health establishment shall be released to the media without the consent of the person with mental illness.
(2) The right to confidentiality of person with mental illness shall also apply to all information stored in electronic or digital format in real or virtual space (Chapter V, Section 24).

Right to Access Medical Records

- All persons with mental illness shall have the right to access their basic medical records. . (Chapter V, Section 25)
- The mental health professional in-charge of such records may withhold specific information in the medical records if disclosure would result in:
    a. Serious mental harm to the person with mental illness; or
    b. Likelihood of harm to other persons (Chapter V, Section 25)
        - When any information in the medical records is withheld from the person, the mental health professional shall inform the person with mental illness of his right to apply to the concerned Board for an order to release such information (Chapter V, Section 25).

"The Mental Healthcare (Rights of Persons with Mental Illness) Rules, 2018" Chapter II Section 6 states that:
- A person with mental illness, shall be entitled to receive documented medical information pertaining to his diagnosis, investigation, assessment and treatment as per the medical records.
- A person with mental illness may apply for a copy of his **basic in-patient medical record** by making a **request in writing in Form-A,** addressed to the medical officer or mental health professional in-charge of the concerned mental health establishment
- **Within fifteen days** from the date of receipt of the request, basic inpatient medical **record**s shall be **provided to the applicant in Form**-B.
- If a mental health professional or mental health establishment, as the case may be, is unable to decide, whether to disclose information or provide basic in-patient medical records or any other records to the applicant for ethical, legal or other sensitive issues, they must inform Board
- The Board shall take final decision after hearing the 'concerned person with mental illness and MHE/MHP.

WHAT CONSTITUTES BASIC MEDICAL RECORD

"The Mental Healthcare (Rights of Persons with Mental Illness) Rules, 2018" Chapter II, Section 6 defines following as graded basic medical record-keeping for different settings **Form B):**

Basic medical record for community outreach register (in hard copy format):

a. Name of the mental health establishment/doctor ....

b. Date ....

c. Hospital registration number ....

d. Advance Directive (YES/NO) ....

e. Patient's name ....

f. Age/Sex ....

g. Father's/Mother's name ....

h. Address, Mobile No. ....

i. Chief complaints ....

Basic Medical Record of all outpatients (at hospitals, nursing homes, private clinics, camps, mobile clinics, primary health care centers and other community outreach programs, and the like matters) (in hard copy format):

a. Name of the mental health establishment/doctor ....

b. Date ....

c. Hospital registration number ....
d. Advance Directive (YES/NO) ....
e. Patient's name ....
f. Age/Sex ....
g. Father's/Mother's name ....
h. Address, Mobile No. ....
i. Chief complaints ....
j. Provisional diagnosis ....
k. Treatment advised and follow-up recommendations ....

Basic medical record of in-Patient:

a. Name of the hospital/nursing home ....
b. Date ....
c. Patient's name ....
d. Father's/Mother's name ....
e. Age/Sex ....
f. Address ....
g. Patient accompanied by (Name, age and nature of relationship) ....
h. Hospital registration number ....
i. Identification marks ....
j. Nominated representative ....
k. Advanced Directive (Yes or No); If yes salient features of the content ....
l. Date of admission/Date of discharge ....
m. Mode of admission (section under Mental Healthcare Act, 2017): Independent/Supported ....
n. Chief complaints ....
o. Summary of Medical Examination Laboratory investigations ....
p. Provisional/differential/final diagnosis ....
q. Course in the hospital (Treatment and Progress) ....
r. Condition at discharge or discharge at request or leave against medical advice or person with mental illness absconding or others ....

s. Treatment advice at discharge ....

t. Follow-up recommendations ....

Basic psychological assessment report (facilities where persons with mental illness undergoes psychological assessment):

a. Clinic record no. ....

b. Name ....

c. Age ....

d. Education ....

e. Occupation ....

f. Gender ....

g. Date of testing ....

h. Referred by: Language tested in ....

i. Reason for referral ....

j. Comments if any ....

Brief background information (e.g. the nature of the problem, when it started, any previous assessments and like details):

a. Informant ....

b. Salient behavioral observations ....

c. Tests/Scales administered *(Standardized tests/scales)* ....

d. Salient scores *(if applicable such as Intelligence Quotient, scores obtained on cognitive function tests, severity rating on psychopathology scales, disability %, etc.)*

e. Impression ....

f. Recommendations ....

g. Assessed by: Name, Date, Qualification ....

h. Verified/supervised by (if applicable): Name, Date, Qualification ....

Basic minimum standard guidelines for recording of therapy report (facilities where persons with mental illness are provided with therapy for any mental health problem)

a. Name of the Institute/Hospital/Center with address ....

b. Clinic record no. ....

Therapist Session Notes

a. Psychiatric diagnosis: ....
b. Patient name: ....
c. Age: ....
d. Gender: ....
e. Session number/Duration of session: Session participants and date: ....
f. Therapy objectives of the session: ....
g. Method of therapy given: ....
h. Key issues/themes discussed: (Psychosocial stressors/interpersonal problems/intrapsychic conflicts/Crisis situations/Conduct difficulties/Behavioral ....
i. Difficulties/Emotional difficulties/Developmental difficulties/Adjustment issues/ Addictive behaviors/Others) ....
j. Signature: ....
k. Therapy techniques used: ....
l. Therapist observations and reflections: ....
m. Plan for next session: Date for next session: ....
n. Therapist details: Name, Date, Qualification: ....
o. Supervised by (if applicable): Name, Date, Qualification: ....

Right to Personal Contacts and Communication (Chapter V, Section 26)

- A person with mental illness admitted to a mental health establishment shall have the right to refuse or receive visitors and to refuse or receive and make telephone or mobile phone calls at reasonable times subject to the norms of such mental health establishment.
- A person with mental illness admitted in a mental health establishment may send and receive mail through electronic mode including through e-mail.
- Where a person with mental illness informs the medical officer or mental health professional in-charge of the mental health establishment that he does not want to receive mail or email from any named person in the community, the medical officer or mental health professional in-charge may restrict such communication by the named person with the person with mental illness.
- Nothing contained in above sub-sections shall apply to visits from, telephone calls to, and from mail or e-mail to, and from following:
  a. Any Judge or officer authorized by a competent court;
  b. Members of the concerned Board or the Central Authority or the State Authority;
  c. Any member of the Parliament or a Member of State Legislature;

d. Nominated representative, lawyer or legal representative of the person;
e. Medical practitioner in-charge of the person's treatment;
f. Any other person authorized by the appropriate Government.

Right to Legal Aid (Chapter V, Section 27)
- A person with mental illness shall be entitled to receive free legal services to exercise any of his rights given under this Act.
- It shall be the duty of magistrate, police officer, person in-charge of such custodial institution as may be prescribed or medical officer or mental health professional in-charge of a mental health establishment to inform the person with mental illness that he is entitled to free legal services under the Legal Services Authorities Act, 1987 or other relevant laws or under any order of the court if so ordered and provide the contact details of the availability of services.

Right to Make Complaint about Deficiencies in Provision of Services (Chapter V, Section 28)
Any person with mental illness or his nominated representative, shall have the right to complain regarding deficiencies in provision of care, treatment and services in a mental health establishment to:
a. The medical officer or mental health professional in-charge of the establishment and if not satisfied with the response;
b. The concerned Board and if not satisfied with the response;
c. The State Authority.

▪ MODIFICATIONS IN APPROACH IN ASSESSMENT, ADMISSION, TREATMENT, AND DISCHARGE
- Make diagnosis of mental illness only in accordance with National/International Standards Implantable Cardioverter Defibrillator ((ICD) Latest) (Chapter II, Section 3)
- All MHEs are duty bound to record and maintain Basic Medical Record (mandatory)
- Ask for advance directive and nominated representative (mandatory)
- Assess capacity to make mental health care and treatment decisions
- *Decide locus of treatment:* OP/IPD → Mention the reasons of choice and consider the least restrictive option for treatment
- Accordingly decide type of admission and type of requisition form to be filled
- Ask for Advance directive (ask NR, option to check online at SMHA site with access to MHE)
- Assess AD in following paradigms:
  a. If it Is in contravention to any law
  b. If it appears not made of free will
  c. If it looks it was not anticipated for current situation
  d. If it client was not well informed/
  e. If it looks capacity at time of execution was in doubt
  If yes to any of above, then, apply to board for revocation/alteration.

- Check for availability of NR. Also see if NR acting in best interest, is available, is willing, is acceptable to person with mental illness—if not apply to Board (Board has to address issue within 7 days)
- At time of admission, MHP is duty bound to inform PMI/ NR about:
  - Diagnosis, nature of illness, section of admission
  - Proposed T/t plan, anticipated side effects
  - Right about appealing against admission to Board with contact details of board members and forms
  - Right to complaint about any deficiency in services to in-charge MHE/SMHA/Board
  - If any information when withheld → inform Board citing reasons (Chapter V, Section 22)
- Ensure safeguard of rights during hospital stay
  - Safe, hygienic, comfortable conditions, privacy
  - Facilities for communication, recreation, leisure, religious activity,
  - Not forced for: Hospital uniform/ tonsuring/undertake work without remuneration
  - No abuse
  - Allow leave of absence, visitation rights ((Chapter V, Section 20)
- Recordkeeping during admission

  In-patient Basic Record
  - MHE name, CRF No.
  - Patient details (name, age/sex, address)
  - Accompanying person
  - AD/NR, mode of admission
  - Date of admission/discharge
  - Chief complaints, MSE/physical examination
  - Course during stay, investigation
  - Diagnosis, condition at D/S
  - Advise on D/S, FU recommendation

  Psychological Assessment Report
  - Patient articular, test done /language
  - Score, impression, advise
  - Done by/supervised by (with RCI No.)

  Psychotherapy Notes
  - MHE detail, patient detail, mode of therapy, duration, objective, No. of sessions, issue discussed, Done by/supervised by (with RCI No.)
- Ensure at time of admission, admission authorization and admission criteria for respective sections are fulfilled and documented
- After admission, inform Board of all admissions (Within 3 days of women/ minor patient, within 7 days in rest)
- During admission continuous check for capacity assessment and consider revision of admission section accordingly

Types of admission, related admission criteria/assessments and discharge are tabulated in **Table 3.**

Table 3: Admission and discharge provisions of Mental Healthcare Act, 2017.

Type of admission	Admission criteria and concerned procedures	Discharge

Independent admission of major	- Capacity intact, patient gives consent
	- Chapter XII Section 86
	- Criteria for admission:
	  – A mental illness of a severity requiring admission;
	  – Person likely to benefit from admission and treatment;
	  – Person has understood nature and purpose of admission, and has made the request for his own free will, and has the capacity to make mental healthcare and treatment decisions without support or needs minimal support
	- (Use Form C for admission request of patient)
	- No treatment without patient's informed consent.
	- MHE to admit patient on own request, without need of NR
		- Chapter XII, Section 88: Independent patient may get himself discharged from the mental health establishment without the consent of the medical officer or mental health professional in-charge of such establishment. (Use Form G for discharge request of patient)
		- **If MHP has reasons to believe patient cannot be discharged on patient's request** (due to any of the evolving factors like harm to self or others, inability to take care of self, loses capacity during course of admission) → Admission can be converted to section 89 "admission with high support need" with consent of NR and information to Board
		If NR denies for above MHP has to discharge patient

Admission of minor on request of NR	- Chapter XII, Section 87 - (Use Form D for admission request of NR) - **Admission authorization** based on opinion of 2 Psychiatrist/1 Psychiatrist and other MHP/Medical professional (both should have seen patient on day of admission or in preceding 7days) Admission criteria: - A mental illness of a severity requiring admission; - Person likely to benefit from admission and treatment;© (this is the least restrictive option) **At time of admission check for:** - NR has to be legal guardian of minor - In case of minor girl, female attendant is compulsory to stay with child (either a female NR or in case of male NR, a female attendant appointed by NR) **Where to admit: Separate ward** for children and adolescents **Informing board:** Inform within 3 days of admission and immediately of admission extending beyond 30 days → **Board has to respond within 7 days** **MECT for minor:** Prior approval from Board needed, else a prohibited procedure **Periodic check for age:** If patient turns major, change to Section 86	Chapter XII, Section 88 If the nominated representative no longer supports admission of the minor under this section or requests discharge of the minor from the mental health establishment, the minor shall be discharged by the mental health establishment (Use Form H for discharge request of NR)

Contd...

Contd...

Type of admission	Admission criteria and concerned procedures	Discharge
Admission of a person with mental illness, with high support needs	Chapter XII, Section 89 (Use Form E for admission request of NR) Capacity assessment done → Impaired **Admission authorization** based on opinion of 1 Psychiatrist and other MHP/Medical professional (both should have seen patient on day of admission or in preceding 7days) Admission criteria: • Unable to understand the nature and purpose of his decisions and requires substantial support from NR; or • Has recently threatened or attempted or is threatening or attempting to cause bodily harm to himself; or • Has recently behaved or is behaving violently towards another person or has caused or is causing another person to fear bodily harm from him; or • Has recently shown or is showing an inability to care for himself to a degree that places the individual at risk of harm to himself. Assessed for availability as well as acceptability of AD and NR Admission counseling done **Inform board:** Within 3 days of women/minor patient, within 7 days in rest (Board has to respond within 7days) **Periodic check of capacity:** Weekly → change section accordingly Section 89 permits admission max 30 days → if extending inform board → Section 90	Any patient admitted under Section 89 needing readmission within 7 days of discharge— Direct admission under Chapter XII, Section 90

Continuation of the admission of a person with mental illness with high support needs	• Chapter XII, Section 90
	• (Use Form F for admission request of NR)
	• **Admission authorization** based on opinion of 2 Psychiatrist and other MHP/Medical professional (both should have seen patient on day of admission or in preceding 7days)
	• Admission criteria → illness of a severity that the person:
	  – Has consistently over time threatened or attempted to cause bodily harm to himself; or
	  – Has consistently over time behaved violently towards another person or has consistently over time caused another person to fear bodily harm from him; or
	  – Has consistently over time shown an inability to care for himself to a degree that places individual at risk of harm to himself;
	• Max admission permissible for 90 days
	• **Periodic check for capacity: Fortnightly**
	• **Inform Board within 7 days of admission → Board has to dispose plea within 3 weeks**
	• If need of **extending admission** under section 90:
	  – 1st time: 120 days
	  – Subsequently: 180 days each time	

Contd...

Contd...

Type of admission	Admission criteria and concerned procedures	Discharge
Admission of female with child <3 years • Inform board within 72 hours • Assess risk of harm to child at admission • If mother temporarily separated from child due to risk, still allow supervised meetings periodically • **Assess status fortnightly** • If admission and **separation exceeds 30 days** → **inform board (Chapter V Section 21(2)(3)(4))**		
Leave of Absence (LOA) • MHP at his/her discretion can give LOA of any duration • (Use Form I for LOAn request of NR) (Chapter XII, Section 91)		
Discharge • Involve person with mental illness/NR in discharge planning • Discuss future treatment plan • If patient is being transferred to other MHE, duty of discharging psychiatrist to discuss and inform future psychiatrist about the case and proposed plan (Chapter XII, Section 98)		

Flowchart 1 shows protocol for admission of a person with mental illness under MHCA 2017.

Flowchart 1: Protocal for admission of a person with mental illness under MHCA, 2017 (For non-emergency situation for clinents > 18 years age)

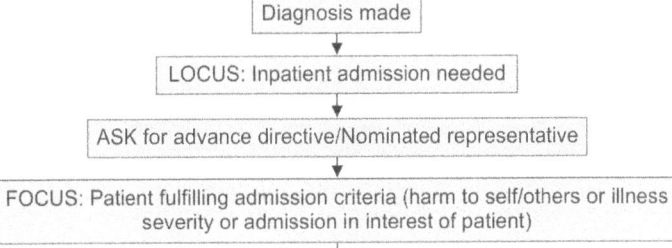

ASSESSING capacity for treatment related decision
Provide adequate & relevant information: Inform about illness/condition, treatment/Care proposed, alternative options of other treatment modality and consequence of no treatment/Care. Inform patient also not just caregiver.
WAY OF PROVIDING INFORMATION: Information should be given in language and manner so that patient and caregiver can understand easily. Aim should be to convey about benefits of treatment without coercing keeping patient's best interest and preferences in mind. Involving patient in **COLLABORATIVE DECISION MAKING** establishes good therapeutic alliance and reduces perceived coercion, promotes autonomy
If patient has not understood, think **can it be done differently or by a different mental health professional** in a better way, try it

Assess capacity by assessing following:
1. Assess **UNDERSTANDING** (It assesses assimilation of FACTUAL knowledge) Ask individual to paraphrase the information explained regarding mental illness/condition and treatment/care options.
2. Does individual **APPRECIATE** consequences (It assesses REASONING and ANALYSIS) Ask individual to describe about medical condition and proposed T/t and likely consequence of taking and not taking treatment
3. **COMMUNICATING** choice (It assesses judgment) Ask individual WHAT **DECISION** individual arrived at and WHAT ARE THE REASONS FOR CHOSING A PARTICULAR OPTION (more important is the reasoning i.e. the process of reaching on this decision than the outcome i.e. the final decision)
   e.g. If person says I DON'T WANT TREATMENT but reasoning behind decision is flawed, CAPACITY IS IMPAIRED and patient is NOT IN A STATE TO GIVE CONSENT
   e.g. If person says I WANT TREATMENT OR I WANT TO GET ADMITTED and reasoning behind is flawed, person may be giving CONSENT, BUT CAPACITY IS IMPAIRED and IT IS NOT A VALID CONSENT
   e.g. And even if person needs admission as per psychiatrist and still with correct reasoning has reached the decision of "OPTING FOR NO TREATMENT" - - >capacity IS INTACT CONSENT FOR NOT TAKING TREATMENT IS VALID and HAS TO BE RESPECTED

Contd...

Contd...

OUTCOME OF CAPACITY ASSESSMENT: Do you have reasons to believe that **PATIENT HAS NOT**
(a) **Understood the information** provided by you relevant to take a decision on the treatment or admission or personal assistance; or
(b) **Appreciated** any reasonably **foreseeable consequence of a decision or lack of decision** on the treatment or admission or personal assistance; or (could not retain information long enough to reach an appropriate decision or could not weigh the risk and benefit of treatment or admission or care or no treatment/care or
(c) Been able to **communicate the decision by any means**

Yes to any of a or b or c : Capacity is impaired   No to all questions: Capacity is intact

Capacity assessment for a client in need of admission

- **Capacity intact**
  - **Consent given** — Admission as independent admission under section 86
  - **Consent denied** — Ask for reasons of refusal, try if any objections can be overcome and consent can be obtained. **If still consent is denied→respect Patient's decision. Document reason for refusal**
- **Capacity impaired**
  - Admission with consent of NR under section 89/90

- In no way coercion should be exercised, autonomy of person with mental illness has to be appreciated. however, one or more mental health professionals may try explaining the medical benefits
- In case of any ambiguity, dilemma (legal/ethical), better to proceed with concurrence of Mental Health Review Board (MHRB)

Inform review board about admission (Within 3 days of women/ minor patient, within 7 days in rest "admissions with high support need")

If admission done with consent of NR (Use form E for section 89/ form F for section 90 for admission request of NR)

Admission authorization has to be based upon opinion of medical officer or mental health professional incharge in section 86; (1) Psychiatrist and Other MHP/Medical professional in section 89; (2) Psychiatrist and Other MHP/Medical professional in section 90 (all professionals authorizing should have seen patient on day of admission or in preceding 7days)

Assess capacity periodically (weekly in section 89/fortnightly in section 90 admissions)→ As soon as capacity regained→ convert it to voluntary admission

Inform persons with mental illness about Right to complain against involuntary admission decision to MHRB and provide contact details for same

During entire hospitalization ensure adequate safeguard of Rights of persons with mental illness (Right to protection from cruel, inhuman and degrading treatment, Right to information, Right to confidentiality, Right to restriction on release of information in respect of mental illness, Right to access medical records)

OTHER IMPORTANT CONCEPTS FOR INPATIENT CARE
Emergency Treatment (Chapter XII, Section 94)
- Any medical treatment, including treatment for mental illness, may be provided by any registered medical practioner in community/hospital with consent of NR in following situations to prevent:
  - Death or irreversible harm to the health of the person; or
  - The person inflicting serious harm to himself or to others; or
  - The person causing serious damage to property belonging to himself or to others where such behavior is believed to flow directly from the person's mental illness.
- The **emergency treatment referred to in this section shall be limited to seventy-two hours or till the person with mental illness has been assessed at a mental health establishment, whichever is earlier.**

Prohibited Treatment (Chapter XII, Section 95)
- Electroconvulsive therapy without the use of muscle relaxants and anesthesia
- Electroconvulsive therapy for minors
- Sterilization of men or women, when such sterilization is intended as a treatment for mental illness
- Chained in any manner or form whatsoever.
  - Notwithstanding anything contained in sub-section
  - If, in the opinion of psychiatrist in-charge of a minor's treatment, if feels electroconvulsive therapy is required, then, prior approval of board and consent of the guardian is needed.

Restriction on psychosurgery for persons with mental illness. (Chapter XII, Section 96)

Psychiatrist in-charge of a person's treatment, if feels psychosurgery is required, then, prior approval of board and consent of the guardian is needed. Central Authority may make regulations for this.

Use of Seclusion and Restrain (Chapter XII, Section 97)
- A person with mental illness shall not be subjected to seclusion or solitary confinement, and, where necessary, physical restraint may only be used when:
  - It is the only means available to prevent imminent and immediate harm to person concerned or to others;
  - It is authorized by the psychiatrist in charge of the person's treatment at the mental health establishment.
- Physical restraint shall not be used for a period longer than it is absolutely necessary to prevent the immediate risk of significant harm.

- The medical officer or mental health professional in-charge of the mental health establishment shall be responsible for ensuring that the method, nature of restraint justification for its imposition and the duration of the restraint are immediately recorded in the person's medical notes.
- The restraint shall not be used as a form of punishment or deterrent in any circumstance and the mental health establishment shall not use restraint merely on the ground of shortage of staff in such establishment.
- The nominated representative of the person with mental illness shall be informed about every instance of restraint within a period of twenty-four hours.
- A person who is placed under restraint shall be kept in a place where he can cause no harm to himself or others and under regular ongoing supervision of the medical personnel.
- The mental health establishment shall include all instances of restraint in the report to be sent to the concerned Board on a monthly basis.
- The Central Authority may make regulations for the purpose of carrying out the provisions of this section.
- The Board may order a mental health establishment to desist from applying restraint if the Board is of the opinion that the mental health establishment is persistently and willfully ignoring the provisions of this section.

Decriminalization of Suicide (Chapter XVI, Section 115)

Notwithstanding anything contained in Section 309 of the Indian Penal Code any person who attempts to commit suicide shall be presumed, unless proved otherwise, to have severe stress and shall not be tried and punished under the said Code.

Insurance for Mental Illness

Every insurer shall make provision for medical insurance for treatment of mental illness on the same basis as is available for treatment of physical illness (as **right to equality and non-discrimination**) **(Chapter V, Section 21)**.

Certain Responsibilities Restricted to Only Public Mental Health Establishments (Chapter XIII) (Table 3)

Table 3: Certain admission provisions specific for public mental health establishments.

Section of MHCA	Provisions for mental health evaluation and treatment
100 Duties of police officers in respect of persons with mental illness	• Every officer in-charge of a police station shall have a duty: – To take under protection any person found wandering within limits of police station whom the officer has reason to believe has mental illness and is incapable of taking care of himself; or – To take under protection any person within the limits of the police station whom the officer has reason to believe to be a risk to himself or others by reason of mental illness.

Contd...

Contd...

Section of MHCA	Provisions for mental health evaluation and treatment
	- Police officer within 24 hours will take the person to a public MHE for assessment and will inform person or NR reasons of taking him/her into protection - If medical assessment does not reveal a mental illness of a nature or degree requiring admission, police officer shall take the person to the person's residence or in case of homeless persons, to a Government establishment for homeless persons - In case of homeless person with mental illness, a First Information Report of a missing person shall be lodged at the concerned police station and the station house officer shall have a duty to trace family and inform them
101 Report to Magistrate of person with mental illness in private residence who is ill-treated or neglected	Every officer in-charge of a police station, who has reason to believe at his own or on reporting of any person that any person with mental illness residing within the limits of the police station is being ill treated or neglected, shall forthwith report the fact to the local Magistrate. Magistrate may cause the person with mental illness to be produced before him and pass order under Section 102
102 Magistrate authorized admission	For a person with mental illness or suspected of mental illness, Magistrate may pass order for: - Assessment and treatment in a public MHE or - Admission order of maximum 10 days for assessment in a public MHE for assessment and treatment if any

103 Prisoners with mental illness	- An order under Section 30 of the Prisoners Act, 1900 or under Section 144 of the Air Force Act, 1950, or under section 145 of the Army Act, 1950, or under section 143 or section 144 of the Navy Act, 1957, or under Section 330 or Section 335 of the Code of Criminal Procedure, 1973, directing the admission of such prisoner with mental illness into any suitable mental health establishment, shall be sufficient authority for the admission of such person in such establishment to which such person may be lawfully transferred for care and treatment therein:
	  – Provided that transfer of a prisoner with mental illness to the psychiatric ward in the medical wing of the prison shall be sufficient to meet the requirements
	  – Provided further that where there is no psychiatric ward in prison, prisoner may be transferred to a MHE with prior permission of the Board.
	- The medical officer of a prison or jail shall send a quarterly report to the concerned Board certifying therein that there are no prisoners with mental illness in the prison or jail.
	- The Board may visit the prison or jail and ask the medical officer as to why the prisoner with mental illness, if any, has been kept in the prison or jail and not transferred for treatment to a mental health establishment.
	- The medical officer in-charge of a mental health establishment wherein any prisoner with mental illness is detained, shall once in every six months, make a special report regarding the mental and physical condition of such person to the authority under whose order such person is detained

104 Persons in custodial institutions	- If it appears to the person in-charge of a State run custodial institution (including beggars homes, orphanages, women's protection homes and children homes) that any resident of the institution has, or is likely to have, a mental illness, then, he shall take such resident of the institution to the nearest mental health establishment run or funded by the appropriate Government for assessment and treatment, as necessary. - The medical officer in-charge of a mental health establishment shall be responsible for assessment of the person with mental illness, and the treatment required by such persons shall be decided in accordance with the provisions of this Act

Implications for Research (Chapter XII, Section 99)

- The professionals conducting research shall obtain free and informed consent from all persons with mental illness for participation in any research involving interviewing the person or psychological, physical, chemical or medicinal interventions.
- In case of research involving any psychological, physical, chemical or medicinal interventions to be conducted on person who is unable to give free and informed consent but does not resist participation in such research, permission to conduct such research shall be obtained from concerned State Authority.
- The State Authority may allow research to proceed based on informed consent being obtained from the nominated representative of persons with mental illness, if the State Authority is satisfied that:
  - The proposed research cannot be performed on persons who are capable of giving free and informed consent;
  - The proposed research is necessary to promote the mental health of the population represented by the person;
  - The purpose of the proposed research is to obtain knowledge relevant to the particular mental health needs of persons with mental illness;
  - A full disclosure of the interests of persons and organizations conducting the proposed research is made and there is no conflict of interest involved; and
  - The proposed research follows all the national and international guidelines and regulations concerning the conduct of such research and ethical approval has been obtained from the institutional ethics committee where such research is to be conducted.
- The provisions of this section shall not restrict research based study of the case notes of a person who is unable to give informed consent, so long as the anonymity of the persons is secured.
- The person with mental illness or the nominated representative who gives informed consent for participation in any research under this Act may withdraw the consent at any time during the period of research.

OFFENCES: CONTRAVENTION OF PROVISIONS OF ACT

Chapter XIV, Section 108. Any person who contravenes any of the provisions of this Act, or of any rule or regulation made thereunder shall for first contravention be punishable with imprisonment for a term which may extend to six months, or with a fine which may extend to ten thousand rupees or with both, and for any subsequent contravention with imprisonment for a term which may extend to two years or with fine which shall not be less than fifty thousand rupees but which may extend to five lakh rupees or with both.

INTERACTION WITH JUDICIARY

Chapter X, Section 69; Appeal in High Court

Any mental health establishment aggrieved by an order of the Authority refusing to grant registration or renewal of registration or cancellation of registration, may, within a period of thirty days from such order, prefer an appeal to the High Court in the State.

Provided that the High Court may entertain an appeal after the expiry of the said period of thirty days, if it is satisfied that the appellant had sufficient cause for not preferring the appeal within the period of thirty days.

Chapter XIII, Section 105; Question of Mental Illness in Judicial Process

If during any judicial process before any competent court, proof of mental illness is produced and is challenged by the other party, the court shall refer the same for further scrutiny to the concerned Board and the Board shall, after examination of the person alleged to have a mental illness either by itself or through a committee of experts, submit its opinion to the court.

Chapter XVI, Section 116; Bar of Jurisdiction

No civil court shall have jurisdiction to entertain any suit or proceeding in respect of any matter which the Authority or the Board is empowered by or under this Act to determine, and no injunction shall be granted by any court or other authority in respect of any action taken or to be taken in pursuance of any power conferred by or under this Act.

CONCLUSION

MHCA is a patient centric Act that will:
- Increase patient /Caregiver involvement
- Produce Accountable Mental Health Systems
- Standardized operating procedures will follow uniformly

But, it puts entire onus more on service provider, it will:
- Increase cost of Mental Health Services
- More legalities may lead to defensive practice
- More paper work.

REFERENCES

1. Jiloha RC. The Mental health act of india, in developments in psychiatry in India. Edited by Malhotra S, Chakrabarti S. Springer India, 2015;611-22.
2. Indian Lunacy Act, 1912. Ministry of Health and Family Welfare, Government of India Publication, New Delhi.
3. Mental Health 1987. Ministry of Health and Family Welfare, Government of India Publication, New Delhi.
4. Mental Healthcare Act, 2017. Government of India Publication, New Delhi.
5. The Mental Healthcare (Central Mental Health Authority and Mental Health Review Boards) Government of India Publication, New Delhi.
6. The Mental Healthcare (State Mental Health Authority) Rules, 2018. Government of India Publication, New Delhi.
7. The Mental Healthcare (Rights of Persons with Mental Illness) Rules, 2018. Government of India Publication, New Delhi.

CHAPTER 26

Legislation Related to Addiction Psychiatry in India

> **LEARNING OBJECTIVES**
> - Narcotic Drugs and Psychotropic Substances Act 1985
> - Legal position of OST medications
> - Guidelines for stocking and dispensing essential narcotic drugs
> - Laws related to alcohol
> - Laws concerning criminal responsibility of intoxicated person
> - Gambling laws in India

WHAT IS A DRUG?

Chemically: Any chemical substance that affects normal functioning of body and/or brain.

In medicine: Any substance with potential to prevent or cure disease or enhance physical or mental welfare.

In pharmacology: Any chemical agent that alters physiological or biochemical processes of tissues or organisms.

In Legal terms: Any substance listed in Schedule I and II of the 1961 Single Convention on Narcotic Drugs, whether natural or synthetic.

Classification of Drugs on Basis of Legality of Use
- *Licit drugs:* use is sanctioned legally e.g. alcohol, tobacco
- *Illicit drugs:* use is contravened by law e.g. cocaine.

Drug Abuse and Crime
- Crimes related to cultivation, manufacture, supply and possession of illicit substances
- Crimes committed to procure substance
- Crimes related to effect of altered mental state due to use of drug

International law governing the control of drugs is composed primarily of UN conventions:
- The Single Convention on Narcotic Drugs of 1961 (as amended in 1972)
- Convention on Psychotropic Substances of 1971

- United Nations Convention against illicit traffic in Narcotic Drugs and Psycho- tropic Substances of 1988.

Drug abuse and Indian legislation: It is based on multipronged approach to:
- Control supply of drugs
- Suppress illicit trafficking
- Demand reduction
- Treatment and rehabilitation
- Awareness building measures.

Indian Legislation and Policies Concerning Narcotic and Psychotropic Use

National Policy on Narcotic Drugs and Psychotropic Substances is based on the directive Principles, contained in Article 47 of the Indian Constitution, which direct the State to endeavor to bring about prohibition of the consumption, except for medicinal purposes, of intoxicating drugs injurious to health.

Narcotic Drugs and Psychotropic Substances (NDPS) Act 1985

This is an Act to provide a comprehensive legislation on narcotic drugs and psychotropic substances which, inter alia, should consolidate and amend the then existing laws relating to narcotic drugs, make provisions for exercising effective control over psychotropic substances, make provisions for the implementation of international conventions relating to narcotic drugs and psychotropic substances, the Narcotic Drugs and Psychotropic Act 1985 came into force.[1]

Act was amended once in 1989 and subsequently in 2001 and 2014. It has been tabled in Lok Sabha as private member bill since 2016, any amendment is yet to take place officially.[2,3]

Purpose of Act: An act to consolidate and amend the law relating to narcotic drugs, to:
- Make stringent provisions for the control and regulation of operations relating to narcotic drugs and psychotropic substances.
- Provide for the forfeiture of property derived from, or used in, illicit traffic in narcotic drugs and psychotropic substances.
- Implement the provisions of the International Conventions on Narcotic Drugs and Psychotropic Substance and for matters connected therewith.

Scope: It extends to the whole of India and to all citizens of India outside India including those on ships and aircrafts registered in India, wherever they may be.

Organization of NDPS Act[1-3]

1985 Act was spread over six chapters comprising 83 sections, after 1989 amendment it has now 8 chapters, which are tabulated in **Table 1**.

Table 1: Organization of NDPS Act.

Chapter No.	Title of chapter	Special remarks of provisions of each section with relevance to psychiatry
I	Preliminary (Definitions)	Defines **"Addict"** means a person who has dependence on any narcotic drug or psychotropic substance **"Narcotic drug"** means coca leaf, cannabis (hemp), opium, poppy straw and includes all manufactured drugs **"Psychotropic substance"** means any substance, natural or synthetic, or any natural material or any salt or preparation of such substance or material included in the list of psychotropic substances specified in the Schedule **"Controlled substance"** means any substance which the Central Government may, having regard to the available information as to its possible use in the production or manufacture of narcotic drugs or psychotropic substances or to the provisions of any International Convention, by notification in the Official Gazette, declare to be a controlled substance **"Cannabis (hemp)"** means- Charas, Ganja and Any mixture of two. Act excludes Bhang, Alcohol and Nicotine **"Licenced chemist"** means a person who has obtained a licence to possess, sell, exhibit or offer for sale or distribution by retail, essential narcotic drugs **"Licenced dealer"** means a person who has obtained a licence to possess, sell, exhibit or offer for sale or distribution by wholesale, essential narcotic drugs **"Medical institution"** means a hospital, dispensary, clinic or an institution by whatever name called that offers services or facilities requiring diagnosis; treatment or care of illness, disease, injury, deformity or abnormality, established and administered or maintained by the Government or Municipal Corporation or Municipal Council or Zila Parishad or any person or body of person **"Prescription"** means a prescription given by a registered medical practitioner for the supply of any of the essential narcotic drugs to a patient for medical use **"Recognized medical institution (RMI)"** means a medical institution recognized under these rules **"Registered medical practitioner (RMP)"** means any person registered as a medical practitioner under the Indian Medical Council Act, 1956 (102 of 1956) or dentist under the Dentists Act, 1948 (16 of 1948) or under any law for the registration of RMP dentists for the time being in force and has undergone training in pain relief and palliative care for prescription of essential narcotic drugs for pain relief and palliative care or training in opioid substitution therapy for prescription of essential narcotic drugs for treatment of opioid dependence **"Essential narcotic drugs"** the opioids identified for medical use (pain relief or opioid substitution therapy, approved by the Drug Controller General of India. includes - Morphine, Methadone, Codeine, Hydrocodone, Oxycodone, and Fentanyl (which central government can notify on the basis of expediency in medical practice).

Contd...

Contd...

Chapter No.	Title of chapter	Special remarks of provisions of each section with relevance to psychiatry
II	Authorities and Officers	Authorizes **central government to take measures** necessary to prevent and combat drug abuse and illicit trafficking, including identification, treatment, education, aftercare, rehabilitation and social reintegration of addicts. The **"Narcotic Drugs and Psychotropic substances Consultative committee"** to tender advice on above matters **Narcotics Control Bureau** is the chief law enforcement and intelligence agency of India responsible for fighting drug trafficking and the abuse **Central Bureau of Narcotics (CBN).** Prior to 1950, the administration of the Narcotics Laws, namely, the Opium Act of 1857 and 1878 and the Dangerous Drugs Act 1930 vested with the Provincial Government. The amalgamation of these Agencies laid foundation of the Opium Department in November, 1950 which is presently known as CBN. The **Narcotics Commissioner (NC)** is assisted by three Deputy Narcotics Commissioners (DNCs) in charge of the Units in the opium growing states i.e. Madhya Pradesh, Rajasthan and Uttar Pradesh. Responsibilities of CBN are: 1. Supervision over licit cultivation of opium poppy In India. 2. Preventive and enforcement functions. 3. Investigation of cases under the NDPS Act, 1985 and filing of complaint in the Court 4. Action for tracing and freezing of illegally acquired property as per NDPS Act.
IIA	National fund for control of drug abuse	Funded with government/public contributions and sale of forfeited property derived from or used in illicit traffic. Fund is for preventing and combating drug abuse and illicit trafficking, promoting identification, treatment, education, aftercare, rehabilitation and social reintegration of addicts.
III	Prohibition, control and regulation	State government to make rules for prohibiting cultivation, production and sale of narcotic and psychotropic substance except for medicinal use and that too with prior sanction.
IV	Offences and penalties	Offense related to violations of the various prohibitions imposed under the Act on the cultivation, production, manufacture, distribution, sale, import and export etc. of narcotic drugs and psychotropic substances. All these offences are triable by Special Courts. Difference in punishment (6 months to 1 year for small quantity for personal consumption to 15–20 years for other serious offenses) **Section 39. Power of court to release certain offenders on probation for** offences relating to small quantity regard being had to the age, character, antecedents or physical or mental condition of the offender court may, instead of sentencing him, may direct release for **undergoing medical treatment for de-toxification or deaddiction** with his consent from a government hospital and to appear before the court within a year with medical a report and meantime, to abstain from the commission of any offence.
V	Procedure for investigation and prosecution	Lays down procedures for all above mentioned sections
VA	Forfeiture of property involved in, illicit traffic	To provide for the investigation, freezing, seizure and forfeiture of property derived from or acquired through illicit trafficking in narcotic drugs and psychotropic substances.

Contd...

Contd...

Chapter No.	Title of chapter	Special remarks of provisions of each section with relevance to psychiatry
VI	Miscellaneous	**Section 64A. Immunity** from prosecution to **addicts found with small quantity** who volunteer for treatment **Section 71 (1):** Establish centers for identification, treatment, education, after care, rehabilitation, social reintegration of addicts and for supply, of any medicinal use NDPS (as prescribed by concerned Government) to the addicts registered with government institutes. **Section 71 (2):** Government may make rules consistent with this Act providing for the **establishment, appointment, maintenance, management and superintendence of, and for supply of** NDPS for above mentioned Section 71 (1)

Offenses and Penalties Under NDPS Act

Section 37: Offenses are non-bailable and non-cognizable

The quantum of sentence and fine varies with the offence. For many offences, the penalty depends on the quantity of drug involved - small quantity, more than small but less than commercial quantity or commercial quantity of drugs. Small and Commercial quantities are notified for each drug. The quantities for some common drugs are tabulated in **Table 2**.

Table 2: Offence and penalties under NDPS Act.

Drug	Small quantity	Commercial quantity
Amphetamine	2 g	50 g
Buprenorphine	2 g	20 g
Charas/hashish	20 g	500 g
Cocaine	1 kg	20 kg
Ganja	5 g	250 g
MDMA	0.5 g	10 g
Methamphetamine	2 g	50 g
Morphine	5 g	250 g
Poppy straw	1 kg	50 kg

Punishment:
For small quantity 1 year rigorous imprisonment or a fine up to ₹ 10,000 or Both.
For commercial quantity: 5–10 years rigorous imprisonment or a fine of 1–2 lac or Both

Legal Provisions Pertaining to Opioid Substitution Therapy (OST)

Currently two drugs are available for OST in India, Buprenorphine and methadone
- Buprenorphine is a "psychotropic"
- Methadone is a "Narcotic"

Buprenorphine
- Being psychotropic is covered under NDPS Act
- Being a pharmaceutical product, is covered under Drugs and Cosmetics Act, 1940 and Rules
- Buprenorphine naloxone being a fixed drug combination (FDC) is also subject to FDC regulations of Central drugs standard control organization.

Drug Controller of India has imposed a condition that these tablets be supplied only to "de-addiction centers" supported or authorized by the government, without defining the phrase "de-addiction center". So, unfortunately, Buprenorphine despite being psychotropic, a less stringently controlled drug as compared to a narcotic drug, due to being caught in poorly coordinated multiple web of regulatory agencies, has become difficult to procure, stock and dispense.

Guidelines for Stocking and Dispensing Essential Narcotic Drugs in Medical Institutions as per NDPS Act[4-7]

Narcotic of relevance to deaddiction psychiatry practice: Methadone, Tramadol.
Background of problem statement: In India, despite need of opioids for good palliative care and opioid substitution therapy, use is not much preferred by health professionals. Complicated rules and regulations along with problems related to attitude and knowledge regarding pain relief and opioids substitution therapy among medical professionals and public are major hindrances for poor access to opioids.

Contributors to Poor Access and Availability of Opioids for Medical Use in India[6]

- Historical origins of regulations are from the archaic legislature for British India for narcotics as a trade crop. It emphasized heavy restrictions to safeguard their commercial interests. The NDPS Act 1985, reflected the same prohibitory tone and language.
- The state NDPS rules were non-uniform, preventing movement of legitimate opioids for medical use across the country.
- The mandates given to government offices were prohibitory. All efforts were geared to eliminate any form of action involving narcotics and hence there was deep-rooted resistance to incorporate medical and scientific use.
- Medical Institutions faced stringent regulations - maintaining multiple licenses for acquiring, stocking, prescribing and using opioids.
- Harsh punishment prescribed in the NDPS Act 1985 (e.g. possible 10 years of rigorous imprisonment even for clerical errors) alienated institutions and pharmacists from stocking these medicines.
- Attitude and knowledge of professionals towards using opioids were negative
- Lack of availability of opioid formats at medical colleges and hospitals, prevented exposure and training of professionals in using them for managing chronic pain. This developed into unfounded fears opiophobia.

- The public associated opioids with addiction or as the last resort and are reluctant to use the drug even if it meant great degree of suffering. This fear was often reinforced by professionals.

Basis for the NDPS Amendment 2014: Opioids are safe, economical and effective for management of severe pain and deaddiction as opioid substitution therapy (OST) in selected groups of patients. There is need to facilitate and improve access to opioids for medical use while maintaining, strengthening and integrating programs to control misuse and diversion. Uniform and simple procedures are required for procurement of opioids for medical use across the country. The NDPS Rules pertaining to the Act are now applicable uniformly across India.

A Glimpse: The Amended NDPS Act 2014
- Expanded the scope of the Act to include Medical and Scientific Use
- Prepared a notified list of **Essential Narcotic Drugs [ENDs]**, i.e. the opioids identified for medical use, approved by the Drug Controller General of India.
- The notified list of ENDs currently includes - Morphine, Methadone, Codeine, Hydrocodone, Oxycodone, Tramadol and Fentanyl
- It defined **'Recognized Medical Institutions'** (RMIs) with criteria for stocking and dispensing opioids for medical use.
- Conferred the powers for **authorizing medical institutions as RMIs, for stocking and dispensing ENDs, to a single state agency** - the State Drug Controller-SDC/Commissioner, Food & Drug Administration-FDA
- Those Institutions fulfilling the criteria to be RMIs, may apply to the State Drug Controller-SDC/Commissioner, Food and Drug Administration - FDA, to procure and dispense ENDs.
- The **authorization of RMIs is for periods of 3 years**, and renewable from the same agency. This removes the need for renewing multiple licenses from different government agencies every few months. Implicitly this requires strengthening the awareness, education and monitoring systems of licit narcotic usage - to prevent misuse and diversions.

Prerequisites for Registered Medical Institute (RMI): The concept of RMI [defined above] came into existence within the Rules, to ensure safe medical usage of the ENDs. It links training and competency in safely using ENDs, with the authorization for stocking/dispensing them. Any Institution as defined above, can purchase, store and dispense methadone once it conforms to the NDPS Rules 2015. They are as follows:
- The institution must have an Officer in-charge of Essential Narcotic Drugs within the RMI responsible for managing Essential Narcotic Drugs at the RMI
- The Office in-charge must be a qualified doctor and registered with the Medical Council of India or the Dental Council of India and be trained in the medical use of opioids.
- The institution must have the facility for safe storage for ENDs; a double locking system e.g. a cupboard with two locks.
- The facility should have basic infrastructure facilities and staff for evaluating and managing the treatment of the patients who would need ENDs.
- The facility should provide proof of space and personnel for the mandated record keeping

- The facility should have capacity to maintain a register of consumption for each opioid as given in Forms provided with the Rules.[6]

Responsibilities of RMIs
- RMI shall ensure and maintain the Minimum Mandatory Requirements as listed above.
- Government hospitals are deemed RMIs provided they follow all mandated requirements mentioned above and must submit the annual consumption report.
- The drugs shall be prescribed only by Registered Medical Practitioners
- Every RMI shall designate one or more RMP who shall be using essential narcotic drugs. When there are more than one registered medical practitioners, one of them shall be designated as Overall officer-in-charge.
- The RMI shall ensure that the RMP, designated as the Medical Officer in Charge has completed the certified training in medical use of ENDs as per the Rules. This officer shall be responsible for the safe use of ENDs at the institution.
- The drugs shall be purchased only from authorized chemists/dealers. The list for the same should be available with the authorising State agency. The list of licensed manufacturers would be available with the Narcotic Commissioner at the centre.
- ENDs shall be prescribed as per the rules and dispensed only to selected patients, registered with the RMI.
- END stock with the RMI shall not be transferred, loaned or sold to other institutions except with the written permission of the Drugs Controller of the state.
- All records and registers shall be maintained as indicated in the Rules, for a period of two years from the last entry. They should be made available for inspection for the Commissioner of Food and Drugs Control Administration or any other officer authorized by him in this regard
- The expired stock of ENDs shall be destroyed in the presence of an official designated by the State Drug Controller/Commissioner of Food and Drugs Control Administration.
- The unused ENDs returned by the patients, shall be considered as receipts, provided the drugs are not damaged or otherwise unacceptable for use.
- RMI shall submit the annual return [Form 3 I] before 31st of March every year even if they have not used any ENDs in the preceding year.
- If there is a change in the 'Officer-in-charge', the details with date of change shall be intimated to the State Drug Controller/Commissioner of Food and Drugs Control Administration, within seven days for re-issue of the RMI certificate with endorsement of the newly employed doctor in charge of the RMI. The RMI shall inform the State Drug Controller/ Commissioner of Food and Drugs Control Administration, in writing, in the event of any change in the constitution of the RMI operating under this approval.
- Where any change in the constitution of the RMI takes place, the current approval shall be deemed to be valid for a maximum period of 90 days from the date on which the change takes place, unless, in the meantime a fresh approval has been taken from the State Drug Controller/Commissioner of Food and Drugs Control Administration, in the name of the Institution with the changed constitution.

- The designated medical officer in charge, shall inform the Commissioner of Food and Drugs Control Administration in writing within thirty days from the date of such change, for issue of fresh Certificate of Recognition.
- If an RMI ceases to exist, the matter shall be informed with details of balance stock of ENDs, if any, and the authorisation certificate surrendered to the State Drug Controller/Commissioner of Food and Drugs Control Administration within 30 days, who will then issue orders for the disposal of the balance ENDs.[6]

Responsibilities of Medical Officer in-charge of RMI

- Ensure that ENDs shall be dispensed to the selected patients who are registered with the RMI.
- Ensure that RMI uses ENDs in the licit manner specified in the Rules.
- Ensure that prescriptions from the RMI are made rationally on valid clinical grounds
- Ensure that the stock of ENDs in the RMI are uninterrupted and adequately available for medical needs of its patients, by sending estimates, and other details to the office of FDA/SDC in time.
- Ensure that ENDs are kept under safe custody to prevent possible misuse and diversion.
- Maintain record in Form No. 3E for each patient, which shall be preserved for a minimum period of two years from the date of last entry.
- Maintain record of all receipts and disbursements of essential narcotic drugs in Form No. 3H which shall be preserved for a minimum period of two years from the date of last entry.
- Shall authorize the deputed qualified personnel to carry such quantity of ENDs as may be required for treatment of home care patients registered with the RMI.
- Maintain the record of issue and receipt of ENDs used for such home care patients
- File return for a calendar year on or before the 31st of March of the subsequent year in Form No. 3-I to the Controller of Drugs. Ensure that all records are available to inspectors from the DC office, for a period of two years from the date of last transaction.
- Ensure that the expired stock of ENDs is destroyed in the presence of a representative of the State Drug Controller/Commissioner of Food and Drugs Control Administration. In the event of any change in the constitution of the RMI, the designated Officer in charge, shall inform the State Drug Controller/Commissioner of Food and Drugs Control Administration in writing within thirty days from the date of such change for issue of fresh Certificate of Recognition.[6]

Process of Recognizing Medical Institution to Stock and Dispense ENDs

Step 1—Training: The Medical Institution ensures that a Registered Medical Practitioner is trained in the medical use of opioids.

Step 2—Applying to the state drugs controller for RMI status: The application is sent in the format of Form 3F to the State Drugs Controller/FDA by the authority in-charge of the institution with

details of the facility and with the name of the trained doctor who will be in-charge of the stocking and dispensing. The following documents are also required:
- Covering letter stating the purpose
- Filled application - Form 3-F.
- Completed Form 3-J which specifies the Annual Requirement of the ENDs and source(s) for purchase
- Name of the employed doctor who would be the Officer in-charge and copy of her/his; a. Medical graduation certificate, b. Certificate of registration, and c. Certificate of training in medical use of opioids
- Self-addressed stamped envelope [Stamp worth ₹ 27/-]

Step 3—Inspection and authorisation for RMI purpose: The drugs controller or designated person on his behalf will inspect the institution.
- If all the prerequisites are appropriately met, the Drug Controller will authorize it as a RMI through a letter of recognition; in the format given in Form 3G, within 60 days from the date of receipt of application.
- If the RMI status is denied – the reasons are to be provided within 60 days from the date of receipt of application.

Step 4—Order of Purchase of ENDs
- The order for purchase of each opioid and each formulation that is required, is then filled by the RMI and submitted to the licensed pharmaceutical agency along with a copy of RMI certificate.
- If the annual estimate is utilized before time, the RMI can repeat the order of purchase of that amount, during the year as per the need, in case of unexpected increase in the number of patients needing ENDs.
- The repeat order of purchase is best done with at least 3 months remaining for the existing stock of the drug to run out. This can prevent interruption in the availability of pain medication for the patients registered with the RMI.

Step 5—Receipt of the consignment
- The applicant will get the original consignment of ENDs along with a copy in the format of Form No 3C which contains the details of the consignment and the time of receipt.
- Retain the original.
- One copy is returned to the supplier and one copy is sent to the State Drug Controller.

Step 6—Maintaining stock and records
- The consignment of ENDs is kept in a cupboard or locker safely under the supervision of the doctor in charge of the RMI.
- Record of the consignment notes is maintained for two years
- The quantity of each formulation of individual drug should be entered in a specified section of the END register which is prepared as per Form 3H. For e.g. if the RMI procures 10 mgs and 20 mgs tablets of oral Morphine, the stock of each should go into separate sections. Separate registers may also be maintained for each formulation.

- The name and address of each patient for whom END was prescribed is entered in the register along with the quantity disbursed. Record of every patient to whom END was dispensed is maintained in the format of Form 3E
- At the end of the day the total quantity of END disbursed that day, should be subtracted from the initial quantity with which the register was started. This amount naturally forms the initial quantity for the next day.
- Record of day-to-day accounts of every transactions in END is maintained in the format of Form 3D
- Once verified, the doctor in charge signs below the last entry of the day in the register.
- All records are kept for period of two years from the date of last entry.
- Although support staff may manage the day-to-day entries, the medical officer in-charge has primary responsibility of the stock and dispensing ENDs.
- The total quantity possessed by the RMI at any one time, should not exceed the submitted estimate (or revised estimate, if any). This quantity may be ordered repeatedly during the year, if the need for ENDs scales up during the year.
- If the requirement for ENDs has increased during the course of the year, the officer in charge of the RMI can submit the revised estimate for the same year by the 31st August. A brief justification for the same is provided while filing the annual return in Form-3 I.
- File annual return to the Controller of Drugs, for the calendar year on or before 31st of March of the subsequent year in the format of Form 3 I.

Maintaining vigilance of left over stock by the officer in-charge, and early action for replenishing stocks, would avoid the most distressful state for patients, resulting from interrupted stocks. This would avoid suffering of patients due to non-availability of essential medicines in the RMI.

Renewal of RMI: The Recognition of RMI is valid for three years. The application for renewal [Form 3-F] is sent from the RMI, at least 60 days prior to the date of expiry of recognition—to the State Drug Controller stating the following:
- Balance of each END from the year's stock
- The total quantity purchased during the year
- The total quantity disbursed in the current year and the balance quantity
- The quantity needed for next year
- If the RMI requires to revise the annual estimate, application for the same should be submitted to the Controller of Drugs by 31st of August of the calendar year. The Medical Officer in charge shall record the justification for the same while filing the annual return in Form 3-I. It is recommended that the RMI should keep enough END stock, to cover requirements for at least 3 months to ensure uninterrupted supply. The order of purchase for the next consignment is readied and sent accordingly to the supplier to ensure at-least 3 month's buffer stock.

Guidelines for individual Registered Medical Practitioners: Any individual Registered Medical Practitioner [RMP] may hold a small stock of ENDs as indicated below, for emergency purposes in her/his own practice, without any special authorisation.[1,6]

- Morphine formulations—total quantity not > 500 mg
- Codeine formulations—not > 2000 mg
- Hydrocodone—total quantity not > 320 mg
- Fentanyl—2 TD patches one each of 12.5 µg/h and 25 µg/h
- Oxycodone—total quantity not > 250 mg
- Methadone—the upper limit of quantity is not yet mentioned in the Rules. If the RMP requires to stock more than the quantity mentioned, she/he can apply using Form 3B to the state drug controller/FDA officer to request for the same and receive special permission for period of three years.

Prescribing ENDs
- Prescriptions must be in capital writing, dated and signed by the RMP with full name, address and her/his registration number
- Prescriptions must specify name, and the address of the person to whom prescription is given
- Prescriptions must mention the total quantity of the END, daily dose and the duration of the prescription.

Home care treatment shall not be provided for treatment of opioid dependence, it can be given for narcotic analgesia.[1]

Laws Relevant to Alcohol
Alcohol is not included in NDPS Act, 1985. The reasons for not including alcohol in the NDPS Act are many, the important ones being:[8]
- Prevailing social acceptance;
- Source of high revenue for Government;
- High prevalence of illicit alcohol available locally with ease being high in society, and
- Large individual variation in clinical course of alcohol dependence contrary to other drugs like opium covered under NDPSA

Alcohol is a subject of State List under the Seventh Schedule of Indian Constitution. Therefore, laws concerning drinking, regulation of sale, consumption and legal age for drinking varies across states. In India, consumption of alcohol is prohibited in states of Gujarat, Manipur, Mizoram and Nagaland, as well as the union territory of Lakshadweep. All other Indian states permit alcohol consumption but have fixed a legal drinking age varying from 18 to 25 years.[9]

Drunk Driving: Alcohol Limit and Punishment in India[10]
Section 185 of the Motor Vehicles Act, 1988 states "Whoever, while driving, or attempting to drive, a motor vehicle":
- Has, in his blood, alcohol exceeding 30 mg. per 100 ml. of blood detected in a test by a breath analyser, or
- Is under this influence of a drug to such an extent as to be incapable of exercising proper control over the vehicle, shall be punishable for the first offence with imprisonment for

a term which may extend to six months, or with fine which may extend to two thousand rupees, or with both; and for a second or subsequent offence, if committed within three years of the commission of the previous similar offence, with imprisonment for a term which may extend to two years, or with fine which may extend to three thousand rupees, or with both.
(One Standard Drink = ½ bottle of Standard Beer = ¼ bottle of Strong Beer = 1 peg (30 mL) Spirits = ½ packet of Arrack = 1 glass (125 mL) of table wine = 1 glass (60 mL) fortified wine.
- One drink (one standard unit of alcohol is 10 mL of absolute alcohol, i.e. 7.87 g) is likely to raise the BAC to approximately 15 to 20 mg/dL)

Motor Vehicle (Amendment) Bill 2016[9]

The Union Cabinet has given its approval for Motor Vehicle (Amendment) Bill 2016 recently. The Amendment bill aims to improve road safety and provides for higher level of fines and penalty for drunk driving. The penalty for drunk driving under the Motor Vehicle (Amendment) Bill 2016 has been increased from ₹ 2000 to ₹ 10,000.

THE DRUGS AND COSMETICS ACT, 1940; THE DRUGS AND COSMETICS RULES, 1945

- This act provide control of sale, supply and distribution of drugs.
- *Schedule H:* List of substances that could be sold by retail on the prescription of a Registered Medical Practitioner only (Prescription Drugs).
- *Schedule X:* Schedule X contains list of drugs whose import, distribution, manufacture, sale, packing and labelling are to be carried out under special provisions. Examples include Amphetamine, Cyclobarbital, Methamphetamine, Pentobarbital, Secobarbital, Methylphenidate etc. List of drugs for which the retailer is to preserve prescription for a period of two years.
- *Schedule G:* List of drugs that could be dangerous to take except under medical supervision, e.g. Cyclophosphamide, Insulin etc.
  - **If drugs fall under NDPS Act** (addiction forming substances) with a symbol **NRx on the left hand corner**[11,12]

Mental Health Care Act 2017

It defines mental illness as "a disorder of mood, thought, perception, orientation and memory which causes significant distress to a person or impairs a person's behavior, judgment and ability to recognize reality or impairs the person's ability to meet the demands of daily life and includes mental **conditions associated with the abuse of alcohol and drugs**, but does not include mental retardation, it **mandates all drug deaddiction and rehabilitation centers also now to be classified as mental health establishment** and to follow same norms and standards of care as defined in MHCA Rules.[13]

Food Safety and Regulation (Prohibition) Act 2011

Gutka is banned under the provision to ban any food product containing harmful adulterants in the centrally enacted Food Safety and Regulation (Prohibition) Act 2011. Offenders can be fined INR200 according to the *Control of Tobacco Products Act (COTPA)*. The Food Safety and Standards Authority of India (FSSAI), under which the ban has been regulated, said offenders can face six months to three years in jail. The law has provisions of imposing fines up to ₹ 25,000 on selling of products that are injurious to health. Karnataka became the 26th state to ban sale, manufacture, storage and distribution of Gutka. It is also in place in five union territories.[14]

Laws Concerning Criminal Responsibility of Intoxicated Person

As per Section 85 of IPC, "Nothing is an offence which is done by a person who, at the time of doing it, is, by reason of intoxication, incapable of knowing the nature of the act, or that he is doing what is either wrong, or contrary to law; provided that the thing which intoxicated him was administered to him without his knowledge or against his will."[15]

Under Section 86 of Indian Penal Code, In cases where act done is not an offence unless done with a particular knowledge or intent, a person who does the act in a state of intoxication shall be liable to be dealt with as if he had the same knowledge as he would have had if he had not been intoxicated, unless the thing which intoxicated him was administered to him without his knowledge or against his will.[15]

However, if the intoxication is induced voluntarily, the act done is an offence even if the person is incapable of knowing the nature of the act or that what he is doing is either wrong or contrary to law.

Gambling Laws in India

The following are the various laws which regulate/restrict gambling in India:[16]
- *The Public Gambling Act, 1867:* This Central legislation provides for the punishment of public gambling. The penalty for breaking this law is a fine of ₹ 200 or imprisonment of upto 3 months.
- *The Lotteries (Regulation) Act, 1998:* This Central Legislation lays down guidelines and restrictions in conducting lotteries.
- *Section 294-A of the Indian Penal Code, 1860:* This Section lays down punishment for keeping a lottery office without the authorisation of the State government.
- *Section 30 of the Indian Contract Act, 1872.*
    - Other than lotteries, legal gambling in India is limited to betting on horse racing.
- Sikkim and Goa are the only two states in India which currently permit gambling (other than horse-racing, dog-racing and lotteries).
- The Information Technology Act 2000 regulates cyber related gambling activities in India.[16]

REFERENCES

1. The NDPS Act Published in the Gazette of India, Extraordinary, Pt. II, Sec. 1, No. 75, dated 16th September, 1985.

2. Act 2 of 1989 enforced w.e.f. 29th May, 1989, Published in the Gazette of India Extraordinary, Pt. II, Sec. 2, No. 59, dated 6th December, 1988, vide S.O. 379 (E), dated 29th May, 1989, published in the Gazette of India, Extraordinary, Pt. II, Sec 3 (ii), No. 300, dated 29th May, 1989.
3. The NDPS Act Amendment 2014 by the Central Department of Revenue – 10th March 2014 http://mpsja.mphc.gov.in/ Joti/pdf/ LU/NDPS% 20SINGH%20SIR.docx%20corrected.pdf.
4. The NDPS third Amendment Rules 2015 by the Central Department of Revenue- in Hindi and English [page 17]- 5th May 2015 http://dor.gov.in/sites/default/files/NDPS%20Third%20Amendment%20Rules%20201 5%20dated%2005%2005%202015_0.pdf.
5. Notification on the Essential Narcotic Drugs by Department of Revenue – 5th May 2015 http://dor.gov.in/sites/default/files/Essential% 20Narcotic% 20Drug%20Notification%2 0dated%2005%20 05%202015_0.pdf.
6. Circular notification by Sri B.N. Sharma to Chief Secretaries/Administrators of all States and UT – 22nd July 2016 http://neigrihms.gov.in/Institute,%20Circular,%20Order,%20Format/Store/circular%2 0notification%20narcotic%20drugs.pdf.
7. Vallath N, Rajagopal MR, Tandon T. Guidelines for Stocking and Dispensing Essential Narcotic Drugs in Medical Institutions. NCG Palliative Care Committee, August 2017.
8. Sahoo S, Manjunatha N, Prasad Sinha BN, et al. Why is alcohol excluded and opium included in NDPS act, 1985? Indian J Psychiatry. 2007;49:126-8.
9. Available at: https://en.wikipedia.org/wiki/Alcohol_laws_of_India. Last accessed on 07.02.18
10. Indian Motor Vehicle Act. Bare Act. Gazette of India. Available at: www.tn.gov.in/sta/Mvact1988.pdf.Last accessed on 07.02.18.
11. The Drugs and Cosmetics act, 1940. Bare Act. Gazette of India. Available at: https://indiankanoon.org/doc/16293633. Last accessed on 07.02.18.
12. The Drugs and Cosmetics Rules, 1945. Available at: https://indiankanoon.org/doc/16293633. Last accessed on 07.02.18.
13. The Mental Health Care Act 2017, Gazette of India, 07.04.2017. Available at: http://www.prsindia.org/uploads/media/Mental% 20Health/Mental%20 Healthcare %20Act,%202017.pdf. [Last accessed on 02.010.18].
14. Food Safety and Regulation (Prohibition) Act 2011. Available at: fsdaup.gov.in/fss-regulation-2011.htm [Last accessed on 02.010.18].
15. BM Gandhi. Indian Penal Code (Paper Back) (2013 ed.). EBC. pp. 1–832. ISBN 81-7012-892-7.
16. Suthar S, Khatija Y. Available at: https://www.slideshare.net/ drsunilsuthar/acts-related-to-addiction-psychiatry. [Last accessed on 02.010.18].

CHAPTER

27

Rights of Persons with Disabilities Act, 2016

> **LEARNING OBJECTIVES**
> - Conditions of relevance for mental health covered in Act
> - Benchmark disabilities
> - Limited guardianship
> - Rights and entitlements provided under the Act
> - Critical appraisal of Rights of Persons with Disabilities Act, 2016
> - Intellectual disability certification guidelines
> - SLD certification guidelines
> - Certification guidelines for mental illness related disability
> - Critical appraisal of Rights of Persons with Disabilities Rules, 2017

INTRODUCTION

This Act repealed Persons with Disabilities Act, 1995 (PWD Act, 1995). It was notified on December 28, 2016 after receiving the presidential assent.

Division: It has 17 chapters and 102 sections.

Principles: Based on following principles:
(a) Respect for inherent dignity, individual autonomy including the freedom to make one's own choices, and independence of persons;
(b) Non-discrimination;
(c) Full and effective participation and inclusion in society;
(d) Respect for difference and acceptance of persons with disabilities as part of human diversity and humanity;
(e) Equality of opportunity;
(f) Accessibility;
(g) Equality between men and women;
(h) Respect for the evolving capacities of children with disabilities and respect for the right of children with disabilities to preserve their identities.

Disabilities covered: The types of disabilities have been increased from existing 7 (in previous PWD Act) to 21 and the Central Government will have the power to add more types of disabilities. The 21 disabilities are given below:
1. Blindness

2. Low-vision
3. Leprosy cured persons
4. Hearing impairment (deaf and hard of hearing)
5. Locomotor disability
6. Dwarfism
7. Intellectual disability
8. Mental illness
9. Autism spectrum disorder
10. Cerebral palsy
11. Muscular dystrophy
12. Chronic neurological conditions
13. Specific learning disabilities
14. Multiple sclerosis
15. Speech and language disability
16. Thalassemia
17. Hemophilia
18. Sickle cell disease
19. Multiple disabilities including deaf blindness
20. Acid attack victim
21. Parkinson's disease.

DISABILITY CONDITIONS OF RELEVANCE FOR MENTAL HEALTH

- Intellectual Disability
- Mental Illness
- Autism Spectrum Disorder
- Specific Learning Disabilities

Persons with "benchmark disabilities" are defined as those certified to have at least *40 percent of the disabilities* specified above.

Rights and Entitlements Provided Under the Rights of Persons with Disabilities Act, 2016[1]

1. *Government responsibility:* Responsibility has been cast upon the appropriate governments to take effective measures to ensure that the persons with disabilities enjoy their rights equally with others.
2. *Reservation:* Additional benefits such as reservation in higher education (not less than 5%), government jobs (not less than 4%), reservation in allocation of land, poverty alleviation schemes (5% allotment), etc. have been provided for persons with benchmark disabilities and those with high support needs.
3. *Right to education:* Every **child with benchmark disability** between the age group of **6 and 18 years** shall have the **right to free education**.

4. *Inclusive government funded education:* Government funded educational institutions as well as the government recognized institutions will have to provide inclusive education to the children with disabilities.
5. No discrimination against Women and children with disabilities.
6. *Right to live in the community:* Not to be forced to live in shelter homes.
7. *Right to protection from cruelty and inhuman treatment.*
    - *Prevention from torture Section 6 (1):* The appropriate Government shall take measures to protect persons with disabilities from being subjected to torture, cruel, inhuman or degrading treatment.
    - *Research-related provisions—Sections 6(2)* No person with disability shall be a subject of any research without,—
        (i) His or her free and informed consent obtained through accessible modes, means and formats of communication; and
        (ii) Prior permission of a Committee for Research on Disability.

Central Committee for Research on Disability as defined in RPWD Rules shall consist of the following persons, namely:
(i) An eminent person having vast experience in the field of science or medicine, to be nominated by the Central Government, ex officio-Chairperson;
(ii) Nominee of the Director General of Health Services not below the rank of Deputy Director General-Member;
(iii) Four persons drawn from National Institutes representing physical, visual, hearing and intellectual disabilities, to be nominated by the Central Government-Members;
(iv) Five persons as representatives of the registered organisations, from each of the five groups of specified disabilities in the Schedule to the Act, to be nominated by the Central Government-Members:
   Provided that at least one representative of the registered organizations is a woman;
(v) The Director, Department of Empowerment of Persons with Disabilities, New Delhi shall be the Member Secretary.

8. *Protection from abuse, violence and exploitation:* Section 7 (2)—Any person or registered organization who or which has reason to believe that an act of abuse, violence or exploitation has been, or is being, or is likely to be committed against any person with disability, may give information about it to the Executive Magistrate or police within the local limits of whose jurisdiction such incidents occur.
   Section 7 (3)—The Executive Magistrate on receipt of such information, shall take immediate steps to stop or prevent its occurrence, as the case may be, or pass such order as he deems fit for the protection of such person with disability including an order—
   (a) To rescue the victim of such act, authorizing the police or any organization working for persons with disabilities to provide for the safe custody or rehabilitation of such person, or both, as the case may be;
   (b) For providing protective custody to the person with disability, if such person so desires;
   (c) To provide maintenance to such person with disability.

9. *Section 9—Right to home and family:* Section 9—(1) No child with disability shall be separated from his or her parents on the ground of disability except on an order of competent court, if required, in the best interest of the child.
(2) Where the parents are unable to take care of a child with disability, the competent court shall place such child with his or her near relations, and failing that within the community in a family setting or in exceptional cases in shelter home run by the appropriate Government or non-governmental organization, as may be required.
10. *Section 10—Reproductive rights:* Section 10(1) The appropriate Government shall ensure that persons with disabilities have access to appropriate information regarding reproductive and family planning.
(2) No person with disability shall be subject to any medical procedure which leads to infertility without his or her free and informed consent.
11. *Section 11—Accessibility in voting:* The Election Commission of India and the State Election Commissions shall ensure that all polling stations are accessible to persons with disabilities and all materials related to the electoral process are easily understandable by and accessible to them.
12. *Section 12—Access to justice:* Section 12(1) The appropriate Government shall ensure that persons with disabilities are able to exercise their legal capacity at par with others and they have right to access any court, tribunal, authority, commission or any other body having judicial or quasi-judicial or investigative powers without discrimination on the basis of disability.
(3) The National Legal Services Authority and the State Legal Services Authorities constituted under the Legal Services Authorities Act, 1987 shall make provisions including reasonable accommodation to ensure that persons with disabilities have access to any scheme, programme, facility or service offered by them equally with others.
13. *Section 13—Right to exercise equal legal capacity:* Section 13(1) The appropriate Government shall ensure that the persons with disabilities have right, equally with others, to own or inherit property, movable or immovable, control their financial affairs and have access to bank loans, mortgages and other forms of financial credit.
14. *Section 14—Provision for guardianship:* Section 14(1) District Court may offer **"limited guardianship"** means a system of joint decision which operates on mutual understanding and trust between the guardian and the person with disability, which shall be limited to a specific period and for specific decision and situation and shall operate in accordance to the will of the person with disability.
Where the limited guardianship is to be granted repeatedly, in which case, the decision regarding the support to be provided shall be reviewed by the Court or the designated authority, as the case may be, to determine the nature (limited guardianship or total support) and manner of support to be provided
15. *Reservation in job:* Every appropriate Government shall appoint in every Government establishment, not less than 4% of the total number of vacancies in the cadre strength in each group of posts meant to be filled with persons with benchmark disabilities of which, 1% each shall be reserved for persons with benchmark disabilities under clauses (a), (b) and (c) and 1% for persons with benchmark disabilities under clauses (d) and (e), namely:

a. Blindness and low vision;
b. Deaf and hard of hearing;
c. Locomotor disability including cerebral palsy, leprosy cured, dwarfism, acid attack victims and muscular dystrophy;
d. Autism, intellectual disability, specific learning disability and mental illness;
e. Multiple disabilities from amongst persons under clauses (a) to (d) including deaf-blindness in the posts identified for each disabilities.

16. *Penalties for offences*
    - The Act provides for penalties for offences committed against persons with disabilities and also violation of the provisions of the new law.
    - Any person who violates provisions of the Act, or any rule or regulation made under it, shall be punishable with imprisonment up to six months and/or a fine of ₹ 10,000, or both. For any subsequent violation, imprisonment of up to two years and/or a fine of ₹ 50,000 to ₹ 5 lakh can be awarded.
    - Whoever intentionally insults or intimidates a person with disability, or sexually exploits a woman or child with disability, shall be punishable with imprisonment between six months to five years and fine.
    - *Special Courts* will be designated in each district to handle cases concerning violation of rights of PWDs.

CRITICAL APPRAISAL OF RIGHTS OF PERSONS WITH DISABILITIES ACT, 2016

- *Positive aspects of RPWD Act for mental disabilities:*
  (a) It is a very client centered Act, inclined towards making persons with disability in possession of requisite rights to exercise their true potential in all walks of life than just providing social welfare measures
  (b) Term mental retardation has been replaced by intellectual disability.
- *Critique of RPWD Act for mental disabilities:*
  Schedule {clause (zc) of Section 2} on specified disabilities section **mentions** in sub-section 2 **intellectual disability including Specific learning disability and autism spectrum disorder.** Three entirely different entities have been erroneously clubbed together.

CERTIFICATION GUIDELINES FOR MENTAL DISABILITIES AS MENTIONED IN RIGHTS OF PERSONS WITH DISABILITY RULE, 2018 AS PER RIGHTS OF PERSONS WITH DISABILITIES RULES, 2017[2]

Rule 17. Application for certificate of disability.
1. Any person with specified disability may apply in Form -IV for a certificate of disability and submit the application to:
   (a) A medical authority in the district of residence of the applicant as mentioned in the proof of residence in the application; or

(b) The concerned medical authority in a government hospital where he may be undergoing or may have undergone treatment in connection with his disability:
- Provided that where a person with disability is a minor or suffering from intellectual disability or any other disability which renders him unfit or unable to make such an application himself, the application on his behalf may be made by his legal guardian or by any organization registered under the Act having the minor under its care.

2. The application shall be accompanied by -
   (a) Proof of residence;
   (b) Two recent passport size photographs; and
   (c) Aadhaar number or aadhaar enrollment number, if any.

Rule 18. Issue of certificate of disability.
   (2) The medical authority shall issue the certificate of disability or reason of rejection within a month from the date of receipt of the application.
   (3) The medical authority shall, after due examination issue a -
       (i) **Permanent certificate,** where there are no chances of variation of disability over time in the degree of disability; or
       (ii) **Certificate of disability indicating the period of validity,** in cases where there is any chance of variation over time in the degree of disability.

19. *Certificate issued under Rule 18 to be generally valid for all purposes,* i.e. facilities, concessions and benefits admissible for persons with disabilities under schemes funded by the Government.

GUIDELINES FOR INDIVIDUAL DISABILITY CERTIFICATION

Intellectual Disability

Diagnosis: Referred to Child/clinical psychologists for adaptive functioning and IQ testing. The tools that can be used for the same include:
(i) Adaptive functioning: VSMS
(ii) IQ testing: BKT/MISIC
    Based on the above the diagnosis of intellectual disability (ID) will be confirmed.

Disability calculation: The disability calculation will be done based on adaptive functioning severity, i.e. VSMS score. The following will be used for disability calculation:
(i)   VSMS score 0-20: Profound Disability—100%
(ii) VSMS score 21-35: Severe Disability—90%
(iii) VSMS score 36-54: Moderate Disability—75%
(iv) VSMS score 55-69: Mild Disability—50%
(v)   VSMS score 70-84: Borderline Disability—25%

Age for certification: The minimum age for certification will be one (01) completed year. Diagnosis as per age will be:
- *Global Developmental Delay (GDD)* for children 1-5 years
- *Intellectual Disability* for children > 5 years.

Medical authority: The Medical Superintendent or Chief Medical Officer or Civil Surgeon or any other equivalent authority as notified by the State Government shall be the head of the Medical Board. The Authority shall comprise of:
(a) The Medical Superintendent or Chief Medical Officer or Civil Surgeon or any other equivalent authority as notified by the State Government
(b) Pediatrician or Pediatric Neurologist (where available)/Psychiatrist or Physician (if age >18 years)
(c) Clinical or Rehabilitation Psychologist
(d) Psychiatrist.

Validity of certificate
(i) *Temporary certificate for children < 5 years:* The certificate will be valid for maximum 3 years/5 years age (whichever is earlier).
(ii) *For children 5–17 years:* The certificate will mention a renewal age. The certificate will have to be renewed at age of 5 years, 10 years and 18 years.
(iii) The certificate issued at 18 years age will be valid lifelong.

Specific Learning Disability (SLD)

Screening: (i) The *teachers of the public and private school* shall carry out the screening in Class III or at eight years of age, whichever is earlier.
(ii) Every school (public and private) shall have a screening committee headed by the principal. After applying the screening test, if an anomaly is detected then, the teacher should bring it to the notice of principal and screening committee of the school. The teachers shall interview the parents to assess their involvement and motivation regarding their child's education. If the parents are motivated and screening questionnaire suggests SLD, then child should be referred for further assessment.
(iii) The child shall be referred to pediatrician for SLD assessment by the principal of the school with the recommendations of the screening committee endorsed.

Diagnosis: The diagnosis will require a *team approach involving a pediatrician and clinical or rehabilitation psychologist.* This would involve three steps:
- *Step 1—Assessment of pediatrician:* The pediatrician will do the initial assessment involving detailed neurological examination including vision and hearing assessment.
- *Step 2—IQ Assessment:* Child/clinical psychologist will do the IQ assessment using MISIC or WISCIII. If the IQ is determined to be >85, then step 3 will be applied.
- *Step 3—SLD Assessment:* This would involve using National Institute for Mental Health and Neurosciences (NIMHANS) battery for diagnosis and rating severity.

Medical authority: The Medical Superintendent or Chief Medical Officer or Civil Surgeon or any other equivalent authority as notified by the State Government shall be head the certification authority. The medical authority will comprise of:
(a) The Medical Superintendent or Chief Medical Officer or Civil Surgeon or any other equivalent authority as notified by the State Government

(b) Pediatrician or Pediatric Neurologist (where available)
(c) Clinical or Rehabilitation Psychologist
(d) Occupational Therapist or Special Educator or Teacher trained for assessment of SLD.

Validity of certificate: The *certification will be done for children aged eight years and above only.* The child will have to undergo *repeat certification* at the age of *14 years and at the age of 18 years.* The certificate issued at *18 years will be valid life long.*

Mental Illness

- *Examination:* The examination process will consist of clinical assessment, Indian Disability Evaluation and Assessment Scale (IDEAS) scale and/or IQ assessment.
- In some cases where there is suspicion of intellectual deficits or additional intellectual evaluation is required for any reason, Standardized IQ test may be carried out. Categories on IQ score will be:
    (i) *Mild Mental Disabilities:* The range of 50–69 (standardized IQ test) is indicative of mild disability.
    (ii) *Moderate Mental Disability:* The IQ is in the range of 35–49
    (iii) *Severe Mental Disability:* The IQ is in the range of 20–34.
    (iv) *Profound Mental Disability:* The IQ in this category estimated to be under 20.
- *In cases where the mental behavioral condition requires only IDEAS*, then only *IDEAS can be administered and degree of disability certified.*
- *In cases where the mental behavioural condition requires only IQ*, then a standardized IQ test shall be used to certify degree of disability.
- In *some cases, only one test may not estimate disability* comprehensively. Such a person may have borderline or normal score on one test with disability score on the other. In such cases *both IQ and IDEAS shall be used, the score indicating more severe disability should be the degree of disability* for that person.

Medical authority: The Medical Superintendent or Chief Medical Officer or Civil Surgeon or any other equivalent authority as notified by the State Government shall be head of the certification authority with the following two other members:
(a) Psychiatrist for clinical assessment,
(b) Trained psychologist to administer IQ tests.

CRITICAL APPRAISAL OF RIGHTS OF PERSONS WITH DISABILITIES RULES, 2017

- **Positive aspects of RPWD Act Rules for mental disabilities:** Very structure guidelines for screening, diagnosis, severity rating, with psychometric scales too mentioned
- **Critique of RPWD Act Rules for mental disabilities:**
    (a) After a huge effort, in last six years, process of certification was eased by allowing it to be issued by single medical authority (SMA) for persons with mental illness and intellectual disability to reduce the distress of clients and families. However, these

rules have again increased it to certification by a board than SMA, increasing paper work and time taken, subsequently causing undue distress to service users.
(b) Psychiatrist has no more any role in SLD certification at any step, neither screening, nor diagnosis, nor certification.
(c) No mention about certification for Autism in entire rules, has it been forgotten or Since in RPWD Act schedule definition of 'intellectual disability' mentions including SLD and Autism, so, has it been clubbed with ID assessment, is not clear
(d) Mental illness (MI) and intellectual disability (ID) seems to have been equated at one erroneously at two places:
  (i) Certification for mental illness mentions three categories. One requiring IDEAS administration alone, second requiring IDEAS and IQ both, which is understood. There is a third category mentioned where only IQ is needed, which suggests the conceptual error of clubbing MI and ID as one.
  (ii) Central research committee for disability will consist of one person from national institute of other physical disabilities and intellectual disability. No mention of other mental disabilities including MI/SLD/Autism, as if MI and ID have been equated erroneously as one.

REFERENCES

1. The Rights of Persons with Disabilities Act, 2016, Gazette of India (Extra-Ordinary); 28 December.2016. [Last accessed on 2018 Jan 27]. Available from:http://www.disabilityaffairs.gov.in/uploaad/uploadfiles/files/RPWD/ACT/2016.pdf.
2. Rights of Persons with Disabilities Rules, 2017, Gazette of India (Extra-Ordinary); 15 June.2017. [Last accessed on 2018 Jan 27]. Available http://www.ccdisabilities.nic.in/page.php?s=&t=yb&p=RPwDRule.

SECTION VIII

Other Medicolegal Issues of Relevance for Mental Health Professionals

CHAPTER 28

Human Rights of Persons with Mental Illness

> **LEARNING OBJECTIVES**
> - Concept of human rights
> - Right to health
> - Global developments and rights of persons with mental illness
> - Indian perspective of human rights of persons with mental illness
> - WHO Mental Health Laws: 10 Basic Principles
> - UNCRPD 2006
> - Post-UNCRPD era: Legislative reforms in India
> - Rights and privileges of persons with mental illness
> - Rights of families and caregivers of persons with mental illness
> - Competence, capacity and guardianship

Every human being inherently possesses certain rights by virtue of being born as a human being. These rights, usually referred as Human Rights, are the moral principles or norms describing certain standards of human behavior regularly protected as legal rights in municipal and international law. These laws are the inalienable fundamental rights of a person regardless of his nation, location, language, religion, ethnic origin or any other status. Applicable everywhere and at every time, these laws are egalitarian in the sense of being the same for everyone. They are regarded as requiring empathy and the rule of law with the obligation on persons to respect the human rights of others. The Universal Declaration of Human Rights[1] 1948, codified the right to life and liberty and right to be free from inhuman, degrading treatment. It defines human rights as those rights, which are inherent in our nature and without which we cannot live as human beings. The right to life in Article 21 of India's Constitution means something more than survival of human existence. Within its ambit, it includes the right to live with dignity, right to health, right to potable water, right to pollution free environment and right to education etc., which have been held to be part of right to life.

Section 2(d) of the Protection of Human Rights Act 1993[2] has defined human rights to mean the rights relating to life, liberty, equality and dignity of the individual guaranteed under the Constitution or embodied in the international covenants and enforceable by the courts in India.

RIGHT TO HEALTH

The preamble of the World Health Organization (WHO) succinctly underscores the enjoyment of the highest standard of health as a fundamental right of every human being. According to Article 25 of the Universal Declarations of Human Rights, everyone has the right to a standard of living, adequate for the health of himself, including food, clothing, housing, medical care, and necessary services.

Health is a unity and harmony within the mind, body, and spirit, which is unique to each person. The level of wellness or health is, in part, determined by the ability to deal with and defend against stressful situations. Health is on a continuum with movements between a state of optimum well-being and illness. It is determined by physiological, psychological, socio-cultural, spiritual, and developmental stage variables.[3]

Studies reveal that individuals' poorer health status, including higher morbidity, lower life expectancy, higher rates of infant mortality, mental ill-health are linked to their social status. Discrimination rooted in social status affects people's health in at least three distinct ways: (a) health status, (b) access to healthcare, and (c) in quality of health services.[4]

Though every man, woman and child is entitled to the fundamental human rights including right to health, mentally challenged persons as a group have always lived a stigmatized existence in all societies across the world, deprived of their legitimate rights. They have not only remained ignored, isolated and side-lined from the mainstream social life, they have been subjected to inhuman treatment of being chained, tortured and physically abused in blatant violation of their human rights. They have faced indignation, discrimination and invisibilization in every walk of life and dumped into the high enclosures of lunatic asylums to vegetate for the rest of their lives. Abandonment of mentally ill has remained a world-wide phenomenon because of socio-cultural reasons and religious belief.[5] The rights of mentally ill include not only their privileges but also the remedial rights of protection against infringement of their human and other statutory rights against any abusive or harmful treatments given under the guise of mental health.[6]

GLOBAL DEVELOPMENTS AND RIGHTS OF PERSONS WITH MENTAL ILLNESS

Global concern of the civil society towards the disabled and the disadvantaged became visible from the beginning of 20th century and mental illness became a subject of scientific scrutiny and humane treatment. With the advent of General Hospital Psychiatry movement in 1930s, there was a paradigm shift in the management of the mentally ill who were, so far slogging in the depressing environment of the lunatic asylums. They no longer remained the subjects of curiosity, fear or affliction by supernatural powers for the general public as they began to be accepted as patients in general hospitals like others. Introduction of electro-convulsive therapy and psychotropic medication made the possibility of treatment a reality.

Post-second World War period was marked by reforms against racial and caste based discrimination, cruelty and injustice against women, children and the disabled, through various international instruments. After the Convention on the Declaration of Human Rights 1948[1], the International Convention on the Elimination of All Forms of Racial Discrimination, 1965[7], the International Convention on Civil and Political Rights, 1966,[8] the International Convention on Economic, Social and Cultural Rights, 1966,[9] the Convention on the Elimination of all forms of Discrimination against Women, 1979,[10] the Convention against Torture and Other Cruel, Inhuman or Degrading Treatment or Punishment, 1984,[11] the Convention on the Rights of the Child, 1989,[12] are some of the international initiatives which brought sweeping reforms in the world social order.

Article 12 of the International Convention on Economic, Social and Cultural Rights, 1966[9] provides "that the state parties to the present Convention recognise the rights of everyone to the enjoyment of highest attainable standards of physical and mental health and the Article 12 of the Convention on the Elimination of all forms of Discrimination against Women, 1979,[10] provides that state parties shall take all appropriate measures to eliminate discrimination against women in the field of health.

The 1971 Declaration on the Rights of Mentally Retarded Persons was adopted by the General Assembly on 20th December 1971, keeping in view the necessity for providing help to mentally retarded persons in order to enable them to develop their ability and promoting their integrity in normal life. The Declaration provides a framework within which the national and international actions should be initiated for the advancement of rights set forth in the Declaration.[13]

Declaration of Hawaii 1992 by General Assembly of World Psychiatric Association (WPA) advocates for the patients' right to treatment and patients' consent for treatment. It also discusses treatment under special circumstances, where if the patient does not have judgment into his condition then treatment is administered in his best interest. As soon as the condition for compulsory treatment is no longer applicable, psychiatrist should obtain voluntary consent and treat the patient.[14]

In 1996, the Committee on Economic, Social and Cultural Rights adopted General Comment 5, detailing the application of the International Covenant on Economic, Social and Cultural Rights (ICESCR) with regard to people with mental and physical disabilities. General Comments, which are produced by human rights oversight bodies, are an important source of interpretation of the articles of human rights conventions. General comments are non-binding, but they represent the official view as to the proper interpretation of the convention by the human rights oversight body.[15]

Post-independence India stayed in-step with the international developments and witnessed the growth of general hospital psychiatry units (GHPUs) and the introduction of post-graduate psychiatry training programme at a large scale in the country. National Mental Health Programme[16] (NMHP) introduced in 1982 brought the mental health services to the community with the aim of providing mental health services to each and every needy person. Integration of mental health services with the general health played a significant role in *reducing the stigma attached to mental illness.*

INDIAN PERSPECTIVE OF HUMAN RIGHTS OF PERSONS WITH MENTAL ILLNESS

Mental Health Act, 1987

Draconian colonial era law, symbol of custodial confinement, the Indian Lunacy Act, 1912, was replaced by Mental Health Act 1987,[17] providing for the first time, the provision of human rights for the mentally ill. Chapter VIII of the Act provides for the Protection of Human Rights of the mentally ill. Under this chapter, Section 81 of the Act provides that no mentally ill person shall be subjected during treatment to any indignity or cruelty. No such patient shall be used for research unless it is of direct benefit to the patient, with no barrier to his communication with the outside world.

It took six years for the Act to come into action and the violation of the rights of the mentally ill continued in the mental hospitals and the community alike.

Persons with Disabilities Act, 1995

Persons with Disabilities (Equal Opportunities and Full participation) Act, 1995 includes mental illness into the ambit of disability. For the first time, mental illness was recognized as a disability in India.[18]

Insurance Regulatory Development Authority Act, 1999

Insurance Regulatory Development Authority (IRDA) Act 1999 endeavors that insurance will be provided to treatment of mental illness at par with that of physical illness as given under Section 21(2) of the Act.[19]

Supreme Court Decisions on Management of Mental Hospitals[20]

There have been several landmark judgments by the Supreme Court of India which have paved path to transform asylums into model psychiatric institutions. Cases of BR Kapoor vs Union of India and PUCL vs Union of India were related to the deplorable conditions in the Hospital for Mental Disease at Shahdara, Delhi. RC Narayan vs state of Bihar case of 1997 is about the functioning of Ranchi Mental Asylum. Supreme Court also intervened to improve the functioning of Mental Hospital at Gwalior in Madhya Pradesh.

India's Constitution empowers both Central and State governments to introduce measures including the authority to legislate. The Mental Health Act, 1987 is civil rights legislation to regulate standards in mental health institutions. However, the effectiveness of this Act is seriously questionable in ensuring protection of the rights of the mentally ill.

The Supreme Court cases clearly demonstrate that until recently many non-criminal mentally ill persons were consigned to jails and those living in mental hospitals were no better off. Sheela Barse vs Union of India case concerns detention of non-criminal mentally-ill persons of West Bengal. The Supreme Court observed that admission of non-criminal mentally ill persons to jails is illegal and unconstitutional. In another case, the Supreme Court denounced the practice of physical restraining and ordered the cessation of the practice of tying up the patients, who were unruly or not physically controllable, with iron chains and ordered medical treatment for these patients.

However, on August 6, 2001, the tragic death of 26 mentally-ill patients in Erwadi, Tamil Nadu showed the callous attitude of private authorities and the state government in implementation of Supreme Court orders. In that incidence, charred dead bodies of 26 patients were found, tied to their beds when the fire engulfed the place they were lodged in. The National Human Rights Commission (NHRC)[22] of India suo moto advised all the states to submit a certificate stating no person with mental illness is kept chained in either government or private institutions.

Under Section 12 of the Protection of Human Rights Act, 1993,[2] the NHRC is mandated to visit government run mental hospitals to study the living conditions of inmates and make recommendations thereon. A project, named Quality Assurance in Mental Health Institutions[23] was initiated in 1997 to analyse the conditions prevailing in 37 government run mental hospitals in the country.

The findings of this study confirm that mental hospitals in the country are still being managed and administered on custodial care model with prison like structure of high walls, watch tower, fenced wards and locked cells. The cases reaching the Supreme Court at different points of time through public interest litigation (PIL), discuss only the deplorable conditions of the institutions and none mentioned the rights of the inmates to minimum standards of care and treatment. However, the cases have demonstrated the need for continued judicial monitoring in order to ensure that the state acts in accordance with the statute and the Constitution.

In 1996, WHO developed the Mental Health Care Law which comprise ten Basic Principles, these are the guidelines for the protection and promotion of human rights of persons with mental illness.[24]

Mental Health Laws: 10 Principles

1. Promotion of mental health and prevention of mental disorders
2. Access to basic mental health care
3. Mental health assessments in accordance with internationally accepted principles
4. Provision of least restrictive type of mental health care
5. Self-determination
6. Right to be assisted in the exercise of self-determination
7. Availability of review procedure
8. Automatic periodic review mechanism
9. Qualified decision-makers
10. Respect of the rule of law.

UN Convention on Rights of Persons with Disabilities, 2006

UN Convention on Rights of Persons with Disabilities, 2006 was adopted on 13th December 2006 and came into force on 3rd May, 2008. It includes mental illness as a disability. India, as a member state, is one of the signatories of this convention and ratified it in October, 2007. The convention provides right to respect for physical and mental integrity on equal basis. Member countries to the convention are required to provide equal rights of all disabled persons to live in the community. Appropriate measures are taken for their inclusion and full participation in the community. State parties shall also protect privacy of the personal health and rehabilitation on an equal basis with others. According to the convention, the persons with disabilities have right to enjoy highest standard of health without discriminzation.[25]

POST-UNCRPD ERA: LEGISLATIVE REFORMS IN INDIA

National Mental Health Policy, 2014

National Mental Health Policy[26] of India was introduced by the then union health minister on 10th October, 2015 with the objective of providing:
1. Universal access to mental health care.
2. Increase access to and utilization of comprehensive mental health services
3. Mental healthcare access to homeless, socially deprived and those living in remote areas
4. Reduce the prevalence and impact of risk factors
5. Reduce risk and incidence of suicide and attempted suicide
6. Respect for the rights of the mentally ill and protection from harm of mentally ill
7. Reduce stigma associated with mental; health problems
8. Enhance availability and equitable distribution of resources
9. Enhance financial allocation financial allocation and improve utilization for mental healthcare
10. Identify social, biological and psychological factors related to mental health.

The Rights of Persons with Disabilities Act, 2016

The Rights of Persons with Disabilities Act, 2016 is the disability legislation passed by the Indian Parliament to fulfill its obligation to the United Nations Convention on the Rights of Persons with Disabilities, which India ratified in 2007. The Act replaces the existing Persons with Disabilities (Equal Opportunity Protection of Rights and Full Participation) Act, 1995.[27]

In view of fast occurring changes at the national and the international scene, working with MHA 1987 became far from satisfying. To devise a strong mechanism to address concerns of persons suffering with mental illness and to ensure compliance with International Instruments such as WHO rules and Convention on Rights of Persons with Disabilities, Draft Bill on Mental Healthcare was prepared by the Ministry of Health and Family Welfare.[28]

The Mental Healthcare Act (No. 10), 2017

Mental Healthcare Bill was passed by the Rajya Sabha in August, 2016 and the Lok Sabha on March 27, 2017. It received President's assent on 7th April, 2017 and became an Act known by the name, Mental Healthcare Act (No. 10) 2017. It provides for Mental Healthcare and services for persons with mental illness, and to protect, promote and fulfill the rights of such persons during the delivery of mental healthcare and services. The Act has 16 Chapters and 126 Sections and provides an explicit and elaborate definition of mental illness which also includes mental conditions arising from alcohol and drug use. It is, a substantial disorder of thinking, mood, perception, orientation or memory that grossly impairs judgment, behavior, capacity to recognize reality or inability to meet the ordinary demands of life; mental conditions associated with the abuse of alcohol and drugs (Mental Retardation not included).

It is a patient friendly Act to undo all the accesses mentally ill have been accorded through the ages. The Act provides that the mental illness shall be determined only by the international standards to prevent exploitation in the name of mental illness. According to the Act every person (not minor) has the right and capacity to make decision regarding his mental healthcare/treatment if he has the ability to understand the information for decision and appreciate foreseeable consequences and is able to communicate his decision. The Act also empowers everyone (not minor) to make an advance directive (AD) in writing for the way he wished to be cared for treatment of mental illness and the way he wished not to be treated for mental illness. He has the right to nominate his representative to make decision on his behalf. Section 18 gives right to access mental healthcare and treatment from mental health services run or funded by the government. The services have to be of affordable cost, good quality, available in sufficient quantity, geographically accessible, without any discrimination on gender, sexual orientation, religion, culture, caste, social/political beliefs, class, disability or any other basis and provided in a manner acceptable to the mentally ill.

The Act puts the responsibility on the government to integrate mental health services with general health services, provide treatment to support patient to live in the community with the family and ensure long-term care. The government has to ensure that no patient travels long distance to access treatment, availability of minimum mental health services in each district should be made. According to Section 19, mentally ill have the right to live in society and not to be segregated for want of or non-acceptance of family. In case the patient needs legal support, it is the duty of the government to provide it. Their treatment shall be at par with physically ill and a woman receiving care in a mental health establishment whether treatment or rehabilitation shall not be ordinarily separated from her baby less than 3 years. Under Section 22, the mentally ill and the nominated representative have right to information about the illness. They also have the right to complain about the deficiencies in treatment to the treating doctor, review board or the state mental health authority. The Act decriminalises attempted suicide. According to the Section 115, notwithstanding anything contained in Section 309 of Indian Penal Code any person who attempts to commit suicide shall be presumed, unless proved otherwise, to have severe stress and should not be tried and punished under said code. It is government's duty to provide care, treatment and rehabilitation to such person to reduce the risk of recurrence.

RIGHTS AND PRIVILEGES OF PERSONS WITH MENTAL ILLNESS

In view of the above developments rights and privileges of the mentally ill can be described as follows.

Confidentiality

Information about their illness and treatment is a personal matter of the patients and it cannot be made public or revealed to third parties without consent. Mental health professionals are bound by professional codes of conduct that generally include rules for confidentiality. All professionals involved in the care of persons with mental disorders have a particular duty to prevent any breach of confidentiality.

According to the Section 24 of the Mental Healthcare Act, 2017, no photograph or any other information of patient undergoing treatment in a mental health establishment shall be released to media without his consent. Right to confidentiality is applicable to all information stored in electronic/digital form.

There are a few exceptional instances when confidentiality may be breached. Legislation may specify the circumstances when information on mental health patients may be released to other parties without the prior consent of the user. These exceptions may include situations such as life-threatening emergencies or if there is likelihood of harm to others. However, the information disclosed should be limited only to that required for the purpose at hand. Also, when courts of law require the release of clinical information to judicial authorities, and if the information is pertinent to the particular case, mental health professionals are obliged to provide the information required.

There are other complicated issues concerning the need to maintain confidentiality and the need to share certain information with primary caregivers who are often family members. Patients and their nominated representatives have the right to ask for judicial review of, or appeal against, decisions to release information.

Access to Information

Mentally ill have a statutory right to free and full access to their clinical records maintained by mental health facilities and mental health professionals. This right is protected by general human rights norms. According to Section 22 of Mental Healthcare Act 2017, persons with mental illness or their nominated representative have the right to know the criteria under which the patients are being admitted and if not satisfied with the answer they has the right to apply to the concerned board for review.

They also have the right to know the nature of the mental illness they are suffering from and the purpose of the treatment. The information should be provided in a language understandable to the patient.

It is possible that in exceptional situations, revealing clinical records of a person may put the safety of others at risk or cause serious harm to that person's mental health. For example, clinical records sometimes contain information from third parties, such as relatives or other professionals, about a severely disturbed patient, which, if revealed to that patient at a particular time may cause a serious relapse or, worse still, cause the patient to do harm to himself or herself or to others. Many jurisdictions therefore give professionals the right (and duty) to withhold such parts of records. Normally, withholding information can only be on a temporary basis, until such time as the persons are able to deal with the information rationally.

Section 25 of Mental Healthcare Act, 2017 provides right to the mentally ill Right to access Basic Medical Record. However, some information may be withheld by the medical officer in charge which if disclosed would result in serious mental harm to patient or likely harm to other persons.

Conditions in Mental Health Establishments and the Rights of Mentally Ill

Mentally ill residing in mental health establishments are often subject to poor living conditions, such as lack of or inadequate clothing, poor sanitation and hygiene, insufficient and poor quality food, lack of privacy, being forced to work, or being subjected to physical, mental and sexual abuse from other patients and staff . Such conditions violate internationally agreed norms for rights and conditions in mental health establishments.

According to the Section 21 of the Mental Healthcare Act 2017, there will be no discrimination against mentally ill and they will be treated at par with the physically ill. They are entitled to emergency services and the ambulance services are provided in the same way as the physically ill get. Environment of the mental health establishments is to be similar to the environment of hospitals for physical ailments. According to the Section 26 of the Act, an admitted patient has the right to refuse or receive visitors. He is also entitled to make phone calls at reasonable times. He may send or receive e-mails. However, a judge, an officer authorised by the government, a member parliament or a member of legislative assembly are entitled to visit a patient. Treating physician and the nominated representative or a legal representative have free access to the patient.

The admitted patients have freedom of communication, which includes freedom to communicate with other persons in the facility; freedom to send and receive uncensored private communications. They enjoy freedom of religion or belief. The environment and living conditions in mental health facilities have to be as close as possible to those of the normal life of persons of similar age.

Patients admitted to mental health establishments have the right to be protected from cruel, inhuman and degrading treatment as set out in Article 7 of the International Convention on Civil and Political Rights (ICCPR).[29]

The provision of a safe and hygienic environment is a health concern, and critical to a person's overall well-being. No individual should be subject to unsafe or unsanitary conditions when receiving mental health treatment.

Privacy is a broad concept limiting how far society can intrude into a person's affairs. It includes information privacy, bodily privacy, privacy of communications and territorial privacy. These rights are frequently violated with regard to people with mental disorders, particularly in psychiatric facilities.

Moreover, if adequate services are provided in the community, deinstitutionalization may in itself become a means towards many people obtaining greater privacy through discharge from crowded and impersonal hospital conditions. However, it is important to note that in mental health establishments the right to privacy does not mean that, in particular circumstances such as those involving a suicidal patient, that person cannot be searched or continually observed for his or her own protection. In these circumstances, the limitation on privacy needs to be carefully considered against the internationally accepted right.

Awareness of the Rights

Although legislation may provide many rights to persons with mental disorders, they are frequently unaware of their rights and thus unable to exercise them. It is therefore essential that legislation include a provision for informing patients of their rights when interacting with mental health services.

Under Section 27 of MHCA 2017, a mentally ill is entitled to free legal services and it is the duty of the magistrate, police officer or the medical officer to inform him of his entitlement for legal services under state legal authority. Under Section 28 of the Act, the patient or his nominated representative have right to complain about the deficiencies in care, treatment and services to the medical officer, the review board or the state mental health authority.

According to the MI Principles following is the Notice of Rights:
1. A patient in a mental health facility shall be informed as soon as possible after admission, in a form and language which the patient understands, of all his or her rights in accordance with these Principles and under domestic law, which information shall include an explanation of those rights and how to exercise them.
2. If and for so long as a patient is unable to understand such information, the rights of the patient shall be communicated to the nominated representative, if any and if appropriate, and to the person or persons best able to represent the patient's interests and willing to do so *(Principle 12(1) and (2), MI Principles).*[30]

The information should include an explanation of what these rights mean and how they may be exercised, and be conveyed in such a way that patients are able to understand it. In countries where various languages are spoken, the rights should be communicated in the person's language of choice.

Provisions can be made for communicating these rights to personal representatives and/or family members in the case of patients who lack the capacity to understand such information.

Rights of Families and Caregivers of Persons with Mental Illness

Family members often bear the brunt of the person's behavior when he or she is ill or relapses, and it is usually the caregivers/family members that fundamentally love, care and worry about the person with the mental disorder. Sometimes they too become targets of stigma and discrimination. In some countries, families and caregivers also carry the legal responsibility for third-party liability arising from actions of persons with mental disorders. The important role of families needs to be recognized.

Family members and caregivers need information about the illness and treatment plans to be better able to look after their ill relatives. Legislation should not arbitrarily refuse information merely on grounds of confidentiality though the extent of an individual's right to confidentiality is likely to vary from culture to culture. For instance, in some cultures a patient's refusal to allow information to be released to family members or carers would need to be fully respected, while in others the family may be regarded as a unified, structured unit, and confidentiality may extend to culturally determined members of that family.

It is likely, in these situations, that patients themselves are more accepting of the need to provide family members with information. In countries where there is more emphasis on the individual, as opposed to the family, it is more likely that the individual himself/herself may be less inclined to share information. Many variations and gradations are possible depending on culturally accepted practices. Families can play an important role in contributing to the formulation and implementation of a treatment plan for the patient, especially if the patient is incapable of doing it alone.

Legislation ensures involvement of families in many aspects of mental health services and legal processes. For example, family members may have the right to appeal against involuntary admission and treatment decisions on behalf of their relative, if the latter lacks the capacity to do so himself/herself. Similarly, they may be able to apply for the discharge of a mentally ill offender. Countries may also choose to legislate that family groups should be represented on review bodies.

Legislation also ensures that family members are involved in the development of mental health policy and legislation, as well as mental health service planning

Key issues related to families and caregivers of mentally ill:
- It is common for families and carergivers to assume major responsibility for looking after persons with mental illness, and legislation needs to reflect this. Legislation should not arbitrarily refuse information merely on the ground of confidentiality though the extent of an individual's right to confidentiality is likely to vary from culture to culture.
- Families and carergivers can play an important role in contributing to the formulation and implementation of a treatment plan for the patient, especially if the patient is incapable of doing this alone. Legislation ensures that families and caregivers have access to the support and services they require in caring for a person with a mental disorder.
- Legislation ensures involvement of families and caregivers in many aspects of mental health services, as well as the legal processes such as involuntary admission and appeal. Legislation also ensures that family members and caregivers are involved in the development of mental health policy and legislation, as well as mental health service planning.

Competence, Capacity and Guardianship

Most persons with mental disorders retain the ability to make informed choices and decisions regarding important matters affecting their lives. However, in those with severe mental disorders, this ability might be impaired. In these circumstances, there must be suitable provisions that allow managing the affairs of people with mental illness in their best interests.

Two concepts that are central to decisions about whether or not a person may make choices concerning various issues are *"competence"* and *"capacity"*. These concepts affect treatment decisions in civil and criminal cases, and the exercise of civil rights by persons with mental disorders.

There is often a tendency to use the terms "capacity" and "competence" interchangeably in relation to mental health; however, they are not the same. Generally, *capacity* refers specifically to the presence of mental abilities to make decisions or to engage in a course of action, while *competence* refers to the legal consequences of not having the mental capacity. In these definitions, "capacity" is a health concept, whereas "competence" is a legal concept. Capacity refers to individual levels of functioning, and competence to their impact on legal and social standing.

Assessment of Incapacity

Ordinarily, there is a presumption of capacity and, consequently, of competence. Thus, a person is assumed to be capable and competent to make decisions unless proven otherwise. The presence of a major mental disorder does not in and of itself imply incapacity in decision-making functions. Hence, the presence of a mental disorder is not the overall determining factor of capacity, and certainly not of competence.

In addition, despite the presence of a disorder that may affect capacity, a person may still have the capacity to carry out some decision-making functions. Capacity and competence are thus function- specific. Therefore, because capacity may fluctuate from time to time, and is not an "all or nothing" concept, it needs to be considered in the context of the specific decision or function to be accomplished.

Some examples of specific capacities are as following:
- *Capacity to make a treatment decision requires* the person must have the ability to: (a) understand the nature of the condition for which the treatment is proposed; (b) understand the nature of the proposed treatment; and (c) appreciate the consequences of giving or withholding consent to treatment.
- *Capacity to select a substitute decision-maker requires* the person must have the ability to: (a) understand the nature of the appointment and the duties of the substitute decision-maker; (b) understand the relationship with the proposed substitute; (c) appreciate the consequences of appointing the substitute decision-maker.
- *Capacity to make a financial decision requires* the person must have the ability to(a) understand the nature of the financial decision and the choices available;(b) understand the relationship to the parties to, and/or potential beneficiaries of , the transaction; and (c) appreciate the consequences of making the financial decision. A finding of lack of capacity should be time-limited (i.e. it will have to be reviewed from time to time), because a person may regain some or complete functionality over time, either with or without treatment of the mental disorder.

Determining incapacity and incompetence:
Determination of *incapacity* may be made by a health professional, but a judicial body would determine *incompetence*. Capacity is the test for competence, and people should be judged as lacking competence only if they are actually incapable of making specific kinds of decisions at a specific time.

CONCORDANCE OF MENTAL HEALTHCARE ACT WITH MI PRINCIPLES FOR TREATMENT OF PERSONS WITH MENTAL ILLNESS

Voluntary and Involuntary Mental Healthcare

Voluntary admission and voluntary treatment requires free and informed consent that forms the basis of the treatment and rehabilitation of people with mental illness. All patients must be assumed initially to have capacity and every effort should be made to enable a person to accept voluntary admission or treatment, as appropriate, before implementing involuntary procedures.

MI Principles: Informed consent

No treatment shall be given to a patient without his or her informed consent, except as provided for in paragraphs 6, 7, 8, 13 and 15 [of the present principles]. *(Principle 11(1), MI Principles)*[30]

Consent to be valid, must satisfy the following criteria *(MI Principle 11)*:
- The person/patient giving consent must be competent to do so, and competence is assumed unless there is evidence to the contrary.
- Consent must be obtained freely, without threats or improper inducements.
- There should be appropriate and adequate disclosure of information. Information must be provided on the purpose, method, likely duration and expected benefits of the proposed treatment.
- Possible pain or discomfort and risks of the proposed treatment, and likely side-effects, should be adequately discussed with the patient.
- Choices should be offered, if available, in accordance with good clinical practice; alternative modes of treatment, especially those that are less intrusive, should be discussed and offered to the patient.
- Information should be provided in a language and form that is understandable to the patient.
- The patient should have the right to refuse or stop treatment.
- Consequences of refusing treatment, which may include discharge from the hospital, should be explained to the patient.
- The consent should be documented in the patient's medical records.

The right to consent to treatment implies also the right to refuse treatment. If a patient is judged as having the capacity to give consent, then refusal of such consent must also be respected. If admission is needed, one should aim to promote and facilitate voluntary admission to a mental health facility, after obtaining informed consent and treatment.

MI Principles: Voluntary admission and treatment

Where a person needs treatment in a mental health facility, every effort shall be made to avoid involuntary admission. *(Principle 15(1), MI Principles)*

Voluntary admission brings with it the right to voluntary discharge from mental health care facilities.

The MI Principles state that patients not admitted involuntarily have the right to leave the facility at any time unless the criteria for involuntary admission are met.

Chapter XII of the MHCA 2017 deals with admission, treatment and discharge of mentally ill for independent admission. Sections 85, 86 provide that any person with capacity to make health care decision requesting admission of his own free will and has understood nature and purpose of admission shall be admitted and have treatment with informed consent. Such a patient shall be immediately discharged if he requests, and cannot be refused by the medical officer incharge. However, he may prevent discharge for 24 hours to allow assessment for supported admission. Section 87 deals with admission of a minor.

A problem which sometimes arises is when patients who lack the capacity to consent are "voluntarily" admitted to a hospital simply because they do not protest against the admission.

One example of this would be a patient who is admitted "voluntarily" but has no understanding of either the fact or the purpose of the admission.

Other people may "accept" treatment or admission without protest merely because they are intimidated or because they do not realize they have the right to refuse. In these cases, their lack of protest should not be construed as consent, since consent must be voluntary and informed.

The concept of "voluntary" precludes the use of coercion; it implies that choices are available and that the individual has the ability and right to exercise that choice.

Key issues related to independent admission and treatment:
- Where a person needs inpatient treatment, legislation should support voluntary admission and every effort shall be made to avoid involuntary admission.
- If the law permits the authorities to retain voluntary patients when they attempt to leave, this should only be possible if the criteria for involuntary admission are met.
- On admittance to the mental health establishment, voluntary patients may be informed of the fact that mental health professionals of the facility may exercise the authority to prevent their discharge should they meet involuntary admission criteria.
- Voluntary patients must be treated only after obtaining informed consent. Where the patient has the capacity to give informed consent, such consent is a prerequisite for treatment.

Supported/Involuntary Admission

Supported or involuntary, or compulsory, admission to mental health establishment and involuntary treatment are controversial topics in the field of mental health as they impinge on personal liberty and the right to choose, and they carry the risk of abuse for political, social and other reasons.

On the other hand, such a admission and treatment can prevent harm to self and others, and assist some people in attaining their right to health, which, due to their mental disorder, they are unable to manage voluntarily.

Several international human rights documents, such as the MI Principles (1991), [30] European Convention for the Protection of Human Rights and Fundamental Freedoms (1950)[31] and The Declaration of Hawaii (1983),[14] accept the need, at times, for involuntary admission and treatment of persons with mental disorders.

However, it is important to stress that supported or involuntary admission and treatment is required only for a minority of patients who suffer from mental disorders; in many instances where patients are admitted and treated involuntarily, if humane treatment and a proper opportunity for voluntary care were provided, such admission and treatment could be reduced further. MHCA 2017 provides for supported admission under Section 89 of the Act. Admission is done on the request of the nominated representative.

For this purpose, an independent examination by two psychiatrists should confirm the risk of bodily harm or violence to self or to others and the patient lacks the capacity to care for self. Such an admission is done with least restrictive care option possible. Very high support from nominated representative. Treatment is done as per advance directives or informed consent. Admission under this Section will be valid for 30 days, Following this treatment patient can be discharged or continue as an independent patient as in the above Section. Under Section 90 of the Act supported admission beyond 30 days is done. All the supported admissions are informed to the review board within a week, and in case of women and minors within three days.

Under a fully "separate" approach, the admission and treatment procedures are independent of each other. First, the person is assessed for involuntary admission, then, if an involuntarily admitted patient requires involuntary treatment, the treatment need has to be assessed and a separate procedure for sanctioning such treatment is necessary.

Many individuals and organizations, especially user groups, object to combining involuntary admission and involuntary treatment and argue that a person's consent or refusal to admission and to treatment, are separate issues. Persons may require involuntary admission but not involuntary treatment, or, indeed, involuntary treatment without having to be placed outside their homes or communities. Moreover, it is argued that capacity is issue-specific, in that a person who is judged to be lacking capacity to make decisions regarding admission to a mental health facility may still retain the ability (capacity) to make decisions regarding treatment. It is argued that involuntary treatment violates fundamental human rights principles. For example, General Comment 14 to Article 12 of the ICESCR provides that the right to health includes the right to be free from non-consensual medical treatment. It is further argued that it is possible that an independent authority, for example a court or a review board, may commit a person to a psychiatric facility due to a mental illness, but this same authority, or a separate one, may find that the person has not lost his/her capacity to make treatment decisions. Assessment to determine incapacity to consent to treatment is thus necessary.

Furthermore, advocates of a separate approach argue that the provision of two independent procedures for invoking involuntary admission and involuntary treatment ensures an extra layer of rights protection for persons with mental disorders.

On the other hand, advocates of the combined approach contend that with the separate approach there is a risk that if too much time elapses between the two processes, treatment can be seriously delayed, with detrimental effects for the individual concerned, as well as, possibly, to healthcare workers and other patients if the person is highly aggressive. In addition, due to the unavailability of human and financial resources in many low-income countries, it can be difficult to institute two separate procedures for involuntary admission and involuntary treatment.

Involuntary admission: Key issues:

Involuntary admission is generally permitted only if *all* the following criteria are met and the patient is refusing voluntary admission:
- There is evidence of a mental disorder of specified severity,
- There is a serious likelihood of immediate or imminent harm to self or others, and/or a deterioration in the patient's condition if treatment is not given,
- Admission includes a therapeutic purpose, and
- This treatment can only be given by admission to a mental health facility.

Procedure to be followed for involuntary admission:
- Two mental health practitioners should certify that criteria for involuntary admission are fulfilled and recommend involuntary admission.
- An application for involuntary admission should be made in accordance with local culture and conditions.
- The mental health facility should be licensed to provide adequate and appropriate care and treatment, and therefore permitted to admit involuntary patients.
- Review Board should endorse involuntary admission within seven days, (three days in case of women and children). The person should be entitled to a legal representative at the hearing.
- Patients, their families and legal representatives should be informed immediately of the grounds for involuntary admission and of the patient's rights.
- Patients, their families and/or their legal representatives have a right to appeal to the review board and/or a court against involuntary admission.

Procedure to be followed for involuntary treatment:
- The treatment plan should be proposed by an approved and registered mental health practitioner having sufficient expertise and knowledge to undertake the proposed treatment.
- A second independent registered mental health practitioner should be required to agree to the treatment plan.
- Review board should be informed about the recommended treatment to review the treatment plan. It should meet again at set intervals to assess the need for continued involuntary treatment.
- Where the sanction for involuntary treatment is for a limited period, continued treatment can only be administered if the sanctioning process is repeated.
  - Involuntary treatment should be discontinued when patients are judged to have recovered their capacity to make treatment decisions, when there is no longer a need for treatment or when the sanctioned time has elapsed which ever happens earliest.
  - Patients and their families and/or personal representatives should be immediately informed of involuntary treatment decisions being made and, as far as is feasible, they should be involved in developing the treatment plan.
  - Once involuntary treatment is sanctioned, patients, families and personal representatives must be informed of their rights to appeal to the review board, tribunal and/or court against the involuntary treatment decision.

Advance directives give patients an opportunity to make decisions for themselves during periods when they are able to give informed consent for periods when they are not so capable. If a law provides for the use of advance directives or other forms of substitute decision-making, it should define such terms clearly and consistently.

Chapter III of MHCA 2017, under Section 5 empowers people to make an advance directive in writing to specify the way he wished to be treated when he gets a mental illness. He can do so irrespective of past mental illness/treatment.

Key Issues during Emergency Situations

An emergency situation is one in which the time required to follow substantive procedures would cause considerable delay, resulting in harm to the concerned person or others. In an emergency, involuntary admission and treatment is permitted on the assessment and advice of a qualified medical practitioner.

Emergency treatment must be time-limited (usually no longer than 72 hours), and substantive procedures for involuntary admission and treatment, if necessary, must be initiated as soon as possible and completed within this period.

Emergency treatment should not include:
- Depot neuroleptics
- ECT
- Sterilization
- Psychosurgery and other irreversible treatment.

Procedure for emergency admission and treatment: A qualified practitioner should examine the person and certify that the nature of the emergency requires immediate involuntary admission and treatment.
- A treatment plan should be drawn up under the supervision of a medical or mental health professional.
- Procedures for involuntary admission and/or involuntary treatment should be initiated immediately if it is assessed that the person is likely to require involuntary care beyond the stipulated time limit for emergency treatment.
- It is inappropriate to reapply emergency powers when a patient has been released following completion of the procedure for involuntary admission, unless there is a substantial change in the nature of the emergency.
- Patients' family members, nominated representatives and/or a legal representative should be immediately informed of the use of emergency treatment.
- Patients, their families and/or personal representatives have the right to appeal to a Mental Health Review Board and Mental Health Authority or courts against emergency admission and treatment.

Special Treatments

Countries enact legislation to protect people against abuses in the use of certain treatments such as major medical and surgical procedures, ECT, psychosurgery or other irreversible treatments. Some countries also specifically ban certain interventions if they are being unjustifiably used as treatments for mental disorders. Sterilization as a treatment for mental illness is an example of this. In addition, the mere fact of having a mental disorder should not be a reason for sterilization or abortion without informed consent.

According to MI Principles, sterilization shall never be carried out as a treatment for mental illness *(Principle 11(12), MI Principles)*[30] nor major medical or surgical procedures. A major medical or surgical procedure may be carried out on a person with mental illness only where it is permitted by domestic law, where it is considered that it would best serve the health needs of the patient and where the patient gives informed consent, except that, where the patient is unable to give informed consent, the procedure shall be authorized only after independent review by the review board. *(Principle 11(13), MI Principles)*.

Key issues related to special treatments
Sterilization is not a treatment for mental disorder, and having a mental disorder should not be a reason for sterilization (or abortion) without informed consent. Ethical standards that govern major medical and surgical procedures that are applicable to all patients should also be applied to persons with mental disorders.

Major medical and surgical procedures should be performed only with informed consent, except under exceptional circumstances. In these circumstances, proposed medical or surgical treatment should either be authorized as involuntary treatment by a review board or by proxy consent.

Emergency medical and surgical treatments for people with mental illness should be treated in the same manner for all patients who need such emergency treatment without consent. Psychosurgery and other irreversible treatments should not be permitted as involuntary treatment, and, as additional protection, all such treatment should be reviewed and sanctioned by an independent review board.

ECT should be administered only after obtaining informed consent. Modified ECT should be utilized. MHCA 2017 (Section 95) does not permit direct ECT to any patient and it bans ECT treatment for children.

Seclusion and Restraint

MI Principles: Seclusion and restraint

Physical restraint or involuntary seclusion of a patient shall not be employed except in accordance with the officially approved procedures of the mental health establishment and only when it is the only means available to prevent immediate or imminent harm to the patient or others. It shall not be prolonged beyond the period which is strictly necessary for this purpose. All instances of physical restraint or involuntary seclusion, the reasons for them and their nature and extent shall be recorded in the patient's medical record. A patient who is restrained or secluded shall be kept under humane conditions and be under the care and close and regular supervision of qualified members of the staff. A personal representative, if any and if relevant, shall be given prompt notice of any physical restraint or involuntary seclusion of the patient. (Principle 11(11), MI Principles).[30]

Seclusion and restraint under MHCA:
Section 97 of the MHCA 2017 does not permit seclusion or solitary confinement of person with mental illness. Physical restrain permitted only when (a) It is the only means available to prevent harm (b) Authorised by the treating psychiatrist. Physical restraint should not be used longer than required.

Procedure for exceptional use of seclusion and restraints:
- Should be authorized by an accredited mental health practitioner;
- The mental health establishment should be licensed as having adequate facilities for undertaking such procedures safely;
- The reasons and duration of seclusion and restraint and the treatment given to ensure speedy termination of these procedures, should be entered in the patients' clinical records by the mental health professional authorizing these procedures.
- Records of all seclusion and restraint should be documented in a register, which is accessible to the review board. Patients' family members and/or their personal representatives may need to be immediately informed when patients are subjected to seclusion or restraint.

Rights of Persons with Mental Illness in Clinical and Experimental Research

No one shall be subjected to torture or to cruel, inhuman or degrading treatment or punishment. In particular, no one shall be subject without his free consent to medical or scientific experimentation. *(Article 7, International Covenant on Civil and Political Rights (ICCPR).*[29] Article 7 of the ICCPR (1966) prohibits clinical and experimental research without informed consent. This Article is an important part of the ICCPR and has been designated as one of the provisions that is non-derogable; it can never be limited even under conditions of national emergency. The UN Human Rights Committee has made it clear that "Article 7 (of the ICCPR) allows no limitation… no justification or extenuating circumstances may be invoked to excuse a violation of Article 7 for any reasons". Article 7 therefore prohibits research on subjects who lack the capacity to consent. *On the other hand, MI Principle 11* states that, "clinical trials and experimental research shall never be carried out on any patient without informed consent, except that a patient who is unable to give informed consent may be admitted to a clinical trial or given experimental treatment, but only with the approval of a competent, review board specifically constituted for this purpose". The *International Ethical Guidelines for Biomedical Research Involving Human Subjects*, prepared by the Council for International Organizations of Medical Sciences (CIOMS, 2002),[32] allows biomedical research with proxy consent, or consent from a properly authorized representative, involving individuals who are incapable of giving informed consent.

MHCA 2017 under Section 99 provides that free and informed consent for conducting any kind of research needs to be obtained from the mentally ill person. If he is unable to give informed consent permission from the state mental health authority should be sought which may permit on the basis of informed consent from nominated representative.

Key issues related to clinical and experimental research:
Informed consent for participation in clinical or experimental research must be obtained from all patients who have the capacity to consent. This is applicable to both voluntary and involuntary patients. In countries where clinical and experimental research is permitted with patients who are unable to consent, legislation should include the following safeguards:
- When patients are lacking capacity to give informed consent, they may participate in clinical and experimental research, provided that proxy consent is obtained from legally appointed guardians and/or family members and/or nominated representatives, or by obtaining consent from an independent review body specifically constituted for this purpose.
- Participation of patients who are lacking capacity to consent, by obtaining consent from proxies or an independent review body, should only be considered when: this research cannot be performed on patients who are capable of giving consent; the research is necessary to promote the health of the individual patient and the population represented; adequate procedural safeguards are followed.

IMPLEMENTATION OF HUMAN RIGHTS IN INDIA

The following activities need to be taken up in the country to fulfil the rights of the mentally ill:
- Required physical facilities for the care of mentally ill are made available.
- Professional man-power
- Infra-structure for treatment facilities
- Constitution of Mental Health Review Boards
- Formation of State Mental Health Authorities
- Licensing of mental health establishments
- Information to patients of their rights
- Informed consent of patients
- Procedure for research
- Outpatient services
- Aftercare as a responsibility of the institution
- Placement for destitute chronically ill
- Regular training and improving staff sensitivity
- Half-way homes.

There is a need to develop institutional mechanisms to achieve these.

THE ROLE OF THE LEGISLATION

The Supreme Court petition by the voluntary organization *Saarthak* triggered off a debate on the treatment of persons with mental disorders in India.

Mental Health Legislation has an important role to play in the protection of human rights. Mental illness may affect decision making capacities and they patients may not always seek or accept treatment for their problems. Rarely, persons with mental disorders may pose a risk to themselves and others due to impaired decision making ability. Persons with mental disorders face stigma, discrimination and marginalization.

Mental Healthcare Act, 2017 strikes a fine balance between the individual's rights to liberty and dignity, and society's need for protection. It addresses the issues such as integration into the community, access to high quality care, and protecting the rights of persons with mental disorders, including in areas such as employment, education and housing.

REFERENCES

1. United Nations. Universal Declaration of Human Rights; 1948. Available from: http://www.un.org/en/universal-declaration human-rights/. [Last accessed on January 20, 2018].
2. Protection of Human Rights Act 199e3. Ministry of Law and Justice. Government of India Publication, New Delhi.
3. Pimpley PN. Problems of Non-Attendance of School Among Scheduled Caste Students. In: Pimpley PN, editor. Reform Protest and social Transformation. New Delhi: Ashish Publishing House; 1987.
4. Ramaiah A. Mumbai: Tata Institute of Social sciences; 2007. Dalits' Physical and Mental Health: Status, Root Causes and Challenges.
5. Demyttenaere K, Bruffaerts R, Posada-Villa J, G, et al. Prevalence, severity, and unmet need for treatment of mental disorders in the World Health Organization World Mental Health Surveys. JAMA. 2004;291:2581-90.
6. Shruthi P, Priyanka C, Deepak D. Disabilities and the law. Human Rights law network, a Division of Sociolegal information centre, New Delhi. June 2005.
7. International Convention on the Elimination of All Forms of Racial Discrimination; 1965. Available from:http://www2.ohchr.org/english/law/cerd.htm. [Last accessed on 2017 Dec 01].
8. International Covenant on Civil and Political Rights; 1966. Available from: http://www2.ohchr.org/english/law/ccpr.htm. [Last accessed on 2017 Dec 01].
9. The International Covenant on Economic, Social and Cultural Rights;1966. Available from: http://www2.ohchr.org/english/law/ccpr.htm. [Last accessed on 2017 Dec 01].
10. Convention on the Elimination of all forms of Discrimination against Women; 1979. Available from: http://www.un.org/womenwatch/daw/cedaw/. [Last accessed on 2017 Dec 01].
11. Convention against Torture and Other Cruel, Inhuman or Degrading Treatment or Punishment; 1984. Available from: http://www2.ohchr.org/english/law/cat.htm. [Last accessed on 2017 Dec 01].
12. Convention on the Rights of the Child; 1989. Available from: http://www2.ohchr.org/english/law/crc.htm. [Last accessed on 2016 Dec 01].
13. The 1971 Declaration on the Rights of Mentally Retarded Persons.
14. Declaration of Hawaii (1992). Approved by the General Assembly of the World Psychiatric Association (http://www.wpanet.org/generalinfo/ethic5.html).
15. International Covenant on Economic, Social and Cultural Rights 1996.
16. National Mental Health Programme. Ministry of Health and Family Welfare, Government of India Publication, New Delhi 1982.
17. Mental Health Act 1987. Ministry of Health and Family Welfare. Government of India Publication, New Delhi.
18. Persons with Disabilities (Equal Opportunities and Full Participation) Act 1995. Ministry of Social Justice and Empowerment. Government of India Publication, New Delhi.
19. Insurance Regulatory Development Authority Act 1999. Ministry of Finance. Government of India Publication, New Delhi.
20. Lakhawat M. Human Rights of Mentally ill Persons. Hidayatullah National Law University Raipur, 2013.
21. Saarthak and ANR vs Union of India and others. Writ Petition (Civil) No. 334 of 2001.Available at: http://www.gujhealth.gov.in/Medi_servi/pdf/Judgements.pdf.

22. Care and Treatment in Mental Health Institutions. Some Glimpses in the Recent Past. National Human Rights Commission, New Delhi.2012. Available from: http://www.nhrc.nic.in/Documents/Publications/Care_and_Mental_Health_2012.pdf.
23. Channabasavanna SM, Isaac M, Chandrashekar CR, Varghese M, Murthy P, Rao K, et al. Quality Assurance in Mental Health. New Delhi: National Human Rights Commission (NHRC); 1998.
24. Mental Healthcare Laws WHO 1996. Guidelines for the promotion of human rights of persons with mental disorders (1996). Geneva, World Health Organization. (http://whqlibdoc.who.int/hq/1995/WHO_MNH_MND_95.4.pdf)
25. UN Convention on the Rights of Persons with Disabilities 2006 Available from:http://www.un.org/disabilities/convention/conventionfull.shtml. [Last accessed on 20167 Dec 01].
26. National Mental Health Policy 2014. Ministry of Health and Family Welfare, Government of India Publication, New Delhi.
27. Nair, Shalini (2016-12-15). "Disabilities Bill passed: New conditions, revised quota and a few concerns". The Indian Express. Retrieved 2017-12-15.
28. Mental Healthcare Act, 2017. Ministry of Health and Family welfare, Government of India, New Delhi.
29. International Covenant on Civil and Political Rights (1966). Adopted by UN General Assembly Resolution 2200A (XXI) of 16 December 1966. (http://www.unhchr.ch/html/menu3/b/a_ccpr.htm)
30. Principles for the Protection of Persons with Mental Illness and the Improvement of Mental Health Care (MI Principles) (1991). UN General Assembly Resolution 46/119 of 17 December 1991.(http://www.unhchr.ch/html/menu3/b/68.htm).
31. European convention for the Protection of Human Rights and Fundamental Freedoms (1950). Adopted by the Council of Europe, 4 November 1950. (http://conventions.coe.int/treaty/en/Treaties/Html/005.).
32. The International Ethical Guidelines for Biomedical Research Involving Human Subjects. Council for International Organizations of Medical Sciences (CIOMS), 2002.

CHAPTER 29

Medicolegal Issues in Suicide Risk Assessment and Management

> **LEARNING OBJECTIVES**
> - Prevalence and risk factors
> - Methods of suicide
> - Laws concerning suicide IPC and MHCA
> - Legal provisions pertaining to complete suicide in healthcare setting
> - Guidelines to follow in case of complete suicide inside healthcare establishment
> - Psychological autopsy
> - Malpractice suits following complete suicide
> - Indian Psychiatric Society Guidelines for responsible reporting of suicide in media

Suicide is the act of intentionally causing one's own death. It is also known as completed suicide: "the act of taking one's own life with the intention to kill oneself".[1] Suicidal behavior is as old as human civilization and there have been several references of incidents of suicide in the ancient world literature viewing suicide variously. In ancient Athens, a person who committed suicide without the approval of the state was denied a dignified burial, and would be buried outside the city in an unmarked grave.[2] However, it was deemed to be an acceptable method to deal with military defeat.[3] In Ancient Rome, while suicide was initially permitted, it was later deemed a crime against the state due to its economic costs.[4] Aristotle condemned all forms of suicide while Plato was ambivalent.[5] In Rome, some reasons for suicide included, guilt over murdering someone, to save the life of another, as a result of mourning, from shame from being raped, and as an escape from intolerable situations like physical suffering, military defeat, or criminal pursuit.

Suicide came to be regarded as a sin in Christian Europe and was condemned as the work of the devil. Because of such a belief and occasional official rulings, Catholic doctrine was not entirely settled on the subject of suicide until the later 17th century. A criminal ordinance issued by Louis XIV of France in 1670 was extremely severe, even for the times: the dead person's body was drawn through the streets, face down, and then hung or thrown on a garbage heap. Additionally, all of the person's property was confiscated.[6,7]

Attitudes towards suicide slowly began to shift during the Renaissance. John Donne's work *Biathanatos*, contained one of the first modern defenses of suicide, bringing proof from the conduct of Biblical figures, such as Jesus, Samson and Saul, and presenting arguments on grounds of reason and nature to sanction suicide in certain circumstances.[8]

During the "Enlightenment" period, when society began to secularize, attitude towards suicide liberalized bringing a more modern perspective. Suicide was denied as a crime and a shift in the public opinion at large was witnessed during the 18th century.[9]

By the 19th century, the view of suicide had shifted from being caused by sin to being caused by insanity.[3] The act remained illegal, and it became a target for satire.[10] By 1879, English law differentiated between suicide and homicide, although suicide still punishable by forfeiture of estate.[11] In 1882, the deceased were permitted more dignified daylight burial in England and by the middle of the 20th century, suicide had become legal in much of the western world.[12]

Religious views of suicide also differ, with most Judaeo-Christian traditions viewing suicide in a negative light. In most forms of Christianity, suicide is considered a sin, based mainly on the writings of the Middle Ages.[10] Islamic religious views are against suicide.[13] The Quran forbids it by stating "do not kill or destroy yourself". The hadiths also state individual suicide to be unlawful and a sin. Stigma is often associated with suicide in Islamic countries.[10]

Sati, or self-immolation on a deceased husband's funeral pyre was a well-accepted practice in Hindu communities before it was outlawed during the British regime.[14] However, even Hinduism looks down upon those who deed by suicide, deeming them to become a part of the spirit world, deemed to wander the earth till all eternity.[14] However, at the same time, Hinduism accepts a man's right to end his life through the non-violent practice of fasting to death, termed *Prayopavesa*. This practice is strictly restricted to people who have no desire or ambition left, and no responsibilities remaining in this life.[14] Jainism has a similar practice named *Santhara*.

PREVALENCE AND RISK FACTORS

Approximately 0.5-1.4% of people die by suicide, a mortality rate of 11.6 per 100,000 persons per year.[15,16] Suicide resulted in 842,000 deaths in 2013 up from 712,000 deaths in 1990.[17] rates of suicide have increased by 60% from the 1960s to 2012,[15] with these increases seen primarily in the developing world.[18] Globally, as of 2008/2009, suicide is the tenth leading cause of death. For every suicide that results in death there are between 10 and 40 attempted suicides.[19]

Suicide rates differ significantly between countries and over time.[20] The percentage prevalence of deaths by suicide in 2008 in different regions was: Africa 0.5%, South-East Asia 1.9%, Americas 1.2% and Europe 1.4%. Rates per 100,000 were: Australia 8.6, Canada 11.1, China 12.7, India 23.2, United Kingdom 7.6, United States 11.4 and South Korea 28.9.[20] Suicide was ranked as the 10th leading cause of death in the United States in 2009 at about 36,000 cases committing suicide during the year and about 650,000 people attending emergency departments for attempting suicide.[21] The country's rate among men in their 50s rose by nearly half in the decade 1999-2010.[22] Lithuania, Japan and Hungary have the highest rates.[12] Around 75% of suicides occur in the developing countries.[23] The countries with the greatest absolute numbers of suicides are China and India, accounting for over half the total suicides committed across the globe. In China, suicide is the 5th leading cause of death.[24]

In the Western world, the ratio of completed suicides for men to women is 4:1. This difference is even more pronounced in those over the age of 65, with ten-fold more males than females dying by suicide.[25] On the other hand, women are 2-4 times more likely to make suicide attempts.[21] These differences have been proposed to result from men using more lethal means in their suicide attempts compared to women.[26] However, most studies assessing suicide do not differentiate between suicide and deliberate self-harm.[27]

These ratios do not necessarily hold true globally. The male to female ratio for suicides in China is 0.9:1, with one of the highest suicide rates among women in the world.[28] In the Eastern Mediterranean region, suicide rates are nearly equivalent between males and females.[16,29] The highest rate of female suicide is found in South Korea at 22 per 100,000, with high rates in South-East Asia and the Western Pacific generally.[19] Social stigma, depression, and gender identity disorder contribute for the higher rates of suicide.[30]

Within the wider spectrum of gender, there is universal agreement that individuals on the lesbian, gay, bisexual, transgender, and queer (LGBTQ) spectrum have much higher rates of suicide than the general population. Among transgender persons, rates of attempted suicide are between 30 and 50%.[31,32]

In many countries, the rate of suicide is highest in the middle-aged[32,37] or elderly.[10] The absolute number of suicides however is greatest in those between 15 and 29 years old due to the number of people in this age group.[12] In young males in the developed world, it is the cause of nearly 30% of mortality. In the developing world, rates are similar, but it makes up a smaller proportion of overall deaths due to higher rates of death from other types of trauma. In South-East Asia in contrast to other areas of the world, deaths from suicide occur at a greater rate in young females than elderly females. Suicide resulted in 828,000 deaths globally in 2015 (up from 712,000 deaths in 1990).[5,11] This makes it the 10th leading cause of death worldwide.[4,12]

More than one lakh persons (1,35,445) in India lost their lives by committing suicide in the year 2012 alone. The number of suicides in the country during the decade (2002-2012) has recorded an increase of 22.7% (1,35,445 in 2012 from 1,10,417 in 2002).[33] Attempted suicides are at least 20 times more common than the completed suicide.[34]

ATTEMPTED SUICIDE

Attempted suicide or non-fatal suicidal behavior is self-injury with the desire to end one's life that does not result in death.[19] Globally, around 10 to 20 million non-fatal attempted suicides occur every year leading to injury and long-term disabilities.[15] In the Western world, attempts are more common in young people and females.[21]

Assisted suicide is when one individual helps another bring about their own death indirectly via providing either advice or the means to the end.[20,25] This is in contrast to euthanasia, where another person takes a more active role in bringing about a person's death.[20] Suicidal ideation is thoughts of ending one's life but not taking any active efforts to do so.[19] In a murder-suicide (or homicide-suicide), the individual aims at taking the life of others at the same time. A special case of this is the extended suicide, where the murder is motivated by seeing the murdered persons as an extension of the own self.[21]

Table 1: Risk factors for suicide.

Risk factors for suicide	
1. Medical conditions	• Chronic pain • Traumatic brain injury • Cancer • Kidney failure • Systemic lupus erythematosus • Adverse effects from a number of medications such as beta blockers and steroids
2. Psychosocial factors	• Hopelessness, loss of pleasure in life, depression, anxiousness, poor ability to solve problems, poor impulse control • Recent life stresses such as loss of a family member or friend, loss of job, or social isolation (such as living alone) • Childhood sexual abuse, time spent in foster care • Poverty
3. Previous attempts and self-harm	Previous history of suicide attempts (**most accurate predictor of completed suicide**)
4. Mental disorders	• History of chronic alcohol abuse in self • History of chronic alcohol abuse in one's spouse • Adjustment disorders • Personality disorder • Depressive disorder • Schizophrenia and psychotic disorder
5. Effect of media	• High-volume, prominent, repetitive coverage glorifying/romanticizing suicide (high impact) • Suicide contagion or copycat suicide is known as the Werther effect

RISK FACTORS FOR SUICIDE

Risk factors for suicide are listed in **Table 1**.

Medical Conditions and Suicide

There is an association between suicide and medical disorders such[35]
a. Chronic pain
b. Traumatic brain injury
c. Cancer
d. Kidney failure
e. Systemic lupus erythematosus

Sleep disturbances such as insomnia and sleep apnea are risk factors for depression and suicide. In some instances, the sleep disturbances may be a risk factor independent of depression.[36] A number of other medical conditions may present with symptoms similar to mood disorders, brain tumors, systemic lupus erythematosus, and adverse effects from a number of medications (such as beta blockers and steroids).[14]

Psychosocial Risk Factors for Suicide

The psychological factors, which increase the risk of suicide, include:[37]
- Hopelessness
- Loss of pleasure in life
- Depression
- Anxiousness
- Poor coping ability
- Loss of ability to solve problems
- Poor impulse control.

Sociodemographic profiles also influence suicide risk. In older adults, the perception of being a burden is a risk factor. Suicide in which the reason is that the person feels that he is not a part of society, is known as egoistic suicide. Rates of suicide appear to decrease around Christmas. One study however found the risk may be greater for males on their birthday.[38]

Recent life stresses such as a loss of a family member or friend, loss of a job, or social isolation (such as living alone) also increase the risk of suicide. Those who have never been married are also at greater risk. Being religious may reduce one's risk of suicide.[10] This has been attributed to the negative stance many religions take against suicide and to the greater connectedness religion may give. Muslims, among religious people, appear to have a lower rate of suicide; however, data does not support a difference in rates of attempted suicide rates.[13] Young women in the Middle East may have higher rates. Some may take their own lives to escape bullying or prejudice. A history of childhood sexual abuse and time spent in foster care are also risk factors. Sexual abuse is believed to contribute to about 20% of the overall risk.[10]

Poverty has also been found to be associated with suicide. It is not just absolute poverty, which increases risk of suicide. Increasing relative poverty compared to those around a person is also known to increases suicide risk.[44] Some other special populations are at increased suicide risk due to socioeconomic disadvantages. In India, over 200,000 farmers have died by suicide since 1997, partly due to issues of debt.[39] In China, suicide is three times as likely in rural regions as urban ones, partly, it is believed, due to financial difficulties in this area of the country.[40] https://en.wikipedia.org/wiki/Suicide - cite_note-89

Previous Attempts and Self-harm

A previous history of suicide attempts is the most accurate predictor of completed suicide in the future. Approximately 20% of suicides have had a previous attempt, and of those who have attempted suicide, 1% complete suicide within a year and more than 5% die by suicide within 10 years. Acts of self-harm are not usually suicide attempts and most who self-harm are not at high risk of suicide. *https://en.wikipedia.org/wiki/Suicide - cite_note-Grey2009-56*. Some who self-harm, however, do still end their life by suicide, and risk for self-harm and suicide may overlap.[10]

Mental Disorders and Suicide

The prevalence of any psychiatric illness among suicide decedents varied based on the source of the data: psychological autopsy studies, which retrospectively assess for any history of psychiatric illness based on interviews with acquaintances of the deceased, reported a 34% prevalence of mental disorders in suicide decedents, case series studies reported a prevalence of 24% and studies based on police records reported a prevalence ranging from 5% to 25%.[41-46] Several studies found that the presence of a current mental disorder increased the risk of suicide (odds ratios range from 3.1 to 19.5).[42-46] Several specific conditions were associated with elevated risk for suicide: alcohol consumption (odds ratio = 4.5, 95% CI = 3.0-6.8), a history of chronic alcohol abuse in self (23.4, 95% CI = 12.9-43.7), a history of chronic alcohol abuse in one's spouse (6.1, 95% CI = 2.5-15.4), alcohol dependence (2.8, 95% CI = 1.0-6.8), adjustment disorders (3.4, 95% CI = 1.2-9.6) and personality disorder (9.5, 95% CI = 2.3-84.1).[41]

Effect of Media on Suicide

The media, including the internet plays an important role in influencing suicidal behavior, depending on how it depicts suicide. If the depiction is high-volume, prominent, repetitive coverage glorifying or romanticizing suicide, it can have a very negative overall impact on the public's understanding of suicide as a serious health issue. When detailed description of a particular method to kill oneself is portrayed, this method of suicide may increase in the population as a whole.[47]

This trigger of suicide contagion or copycat suicide is known as the Werther effect, named after the protagonist in Goethe's The Sorrows of Young Werther who killed himself and then was emulated by many admirers of the book. The Blue whale game is greater risk in adolescents who may romanticize death. It appears that while news media has a significant effect on public perceptions and acts of suicide; that of the entertainment media is equivocal.[48,49] In the age of web searches, it is not clear if searching for information about suicide relates to an increase in risk of suicide.

The opposite of the Werther effect is the proposed Papageno effect, in which coverage of effective coping mechanisms may have a protective effect. The term is based upon a character in Mozart's opera The Magic Flute, who (fearing the loss of a loved one) had planned to kill himself until his friends helped him out. When media follows recommended reporting guidelines as mentioned in another section of this chapter, the risk of suicides can be decreased. Getting buy-in from industry, however, can be difficult, especially in the long-term.[49]

METHODS OF SUICIDE

Global Scenario

The leading method of suicide varies among countries. The leading methods in different regions include hanging, pesticide poisoning, and firearms.[3] These differences are believed to be in part due to the ease of availability of the different methods.[10] A review of 56 countries found that hanging was the most common method in most of the countries, accounting for 53% of the male suicides and 39% of the female suicides. Worldwide, 30% of suicides are estimated to occur from pesticide poisoning, most of which occur in the developing world.[50] The use of this method varies markedly from 4% in Europe to more than 50% in the Pacific region.

It is also common in Latin America due to easy access within the farming populations. In many countries, drug overdoses account for approximately 60% of suicides among women and 30% among men. Many suicides are not planned or foreseen and may occur during an acute period of stress and ambivalence. *https://en.wikipedia.org/wiki/Suicide - cite_note-Yip2012-10* The death rate varies by method: firearms 80–90%, drowning 65–80%, hanging 60–85%, car exhaust 40–60%, jumping 35–60%, charcoal burning 40–50%, pesticides 6–75%, and medication overdose 1.5–4%. The most common attempted methods of suicide differ from the most common successful methods; up to 85% of attempts are via drug overdose in the developed world.[50]

Indian Scenario

Hanging was the most frequently reported method of suicide in most of the studies, accounting for 10–72% of all suicides.[41-46] The second most frequently reported method was self-poisoning (often ingestions of organophosphate pesticides), which accounted for 16–49% of all suicides.[41-46] The proportion of all suicides attributed to drowning ranged from 3 to 39% and the proportion attributed to burning or self-immolation ranged from 6% to 57%. Other reported methods of suicide include jumping off heights (0.5–2% of all suicides), being run over by a train (6–13% of all suicides) and using a firearm (3% of all suicides). Some studies report gender-based differences in method preference. A community-based surveillance study by Prasad and colleagues reported in 2006 found that significantly more women chose drowning and burning as modes of suicide than men, while significantly more men chose hanging.[44] A similar pattern of gender-based method preference was reported by Abraham and colleagues among persons 55 years of age and older.[43] Other studies report higher rates of suicides by hanging in males than females,[42,51] a predominance of males in suicide decedents who use other violent methods[42,52] (e.g. jumping in front of a train), and a predominance of females among suicides by self-immolation.[52,53]

▪ LAWS CONCERNING SUICIDE

Legal Status of Attempted Suicide in India

According to Article 21 of the Indian Constitution, "No person shall be deprived of his life or personal liberty except according to procedure established by the law". While the constitution covers the right to life or liberty, till recently, it did not include the 'right to die'. The attempts at taking one's own life was not considered to fall under purview of constitutional right to life.[54] ***However, on 9th March 2018, while legalizing passive euthanasia, the Supreme Court of India said that right to life includes right to die.***

Section 309 of the Indian Penal Code (IPC) *clearly states as follows: "Whoever attempts to commit suicide and does any act towards the commission of such offence, shall be punished with simple imprisonment for a term which may extend to one year or with fine or both."* It is to be noted that the abetting of the commission of suicide (but not the abetting of attempt to commit suicide) is covered under Section 306 IPC and the abetment of suicide of a child is covered under Section 305 IPC. The punishment for these varies from 1 to 10 years of imprisonment and heavy fines. Repealing of Section 309, *per se*, would not affect or impact the above sections on abetment of completed suicide.[54]

Thoughts favoring criminalization of suicide: Some schools of thought believe that the right to life cannot be equated with the right to die. Such acts, if accepted, will lead to anarchism, especially for individuals in distressed states. Punitive laws against suicide have been presumed to have a deterrent effect on suicidal acts. Internationally, the research on the impact of repeal of anti-suicide legislation has yielded mixed results. In 1992, Lester compared suicide rates in Canada in the 10-year periods before and after decriminalization of suicide, and found no increase in the rate of suicide following decriminalization. Similarly, no change was observed in the New Zealand during the decade before or after decriminalization[55] compared the suicide rates in seven countries (Canada, England and Wales, Finland, Hong Kong, Ireland, New Zealand, and Sweden) 5 years prior and 5 years following decriminalization, with an increase in the suicide rates after decriminalization of suicide. This increase in suicide rates can be possibly explained due to better reporting of such attempts as earlier they could have been reported as accidents to prevent legal hassles.

In Indian context, while the level of awareness about existence of section 309 cannot be deemed to be too high, but a significant proportion are aware of its existence, but not deterred to make a suicidal attempt. A study of 200 attempted suicides in a General Hospital Emergency facility revealed that 46.2% males and 26.6% females were aware of the existing law before making the attempt.[56,57] It remains to be seen how decriminalization of suicide affects the national average suicide rate.

Thoughts favoring decriminalization of suicide: This school of thought believes that decriminalization of suicides can make it easy for people to seek help for mental health issues. Under the fear of a punitive law, to avoid legal hassles, majority of attempted suicides are reported to the authorities as accidental, so with decriminalization, the patients and their families will be in a better position to openly seek mental health care after the attempt. From a societal perspective, decriminalization is a more sensitive and humane way of dealing with the problem compared to prosecution.[56]

Delhi High court in a landmark judgment of 1985 had also commented that "*the continuance of Section 309 I.P.C. (criminalizing suicide) is an anachronism unworthy of a human society like ours.*" The Indian Penal Code had been formulated during British Raj Regime of 1860, and was mainly governed by British law of that time. Ironically, India continues to follow the archaic law even though Britain itself had decriminalized suicide way back in 1961.[56]

Provision for Decriminalization of Suicide in Mental Healthcare Act, 2017
Section 115: "Presumption of Severe Stress in Case of Attempt to Commit Suicide. "

(1) Notwithstanding anything contained in Section 309 of the Indian Penal Code, any person who attempts to commit suicide shall be presumed, unless proved otherwise, to have severe stress and shall not be tried and punished under the said Code.

(2) The appropriate Government shall have a duty to provide care, treatment and rehabilitation to a person, having severe stress and who attempted to commit suicide, to reduce the risk of recurrence of attempt to commit suicide.[58]

MEDICOLEGAL PROVISIONS PERTAINING TO COMPLETE SUICIDE IN A HEALTHCARE SETTING

All suicides happening inside a hospital of an inpatient warrant immediate FIR to be lodged with the concerned local police station of the jurisdiction of the hospital. The body should be handed over to police in presence of family members for postmortem examination for exact cause of death. Death certificate should mention cause of death as "under investigation". Subsequently, the Executive Class Magistrate (Subdivisional Judicial Magistrate) inquest ensues, as per Section 174, Criminal Procedure Code. In case relatives are not willing for autopsy, they need to make a written application to the Subdivisional Judicial Magistrate for further decision. File records should be completed including the clinical case details, details of alleged incidence, resuscitation attempts made, end result and discussions with the family along with time and date with legible signatures.[59]

Guidelines to follow in Case of Complete Suicide Inside Healthcare Establishment

When a suicide occurs in the hospital premises during the care of the patient it raises many issues, which need to be handled appropriately. Following are the guidelines to manage such a situation.

Impact on Mental Health Professionals

For mental health professionals, losing a patient under their care by suicide is an unwanted but one of the known occupational hazard. Results of research interview study[60,61] of several mental health professionals who had lost a patient to suicide showed that shock, grief, guilt, fear of blame, fear of law suit, self-doubt, sense of inadequacy, shame, anger and betrayal were the major emotional reactions of therapists.[61] Unresolved emotional experiences in a professional can have a long-term effect and this may be manifest in many ways:[62]
- Rushed or prolonged hospitalization of suicidal patients
- Delay in a patient's first discharge for the weekend
- Excessive use of medication
- Refusal to work with suicidal patients
- Distrust of patient's claims that he/she is not contemplating suicide
- Burn-out symptoms with loss of motivation for work/change in occupational field itself.

Need of Postvention Guidelines

Usually great emphasis is laid on managing suicide attempt cases during training of psychiatrists, but protocols to be followed after a completed attempt are rarely talked about.

Review of the case with a focus on learning rather than blaming can help the professional deal with the incident constructively. Excessive media attention, professional isolation, legal action may lead to re-traumatization and poor coping for the mental health professional concerned.

Postvention Protocols

Schneidman coined the term "postvention" for the provision of crisis intervention, support and assistance for all those affected by a completed suicide.[63] "Affected" individuals include "suicide survivors" those bereaved who had a personal and close relationship with the deceased (e.g. a friend or a family member) and "suicide exposed" those who did not know the deceased personally but witnessed the death of a stranger (e.g. fellow ward patients) or knew about the death through reports of others or media (e.g. suicide of a celebrity).[64] A good postvention guideline should be able to serve two purposes:

1. From clinical perspective, it should extend help across all those affected by the suicide, both suicide survivors and suicide exposed.
2. From public health perspective, it should be able to prevent contagion in the community.[65]

The Following can be essential components of postvention protocol:

Immediate notifications

It begins with details of death, including verification of the death, who died, when, the circumstances, location and whether or not the death was a suicide. The internet and social media can lead to false information spreading quickly, and such false speculations and rumors should be nipped in the bud. Official information should not be released until the circumstances of death have been confirmed by the appropriate authority: police chief, medical examiner and immediate family members. Following the event, the following entities need to be informed at the earliest:

- Family members of the deceased
- Local police station
- Communicate supervisors
- Crisis intervention team of the institute
- All concerned ward staff
- Ward's other patients and relatives for debriefing session
- Communicate administrative officials
- Ensure provisions for informing subsequent shift staff members
- Assess the need of informing legal counsel of the institute or of individual.
- If news has reached to media, arrange for meeting with media for factual accuracy and responsible reporting.

The notice should contain the basic information about the patient's death by suicide. Plan separate meetings for different groups, moderated preferably a neutral empathic senior supervisor. Ensure complete documentation in the case records.

Whom to offer help

Five vulnerable groups can be identified for the intervention:

1. *Family members of the deceased:* Many clinicians fear meeting family members due to a risk of lawsuits or from a potentially emotionally overwhelming confrontation. However, meeting the family in non-defensive way that connects as fellow human beings who have shared a loss with neutral supervisors is helpful. The family should be allowed to express their grief, guilt, anger and blame. It may be painful for the clinician struggling self with guilt and pain, but family needs to be heard in non-defensive, non-judgmental, blame free, space without counterattack or self-castigation.

2. *Mental health professionals dealing with the case (Psychiatrists or psychologists):* Enable professionals to recognize, understand, accept and express emotions felt for (i)) the deceased patient (sorrow, anger, compassion, disappointment, guilt, etc.); (ii) towards self as the therapist (disappointment, fear, doubt, incompetence, shame, anxiety, etc.). Allow them to verbalize their fears of legal action or being blamed by fellow colleagues and discuss ways to handle the situation. Make them realize again that therapist has limited control over patient's behavior and life. If possible constructive discussion about any such previous experience by a senior colleague may help.

3. *Other health professionals* (e.g. nurses, occupational therapists, other members of the team in the hospital) are also highly affected by the suicidal death of a patient, as they know them very well, know their relatives, know their daily routine and feel responsible for their wellbeing. Many of them may feel a similar degree of incompetence as the therapists do but for different reasons. They tend to spend more time with patient and can often blame themselves for not being able to foresee or prevent the act. A separate session with the current staff to be done to encouraged for ventilation of their emotional reactions towards self (guilty, sorrow, disappointment) and how to handle other ward patients' emotional reactions and queries after the event. Staff working in the subsequent shifts should also be informed, and everyone must be watchful for any contagion effects on other patients in the ward over the next few days.

4. *The individual or group who found the body of the patient:* Finding the body may provoke many repetitive flashbacks, anxiety and even impairment in clinical condition shortly after the event. Conduct a debriefing session, help the client process the event, and consider starting short-term anxiolytics, if needed. Continue supportive sessions and ventilation at regular intervals.

5. *Other patients of ward and relatives:* It is very important to plan how the information about the suicide of a fellow-patient is transferred to the others in the group and who should do this. Time and opportunity should be offered for patients to speak up about their views about patient as a person and as a fellow ward inmate. Some of them would have developed fears regarding their own safety and doubts about treatment. Encourage the open expression and a neutral senior supervisor should handle the responses, should do a group grief work and re-instill the faith in treatment.

Administrative or institutional responsibilities
- Provide guidance and support for all employees affected by the patient's suicide;
- Maintain a high level of service and provide an unchanged working and living environment for the employees, patients and patients' families;
- Define actions to support the family of the deceased patient (meetings, funeral, etc.);
- Give the team the option of reviewing the case with an external or internal consultant aimed at understanding the patient's possible risk factors and motives for suicide, if possible a psychological autopsy (PA) can be conducted;
- Appoint key persons for independent review of the case;
- Enable various explanations and interpretations as to why the patient died by suicide by reviewing short and long-term risk factors. It should, however, be acknowledged that retrospective understanding does not mean that the suicide could have been prevented; limitations of what was known before the suicide should be recognized;
- Provide support and advice for clinicians on how to communicate and help other patients who have been affected by the event;
- Provide education about the "normal" sequelae of suicide loss (for clinicians, family and friends) and optimal interventions for survivors of a suicide;
- Provide educational training on how to recognize risk factors for suicidal behavior and optimal intervention strategies.

Things to avoid
It is important to acknowledge that suicide postvention, when not appropriately implemented does have the potential to do harm (i.e. to increase the risk of contagion). To minimize such risk, it is recommended that these interventions avoid:
- Sensationalizing the death,
- Glorifying or vilifying the suicide victim, and
- Providing excessive details about the suicidal act.

PSYCHOLOGICAL AUTOPSY

What is Psychological Autopsy?

It is a procedure carried out in the aftermath of "equivocal deaths," where the circumstances and the manner of death (e.g. suicide, accident, other) is uncertain or not immediately clear. The procedure involves a thorough and systematic retrospective analysis of the decedent's life, with a particular focus on suicide risk factors, motives, and intentions. The psychological autopsy (PA) has been used for almost 60 years to assist medical examiners, to collect research data, inform suicide prevention efforts, and as a forensic tool in the courts.

Origin of Concept

The Psychological Autopsy originated in approximately 1958 as a result of the Los Angeles County Medical Examiner's Office consulting the Los Angeles Suicide Prevention Center for assistance in distinguishing drug-related accidental overdoses from suicides. This collaboration

CHAPTER 29: Medicolegal Issues in Suicide Risk Assessment and Management

laid down the basic principles for the PA procedure. Edwin Schneidman, a director of the LA Suicide Prevention Center, is credited with coining the term "psychological autopsy." His initial definition of a PA was "a thorough retrospective investigation of the intention of the decedent."[2] Since its inception, the PA has become familiar to most suicidologists, suicide researchers, and homicide investigators.[66]

Utility of Psychological Autopsy

The PA has utility in a variety of situations, including the following[66]:
1. Assisting medical examiners with "equivocal" deaths
2. Research on suicide
3. Insurance claims
4. Criminal cases
5. Estate issues
6. Contested wills
7. Malpractice claims
8. Worker's compensation cases
9. Product liability cases
10. Efforts by organizations to prevent suicide
11. Promoting understanding and grieving among surviving family members.

Goals of Psychological Autopsy

The following are some of the key goals of the PA:[66]
- Identify behavior patterns—reactions to stress, adaptability, changes in habits or routine
- Establish presence or absence of mental illness
- Identify possible precipitants
- Determine presence or absence of motives
- Determine presence or absence of suicidal intent
- Determine suicide risk factors—both mitigating and aggravating
- Perform a postmortem suicide risk assessment
- Establish whether or not the deceased was a likely candidate for suicide.

Ethical Considerations

An important ethical and practical consideration related to gathering collateral data from friends, relatives of deceased is the manner in which collateral sources should be contacted and interviewed. Interviewing surviving family and friends is a very sensitive matter and the investigator must consider the survivors' reactions.

MALPRACTICE SUITS FOLLOWING COMPLETE SUICIDE

In words of famous forensic psychiatrist Robert Simon, "there are only two kinds of clinical psychiaatrists—those who have had patients commit suicide and those who will."[67] When a psychiatrist loses a patient to suicide, he may sometimes face a litigation. In fact, suicides account for the greatest number of malpractice suits filed against psychiatrists. The following four criteria must all be fulfilled for the psychiatrist to be held legally accountable for patient suicide.

1. The psychiatrist had a **duty** of care to the patient
2. The psychiatrist **deviated** from the 'standard of care' (degree of skill and care ordinarily employed in similar circumstances by other psychiatrist)
3. Which led to **damage** to the patient
4. As a **direct result of the deviation** from the standard of care (This one is most difficult one to prove in case of suicide litigation suits).

"Foreseeability of suicide" holds legal value in malpractice lawsuits. From a legal standpoint, psychiatric malpractice cases often hinge on the issue of "**foreseeability**". Furthermore, the law considers two basic types of error when considering the issue of foreseeability and whether the psychiatrist exercised professional judgment: errors of fact and errors of judgment. An error of fact is considered to be a "mistake about a fact that is material to a transaction". For example, an "error of fact" occurs when the psychiatrist bases a clinical judgment on erroneous beliefs, such as might occur when the psychiatrist fails to review a patient's history or lab results before making a substantive clinical decision. Psychiatrists are likely to be found negligent for errors of fact.[68]

In contrast, an "**error of judgment**" occurs when the psychiatrist makes an informed clinical decision in good faith that turns out to have been a mistake. The psychiatrist is less likely to be held liable for mere error in professional judgment. This is sometimes referred to as judgmental immunity or the error of judgment rule, which states, "A professional is not liable to a client for advice or an opinion given in good faith and with an honest belief the advice was in the client's best interests, but that was based on a mistake either in judgment or in analyzing an unsettled area of the professional's business."[68]

It is not possible for mental health professionals to predict an attempt of suicide with certainty. However, suicide risk assessment is a professional responsibility with established standards. The risk assessment can be sufficiently adequate, if not perfect, to set in motion appropriate clinical interventions in a vast majority of cases. The assessment of suicide risk is a clinical probability judgment. Generally, it is considered the psychiatrist's professional liability to adequately assess suicide risk, and to put in place a treatment plan. In litigations, courts scrutinize cases for the reasonableness of risk assessment, and whether the committed suicide was "foreseeable". Legal language, however, seldom equates with medical terminology. Foreseeability is a vague term, which sheds no light on the complexities and nuances of psychiatric diagnosis and treatment. It is not a scientific term. Legally defined, foreseeability is the reasonable anticipation that harm or injury is a likely result from certain acts or omissions. A competent assessment and recording of suicide risk must be sufficient to meet fair legal requirements. Foreseeability should not be confused with predictability, for which no professional standards exist. Nor is foreseeability the same as preventability. In hindsight, a suicide may have been preventable, but was not foreseeable at the time of assessment.[67]

Important Measures for Health Professionals
- Conduct a thorough suicide risk assessment
- Continued monitoring of patients found to be at suicide risk
- Ensure safety by offering admission, keeping such patients in high risk or close supervision wards and continuing high-risk management
- Good documentation
- Following postvention guidelines after the event.

INDIAN PSYCHIATRIC SOCIETY GUIDELINES FOR RESPONSIBLE REPORTING OF SUICIDE IN MEDIA

Since media and its reporting of suicide event has a lot bearing on general mass, so, Indian Psychiatric Society (IPS) has come out with a position statement as detailed below for responsible reporting of such events:

News coverage should be neutral
The vulnerable are sometimes unduly influenced by the content of the news report on suicide. The public discourse and attention paid to suicide sometimes romanticizes the act and those who are not emotionally mature may develop a morbid fascination with suicide. The following measures can be taken in the reporting of suicide to prevent an untoward inducement of such acts:
1. Present facts in matter-of-fact language, without sensationalism; be objective rather than emotional.
2. Do not romanticize or glorify the event, or imply martyrdom.
3. Do not indicate blame unless clearly justified; instead, acknowledge that a combination of triggers and vulnerabilities were probably responsible.

News coverage should be discreet
To ensure that news-coverage does not sensationalize suicide to the emotionally vulnerable. To ensure personal intimate details of victims are not shared to avoid the vulnerable empathizing with the victims. Minutiae of the act must not be shared in detail, to prevent people from formulating active suicide plans.
1. Avoid front-page reporting, presentation in boxes, large headlines, lengthy reports, and photographs of the deceased.
2. Do not provide detailed descriptions of the method of suicide.
3. Do not publish suicide notes.

News coverage should be sensitive
1. Consider how the news coverage might occasion psychological and social harm to the survivors of the event.
2. Respect the privacy of the survivors.

Other matters
1. Do not repeatedly play on the event or theme.

2. Do not allow readers to form the impression that suicide is a way of coping with a personal problem, or a way to teach others a lesson.
3. Exercise particular caution when reporting celebrity suicides.

Positive reporting
1. When reporting suicide, also make it an aim to spread public awareness of suicide and mental health. Helplines and sources of help in cases of emergency must be publicized. People must be made aware of early warning signs of distress and suicidal ideations and behavior.
2. The experience of stress must be spoken about and de-stigmatized. Reporting of depression, anxiety, and suicidal ideation must be encouraged.
3. Promote awareness that these conditions are treatable, and problems can be overcome. Stories of people overcoming their mental health problems and suicidal ideations must also be shared.

Suicide is an important clinical and public health issue. Adequate suicide risk assessment, continued monitoring, thorough documentation, sensitivity about legal statutes, their medicolegal responsibilities, postvention guidelines and media reporting guidelines can help mental health professionals in taking up well-informed decisions.

REFERENCES

1. Stack S. The impact of the media on suicide. In: Shrivastava A, Kimbrel M, Lester D (Eds). Suicide from a Global Perspective: Psycho-social Approaches. New York: Nova Science Publishers. 2012; pp. 115-8.
2. Haas AP, Eliason M, Mays VM, et al. Suicide and suicide risk in lesbian, gay, bisexual, and transgender populations: review and recommendations. J Homosexuality. 2011;58(1):10-51.
3. Virupaksha HG, Muralidhar D, Ramakrishna J. Suicide and suicidal behavior among transgender persons. Indian J Psychological Med. 2016;38(6):505-9.
4. Pitman A, Krysinska K, Osborn D, et al. Suicide in young men. The Lancet. 2012;379(9834): 2383-92.
5. Szasz T. Fatal Freedom: The Ethics and Politics of Suicide. Westport, Conn.: Praeger.1999; p. 11.
6. Maris R. Comprehensive Textbook of Suicidology. New York [u.a.]: Guilford Press. 2000. pp. 97-103.
7. Dickinson MR, Leming GE. Understanding Dying, Death, and Bereavement, 7th edition. Belmont, CA: Wadsworth Cengage Learning. 2010. p. 290. https://en.wikipedia.org/wiki/Suicide - cite_ref-160.
8. Minois G. History of Suicide: Voluntary Death in Western Culture (Johns Hopkins University ed.). Baltimore: Johns Hopkins University Press, 2001.
9. Pickering WSF, Walford G. Durkheim's Suicide: A Century of Research and Debate (1. publ. ed.). London [u.a.]: Routledge. 2000.p. 69.
10. McLaughlin C. Suicide-related Behaviour Understanding, Caring and Therapeutic Responses. Chichester, England: John Wiley & Sons. 2007.p. 24.
11. "Catechism of the Catholic Church – PART 3 SECTION 2 CHAPTER 2 ARTICLE 5". Scborromeo.org. 1941-06-01. Archived from the original on 2009-04-25. Retrieved 2009-05-06.
12. "The Bible and Suicide". Religioustolerance.org. Retrieved 2009-05-06.
13. Gearing RE, Lizardi D. Religion and suicide. J Religion Health.2009;48(3):332-41.
14. Hindu Website. Hinduism and suicide Archived 2008-05-07 at the Wayback Machine.

15. Hawton K, van Heeringen K. Suicide. Lancet. 2009;373(9672):1372-81.
16. Sakinofsky I. The current evidence base for the clinical care of suicidal patients: strengths and weaknesses. Canadian J Psychiatry. 2007;52(6 Suppl 1):7S-20S.
17. Yip PS, Caine E, Yousuf S, et al. Means restriction for suicide prevention. Lancet. 2012;379(9834):2393-9.
18. GBD 2013 Mortality and Causes of Death, Collaborators (17 December 2014).
19. Global, regional, and national life expectancy, all-cause mortality, and cause-specific mortality for 249 causes of death, 1980-2015: a systematic analysis for the Global Burden of Disease Study. Lancet. 2015;388(10053):1459-544.
20. Stedman's Medical Dictionary (28th ed.). Philadelphia: Lippincott Williams & Wilkins, 2006.
21. Dodds TJ. Prescribed Benzodiazepines and Suicide Risk: A Review of the Literature. Prim Care Companion CNS Disord. 2017;19(2).
22. Bottino SM, Bottino CM, Regina CG, et al. Cyberbullying and adolescent mental health: systematic review. Cadernos de Saúde Pública. 2015;31(3):463-75.
23. Maris R. Comprehensive Textbook of Suicidology. New York [u.a.]: Guilford Press. 2000.p. 540.
24. Backscheider PR, Ingrassia C. A Companion to the Eighteenth-Century English Novel and Culture. John Wiley & Sons. 2008.p. 530.
25. Paperno I. Suicide as a Cultural Institution in Dostoevsky's Russia. Ithaca: Cornell University Press. 1997.p.60-28.
26. Norman SJS. Life, Death and the Law: Law and Christian Morals in England and the United States. Beard Books. 2002.p. 233.
27. Lanham D. Criminal Laws in Australia. Annandale, NSW: The Federation Press. 2006.p. 229.
28. Law S, Liu P. Suicide in China: unique demographic patterns and relationship to depressive disorder. Current Psychiatry Reports. 2008;10(1):80-6.
29. Duffy M, Costa M. Labor, Prosperity and the Nineties: Beyond the Bonsai Economy, 2nd edition. Sydney: Federation Press. 1991.p. 315.
30. Putnam CE. Hospice or Hemlock? Searching for Heroic Compassion. Westport, Conn.: Praeger.2002. p. 143. ISBN 978-0-89789-921-5. Archived from the original on 2015-09-28.
31. Hales RE, Simon RI (Eds). The American Psychiatric Publishing Textbook of Suicide Assessment and Management, 2nd edition. Washington, DC: American Psychiatric Pub. 2012. p. 714.
32. Eliason S. Murder-suicide: a review of the recent literature.J Am Acad Psychiatr Law. 2009; 37(3):371-6.
33. Accidental deaths and suicide in India. National Crime Records Bureau. Ministry of Home Affairs. 2012. Available from: http://ncrb.nic.in/CD-ADSI- 2012/ADSIHome2012.htm . [Last accessed on 2014 Sep 18].
34. World Health Organization (WHO) Suicide Prevention. 2012. Available from: http://www.who.int/mental_health/prevention/suicide/suicideprevent /en/ index.html. [Last accessed on 2014Sep 18].
35. Kornblum W. Sociology in a Changing World, 9th edition. Belmont, CA: Wadsworth Cengage Learning. 2011.p. 27.
36. Hall. Alternative Considerations of Jonestown and Peoples Temple. San Diego State University."Archived copy". Archived from the original on January 24, 2011. Retrieved 2011-11-10.
37. Krug E. World Report on Violence and Health, Volume 1. Genève: World Health Organization. 2002. p. 196.
38. Eshun S, Gurung RAR. Culture and Mental Health Sociocultural Influences, Theory, and Practice. Chichester, UK: Wiley-Blackwell. 2009.p. 301.
39. Lerner G. Activist: Farmer Suicides in India Llinked to Debt, Globalization. CNN World. Archived from the original on 16 January 2013. Retrieved 13 February 2013.

40. Stark CR, Riordan V, O'Connor R. A conceptual model of suicide in rural areas. Rural and Remote Health. 2001;11(2):1622.
41. Rane A, Nadkarni A. Suicide in India: a systematic review. Shanghai Archives of Psychiatry. 2014;26(2):69-80.
42. Khan F, Anand B, Devi MG, et al. Psychological autopsy of suicide-a cross-sectional study. Indian J Psychiatry. 2005;47:73-8.
43. Bose A, Konradsen F, John J, et al. Mortality rate and years of life lost from unintentional injury and suicide in South India. Tropical Medicine & International Health. 2006;11:1553-6.
44. Prasad J, Abraham VJ, Minz S, et al. Rates and factors associated with suicide in Kaniyambadi Block, Tamil Nadu, South India, 2000-2002. Int J Soc Psychiatry. 2006;52:65-71.
45. Mohanty S, Sahu G, Mohanty MK, et al. Suicide in India: a four -year retrospective study. J Forensic Leg Med. 2007;14:185-9.
46. Chavan B, Singh G, Kaur J, et al. Psychological autopsy of 101 suicide cases from northwest region of India. Indian J Psychiatry. 2008;50:34-8.
47. Sisask M, Värnik A. Media roles in suicide prevention: a systematic review. International journal of environmental research and public health. 2012;9(1):123-38.
48. Stack S. Suicide in the media: a quantitative review of studies based on non-fictional stories. Suicide Life Threat Behav. 2005;35(2):121-33.
49. Pirkis J. Suicide and the media. Psychiatry. 2009;8(7):269-71.
50. Gross VA, Weiss MG, Ring M, et al. Methods of suicide: international suicide patterns derived from the WHO mortality database. Bulletin of the World Health Organization. http://www.who.int/bulletin/volumes/86/9/07-043489/en/
51. Parkar SR, Dawani V, Weiss MG. Clinical diagnostic and sociocultural dimensions of deliberate self-harm in Mumbai, India. Suicide Life Threat Behav. 2006;36:223-8.
52. Shukla G, Verma B, Mishra DN. Suicide in Jhansi City. Indian J Psychiatry. 1990;32:44-51.
53. Abraham VJ, Abraham S, Jacob KS. Suicide in the elderly in Kaniyambadi block, Tamil Nadu, South India. Int J Geriatr Psychiatry. 2005;20:953-5.
54. Bagcchi S, Chaudhuri P. Suicide and the law in India. BMJ. 2013;347:f6975.
55. Lester D. Decriminalization of suicide in seven nations and suicide rates. Psychol Rep. 2002;91:898.
56. Ranjan R, Kumar S, Pattanayak RD, et al. (De-) criminalization of attempted suicide in India: a review. Industrial Psychiatry Journal. 2014;23(1):4-9.
57. Latha KS, Geetha N. Criminalizing suicide attempts: can it be a deterrent? Med Sci Law. 2004;44:343-7.
58. Available at: www.prsindia.org/uploads/media/.../Mental%20Healthcare%20Act,%202017.pdf. Last accessed on 11 February 2018.
59. Available at: www.crpc.co.in/2016/05/section-174-crpc.html. Last accessed on 11 February 2018.
60. Ruskin R, Sakinofsky I, Bagby RM, et al. Impact of patient suicide on psychiatrists and psychiatric trainees. Acad Psychiatry. 2004;28:104-10.
61. Grad OT, Michel K. Therapists as client suicide survivors. In: K Weiner (Ed.). Therapeutic and Legal Issues for Therapists who have Survived a Client Suicide. The Haworth Press, Binghamton NY. 2005. pp. 71-81.
62. Ruskin R, Sakinofsky I, Bagby RM, et al. Impact of patient suicide on psychiatrists and psychiatric trainees. Acad Psychiatry. 2004;28:104-10.
63. Knieper AJ. The suicide survivor's grief and recovery. Suicide and Life-threatening Behavior. 1999;29:353-64.

64. After a Suicide: A Toolkit for Schools, Newton, MA: Education Development Centre, Inc. 2011. http://www.sprc.org/library/AfteraSuicideToolkitforSchools.pdf.
65. Onja T. Guidelines to assist clinical staff after the suicide of a patient. International Association for Suicide Prevention (IASP), 2012.pp. 1-15.
66. Knoll JL. The psychological autopsy, Part I: applications and method. Journal of Psychiatric Practice. 2006;14(6):393-7.
67. Simon RI. Taking the "Sue" out of suicide: a forensic psychiatrist's perspective. Psychiatric Annals. 2000;30(6):399-407.
68. Knoll JL. Lessons from litigation. Psychiatry Times. 2015;32(5). Available at: www.psychiatrictimes.com/career/lessons-litigation. Last accessed on 11 February 2018.

CHAPTER 30

Violence, Crime and Mental Disorders

> **LEARNING OBJECTIVES**
> - Violence vs aggression?
> - Types of violence
> - Victims of violence
> - Biopsychosocial models of violence
> - Philosophy of violence
> - Genetics and violence
> - Psychological theories of violence
> - Mental illness and violence
> - Association of mental illness and offense
> - Crime in social context
> - Social factors in crime
> - Social factors in crime prevention
> - Forensic psychiatry and crime

VIOLENCE

Right from the beginning of human civilization, people have usually been held responsible and blamed only for those acts that they chose to do, as opposed to acts that are involuntary. Aristotle identified a category of less-blameworthy acts that were chosen in circumstances in which the alternatives open to the individual were worse, such as hitting at a person when that is the only way to stop that person all set to knife him.

"The mental faculty of choosing immediate action is known as volition", as distinct from pursuing long-term goals. Much of philosophy and economics assumes that people rationally choose actions so as to maximize the probability of achieving many of those goals of possible. Evolutionary psychology suggests, however, that although humans have numerous 'reasoning instincts' governing specific situations, there is no general reasoning system capable of overriding other systems, and therefore assumption of rational choice may not hold in all situations.

Determinism, another view, states that all actions are caused by what precedes them, with no room for free will. Despite the fact that at the quantum physical level events are non-deterministic (there is a significant component to apparent randomness), it might still be the case that the brain and the mind function as a deterministic system. If this is the case, most determinants hold that people cannot therefore, meaningfully be held responsible for their actions.[1]

It has been hypothesized that, whereas long-term goals are selected consciously and emotional processing is essential to volition, and that it is discrepancy that explains the common experience of repeatedly choosing something that conflicts with one's goals (overeating when trying to lose weight, or shopping for luxury despite wishing to pay off a hefty debt). Similarly, there are several undesirable behaviors, in contravention with the law of the land, detrimental to the societal growth and adversely affecting the economic growth which plague the human existence. Aggression and violence are such behaviors.

WHAT IS AGGRESSION?

Anger is a normal phenomenon experienced by all species and is defined as an affective state motivated towards warning, intimidating, or attacking those perceived as challenging or threatening. *Aggression* is intentionally hurting or gaining advantage over other person, without necessarily involving physical injury.

Pathological aggression or violence is either excessive in degree or arises from a mental disorder often associated with such a condition. In a given situation, anyone can become violent but most aggression is not violence.[2] Aggression includes psychological assault which occurs due to overt, mostly deleterious, social interaction where the intention is to inflict damage or other unpleasantness upon another person. It may occur either in retribution or without provocation. In humans, aggression can result from frustration because of blocked goal. Human aggression can be categorized into:

- *Direct aggression* which is distinguished by physical or verbal behavior with intention to cause harm to other person
- *Indirect aggression* highlighted by a behavior intended to harm socially.

It is questionable to club aggression as an instinct—genetically determined but modified by environment—or learned. Individuals probably have a normal inborn assertiveness with aggression being secondary to early developmental deprivation and insult and or mental disorder, rather than a primary drive. Aggression often results from frustration and threat, such as to low self-esteem and increasing tension. Aggression can also be displaced from original object onto a symbolic representation of it. It can also be explained as a social phenomenon, such as seen in altruist aggression.[3]

Psychology of Aggression

Aggression includes behavior and actions that display a degree of hostility for motivation, including to gain resources, to intimidate others and as a reaction to intimidation. Aggression, using a biological definition, is intra-species fighting while violence is extra-species fighting. Term violence is used clinically for overt physical aggression.[4]

WHAT IS VIOLENCE?

Violence requires overcoming inhibitions, such as result of failure of control, but can be planned and focused as well. World Health Organization (WHO) defines violence as, "intentional use of physical force or power, threatened or actual against oneself, another person, or a group,

or community, which either results in or has high likelihood of resulting in injury, death, psychological harm, mal-development or deprivation". Violence is conceptualized as follows:
- As a medical disorder or illness
- Morally as a crime or sin
- Educationally as a problem of social learning
- Socially as an expression of deprivation.

Medical causes are often cited to reduce an individual's responsibility for his actions. Violence manifests in the following forms:
- Physical
- Sexual
- Psychological
- Emotional.

Epidemiology

Violence is a public health problem and world-wide is responsible for 1% mortality and 10% injuries. It ranks 21st in the causes of death in males and 47th leading cause of death in females.[5] Violence rates are highest in Latin America, Central America and South Africa all of which are six times the average for the world. Over the years violence is increasing globally. In the year 2013, violence resulted into death of an estimated 1.28 million people, up from 1.13 million in 1990.[6,7]

Men are much more violent than women. Being male and young are the best predictors for violence in addition to alcohol and drug misuse.[1] Violence is generally by the powerful against the weak.

Violence has life-long consequences for physical and mental health and social functioning and slows down social and economic development. Violence in many forms is preventable.

TYPES OF VIOLENCE

The term 'violence' is often interchangeably used for aggression and even criminal violence but they are different. They can be differentiated as follows:

Violence is characterized by display of strong physical force against another person, which may be accompanied by aggression and which may cause harm to others.

Criminal violence is directly injurious behavior which is against the law. It includes murder, manslaughter, assault and robbery. Sexual offence and arson are also included as criminal violence.

Each of these situations infers a potential or actual consequent harm. Violence can be classified on the basis of target as:
- *Self-directed* is the violence which may result into suicide or self-abuse, often seen in patients suffering from depressive disorder.
- *Inter-personal* is the violence between two or more persons.
- *Collective* violence could be structural or economic.

There are different forms of violence which are described as follows:

Instrumental Violence

"It is a type of violence which is used as a mean to achieve a goal". It is usually planned and not precipitated by increased arousal except sadistic violence in which pain and cruelty are inflicted not only to control a victim but also to generate sexual arousal and excitement.

Expressive or Reactive Violence

It is a type of violence which is accompanied by strong emotions such as hostility, anger, fear or loss. The primary goal in harming the victim is the expression of these affects. The violence occurs in response to or in conjunction with, feelings of arousal (due to anger, fear, frustration, hostility, resentment) in the perpetrator. It is usually impulsive (but may be planned).

An act of violence may be seen as expressive or instrumental, in some cases features of both are represented, for example violence used to carry out robbery on a victim (instrumental) but also as an angry reaction of the perpetrator for being abused by the victim.

Gang Violence

"It is the violence in which the peer groups play an important role in development of violence and delinquency". Involvement with the deviant peers is the most proximate influence in development of delinquent behavior, including its escalation to violence.

Organized Violence

It includes *illegal drug trade*. India lies between two major hubs of illicit opium trade in Asia.[8]

India has been a transit point for heroin smuggling from countries like Pakistan and Afghanistan on the west and countries like Burma, Laos and Thailand on the east.[9] Because of such strategic location, India witnesses heavy amount of drug-trafficking through its border.[10] India holds the topmost position for the licit opium production for the pharmaceutical trade,[11] but an undetermined quantity of opium is diverted to illicit international drug market. Smuggling occurs mainly through Pakistan and Burma with minor quantities through Nepal.

Cybercrime: It is another crime which has lately come into great prominence. Indian Information and Technology Act, 2000[12] was passed with the aims to check cybercrime and provide legal framework for disciplining e-commerce transactions.[13] However, it has limitations when dealing with several emerging cybercrimes like cyber harassment, defamation, stalking, etc. Also, most cases are not reported due to lack of awareness.[14] In 2001, India and US came together to set an Indo-US cyber security forum to initiate counter-terrorism dialogue.[15]

Violence Against Strangers

Stranger violence is more likely to occur in public places under the influence of alcohol. Violence against strangers is often less severe compared with violence against those who are known to the perpetrator. Some child sex offenders target children who are not known to them.

Intimate Partner/Domestic Violence

Twenty-five percent women experience some form of domestic violence at sometime in their lifetime. Domestic violence is more common among the younger women than the older ones. Though the domestic violence is seen both in men and women, rate of injuries is much higher in women including the indecent sexual assault. The reasons describing women as victims of domestic violence are, power and control exercised by men. While women are economically dependent on their husbands, men may be emotionally dependent on their wives, this reciprocal relationship contributes to the risk of partner abuse and also reduces the likelihood of separation particularly in Indian society.[16]

Family Violence

Majority of the homicide victims are from within the family who are either spouses or children of the perpetrator. About 80% of the killed children are killed by their parents and the new born are most at risk. Violence between the parents is witnessed by about two-thirds of the children, and the violence between the parents often accompanies violence to children as well. Children are victims of physical abuse in 10–16% families and the physical abuse carries the risk of about 10% mortality rate. Sexual abuse of children occurs in 8–10% of the households; and more common when there is domestic violence or physical abuse of children. Severe abuse in children and witnessing family violence is predictive of late violence, delinquency, as well as mental health problems.[17]

VICTIMS OF VIOLENCE

Anyone can become a victim of violence, man, woman or a child, but the contexts in which one becomes the victim of violence tend to differ. The common factor is their vulnerability, at that time, for victimization by mentally ill offenders within the family setting. Some victims of violence may be strangers to the perpetrator, only less than 10% victims are strangers.[18,19]

BIOPSYCHOSOCIAL MODEL OF VIOLENCE

Causation of violence is multifactorial. "Violence is a biopsychosocial—environmental—cultural—political phenomenon". All behaviors have biochemical basis. While biochemical abnormalities can cause psychological symptoms, including aggression and violence, there is also increasing evidence of psychological events, for example, severe abuse during childhood, and severe psychological trauma during adulthood lead to neurobiological abnormalities, for example, in serotonin (5-HT) metabolism in adults. Violence has been associated with low cholesterol levels. Stress and post-traumatic stress disorder (PTSD) cause shrinkage of hypothalamus.[20]

PHILOSOPHY OF VIOLENCE

One area of philosophical debate is that of free will versus determinism. We are hardwired for competitiveness, aggression, sex and continuation of our species, and favoring of our relatives, that is in keeping with, Neo-Darwinist biological determinism. Darwin wrote of the great delusion of free will. Most of our behavior is largely unconscious, such as braking while driving a car, and our response to phone ringing. Are we all the inevitable outcome of our genes, early development and the environment? Hibbes[21] assigns aggression to nature, Nietzsche[22] believes aggression rose from will to power.

Libet[23] shows that the brain detects tactile stimuli before we are conscious of such stimuli. We therefore, kick out in anger or jump if in pain.

GENETICS AND VIOLENCE

Genes associated with violence have been identified, i.e. *MAO-A* gene on the X-chromosome can result in low levels of monoamines, such as serotonin, but the latter appears to require the presence of environmental factors such as early abuse, antisocial families, and availability of weapons, to result in expression of violence that is , there is a genetic hyper-reactivity to stress. In Italy, identification of such genes for violence has led to a reduction in sentence, while in the United States MAO-A data led to reduction of a first-degree murder charges (a capital offence) to voluntary man-slaughter.[24] Like height, multiple genes with small contribution may increase the probability of violence.

Social and cultural factors are more important than genes, as evidenced by reduction in homicide rate by 35 times since Victorian times in United Kingdom.

PSYCHOLOGICAL THEORIES OF VIOLENCE

Ethological Theory

According to this theory, aggression is considered an instinctive behavior that serves an adaptive behavior in evolutionary terms, i.e. it advances natural selection by survival of genes. Aggression between species increases the survival of the most aggressive group, while aggression within the species establishes hierarchies and ensures groups remain at an optimal size and not in competition for resources. It is, thus, territorial for food and facilitates sex selection of strongest. Caste-system in Hindu society and hierarchies in the institution of caste-system explain the aggression within the species.[25]

An ethological theory of aggression was highlighted by Conrad Lorenz according to which a personal bond and individual friendship are characteristics of animals with highly developed intra-species aggression. Firmer the bond, the higher the chances of aggression in the particular animal or species is. Thus, real intimacy may occur only when individuals share real aggression as well as good feelings. Maternally deprived monkeys became aggressive and poor mothers themselves.[26]

Social Learning Theory

According to Bandura, behavior, including aggression are learned at an early age by observing significant others—parents, teachers and peers. Such behaviors are then modeled and initiated. Children seeing adults striking or violent material on TV makes them perform aggressive behavior. Those predisposed to aggression are more likely to watch violent material, indicating how individual differences interact with situational variables.[27]

Operant Conditioning

Aggressive behavior can result in goal being achieved which is positively reinforced. The pleasure and satisfaction the individual may take from being aggressive or taking revenge can itself be rewarding (through the reward center in the brain and adrenergic responses)—hedonic reward, and can become a goal instead. There is a spectrum in individual tendency to seek revenge, which is increased in males compared to females.[28]

Freudian Theories

Sigmund Freud (1856-1939) initially developed, frustration-aggression hypothesis which means frustration from failure to achieve desired internal goal leads to aggression. Aggression may be displaced to apathy, depression, or emotional distress rather than anger. Later Freud refines his theory and says, rather than frustration directly causing aggression, it only increases its likelihood. In 1922, in his, 'Beyond the pleasure principle', he argues that the primary drive to aggression is not frustration but libido (the pleasure seeking drive, *eros*) and that aggression is a secondary drive in response to their association with the death instinct (thanatos).[29]

Arousal

Specific environmental cues result in existing frustration being translated into aggressive behavior. Through classical conditioning, these cues become associated with anger and aggression, and in turn serve to increase the likelihood of aggression. There is experimental evidence of aggression—congruent cues resulting in increased aggression in frustrated subjects.

Group Hostility

The random allocation of an individual to a group shows that merely being a member of a group results in increased hostility to other groups. Violence is often associated with mental illness and there is increasing concern about the level of violence within mental healthcare setting. Are the mentally ill violent? Are they more at risk of violent outbursts than the people without a mental illness? Is there a risk to public safety due to same. These questions are frequently debated both by the scientific community and the public. Since violence is the most fear inducing factor for the public, it is also a major determinant of social stigma and discrimination surrounding the mentally ill.

■ MENTAL ILLNESS AND VIOLENCE

Fifty percent of psychiatrists involved with the management of psychiatric patients report having been assaulted by a patient at least once.[1] With the advent of actuarial risk assessment tools, violence risk assessments are increasingly promoted as core mental health skills:

expected of psychiatrists, prized in the courts of law and correction settings.[30] While evaluating violence, the focus generally remains on the clinical attributes of mental illness. The social and contextual factors that interact to produce violence are often ignored.[1] With the social change in the practice of psychiatry, only those with severe violence receive treatment in psychiatric hospital setting, rest are treated at clinics or community level. Experiences from the hospital setting indicate that the mental illness is not the sufficient cause for the occurrence of violence.[31] Most of these incidents have social or contextual antecedents such as:
- Ward atmosphere
- Lack of clinical leadership
- Overcrowding
- Restrictions in the ward
- Lack of or unstructured activities.

The general public is also accustomed to experience violence among mentally ill which are mostly viscous through movie depictions. The public most fear violence that is random, senseless and unpredictable and associated with mental illness. People are comfortable to know that someone was stabbed to death in a robbery than someone stabbed to death by a psychiatric patient.[32] Public perception of mentally ill as violent is associated with stigma and discrimination—leading to forced legal action and coerced treatment.[33] This perception justifies bullying and otherwise victimizing the mentally ill.[34] In a study, 25% patients were victims of hitting, pushing, chocking, being beaten up. Six percent of those living with the family members were physically victimized.[34] Many mentally ill live in dangerous and impoverished neighborhood where they are at a high risk of being victimized. In a study 8% mentally ill were criminally victimized, much higher than general populations.[35] Victimization and bullying may provoke a patient to violence.

Prior to 1980, it was believed that mentally ill were no more or no less likely to be violent. Crime and violence in mentally ill were associated with the same criminogenic factors thought to determine crime and violence in any one else: gender, age, poverty, drug-abuse.

Although the factors such as young age, male sex, single, low socioeconomic status, and drug-abuse remain the same, in the recent years it is reported that mental illness is another such factor.[36,37] Prevalence of violence in mentally ill without substance use is indistinguishable from general population. Substance use doubles the risk of violence.

In the past, factors predicting violence (personality disorder, impulsivity, anger, violent family background, and substance abuse) were said to be the same, regardless of the mental status of the offender. However, since 1992, studies have shown that having a diagnosis of mental illness is weakly associated with violence. This can also be narrowed down to subgroups with specific types of symptoms such as paranoid (persecutory) delusions (false beliefs) and delusions of passivity (being under external control). Hence certain symptoms, and not entirely the psychiatric diagnoses alone is associated with violence. Nevertheless, the risk of violence is still considerably more in a young male than with the diagnosis of schizophrenia.[38] Amongst those with a diagnosis of mental illness, affective disorders are underrepresented in forensic psychiatric facilities. Risk of violence is, however, more in people with schizophrenia[39] (especially those who are not compliant to treatment) and in young men with acute schizophrenia compared to those labeled as chronic schizophrenia, but it still accounts for less than 10% of violent offenders. Violence may be secondarily to positive symptoms of mental illness, such as delusions (false beliefs) and hallucinations (e.g. voices). Mental illness, especially schizophrenia, may, also lead indirectly to violence through ongoing deterioration in adaptive and social functioning along with personality, so that individuals end up becoming antisocial and impulsive with a lower tolerance to stress. This often leads to disputes in court about the placement to hospital or prison of such individuals. This sometimes results in, wrongly, getting an additional diagnosis of personality disorder to explain their violence. A mentally ill individual may behave aggressively due to "normal" emotional reasons, such as fear and anger, and then experience accompanying corresponding psychotic symptoms such as hallucinations of aggressive content. Violence, law involvement, and imprisonment may themselves precipitate mental illness. For a mentally ill person, the key issue is whether the individual has a delusion of a content on which he or she might act dangerously, for example, of persecution or infidelity, but even then not all morbidly jealous individuals, for instance, assault their partner. Twenty percent of people presenting to hospital with their first episode of schizophrenia have threatened the lives of others, but among these patients, half have already been ill for a year.[40] Overall, however, it is unusual for a person with schizophrenia to present for the first time with serious violence, including homicide. One established period of higher risk is within a few months of discharge from hospital.[41] People with both schizophrenia and substance abuse have higher rates of violence than those with substance abuse alone, who in turn have higher rates than those with schizophrenia alone. Research has generally, but not universally,[42] shown a consistent association between violence and delusions, particularly of threat/control override (TCO) content (which doubles the risk), for example, persecutory delusions, passivity delusions, and thought insertion,[43] although most such subjects are not violent. These findings are in keeping with social psychology theory that violence in general is associated with the individual feeling under threat or losing control of his or her situation. The presence of hallucinations does not alone increase the risk of violence, but it may do so when delusions are present. This also applies to command hallucinations, which may reflect what the individual is otherwise thinking and feeling and which are often only reported after an individual has been violent. Psychiatric patients tend to peak for violent offending at a later age than the general population. It is important to be aware that the oft-quoted "best predictor of future behavior is past behavior" is based on non-psychiatric populations and, in any case, accounts for only 5% of the variance.[44] A history of previous violence is required for this to be relevant in any case. Among severely (psychotic) mentally ill people, delusions of TCO appear to be better predictors than past behavior. Among all individuals, including mentally ill people, a history of expressed threats (as opposed to generalized anger), substance abuse, and personal deprivation or abuse are associated with violence. Indeed, it has been suggested that homicide rates in general may be reduced in the United Kingdom by coordinated multi-agency responses and more policy and educational initiatives targeted specifically to counter domestic violence, child abuse, alcohol abuse, and the carrying of knives and other weapons.[45] Law-breaking behavior in general, and violence in particular, usually decreases when an individual's basic needs are met. For instance, an individual with schizophrenia who kills may have a characteristic history of not only noncompliance with medication, leading to relapse of his or her mental illness, but also of being in a situation of social isolation and poor home conditions. Some individuals may even offend to remove themselves from their situation in the community to the security of a prison or hospital. The risk of being a victim of serious violence and of self-harm or suicide is, however, greater for people with schizophrenia, even if they have behaved seriously violently in the past, than is the risk of homicide or serious harm to others in the future. In summary, although no mental illness is characterized by serious violence, including homicide, the existing evidence suggests that there is a link between mental illness and violence.

Association of Mental Illness and Offence

It should be noted that offending is not a primary characteristic of any mental disorder. However, there are certain conditions which are particularly associated with offending behavior **(Table 1)**. These are described as follows:

Organic Mental Disorders

Dementia

There are certain organic conditions which may manifest with offending behavior as a characteristic symptom. The onset of minor offending such as shoplifting, minor sex offenses, and fraud at a late age may be due to dementia (e.g. Alzheimer's disease), owing to its reduction of intellectual functioning, judgment, and normal inhibitions in social behavior. Elderly people in general often show coarsening of their personality characteristics and dis-inhibition with increasing age. This may often cause embarrassment in the presence of women when one talks openly about the sexual matters generally avoided in such situations. Individuals with delirium

Table 1: Conditions associated with violent/offending behavior.

Organic mental disorders	• Dementia • Head trauma • Huntington's chorea • Epilepsy • Sleep disorder
Psychiatric disorders	• Schizophrenia • Delusional disorders • Mood disorders • Neurotic and stress-related disorders • Personality disorder • Substance/alcohol abuse • Learning (intellectual) disabilities (mental retardation) • Autistic spectrum disorders (ASDs) • Attention deficit hyperactivity disorder (ADHD) • Conduct disorder and oppositional-defiant disorder • Fire-setting

and dementia may become aggressive, but this seldom results in criminal proceedings. Dementia is a syndrome characterized by cognitive decline. Dementias are classified as follows:
1. Cortical
   - Alzheimer's disease
   - Pick's disease
2. Subcortical
   - Parkinson's disease
   - Huntington's disease
   - Wilson's disease
3. Cortical subcortical
   - Lewy body dementia
   - Multiple Creutzfeldt-Jakob disease (CJD)

About 5–10% of the general population above 65 years of age suffers from dementia. About 19–33% forensic psychiatry patients above 60 years of age suffer from dementia. About 1% of the sentenced prisoners above 59 years of age suffer from dementia. About 20–40% persons suffering from dementia have symptoms of delusions and hallucinations and 50% of them have anxiety and depression.

Dementia and Offending Behavior

Dementia is primarily a disorder of old age and people over 65 years of age are under-represented as a proportion of all violent offenders (less than 05%). Behavioral and psychological symptoms of dementia and neuropsychiatric symptoms are numerous and include agitation and aggression. This may also include shouting and verbal insults but also hitting, biting and other physical violence. These behavioral symptoms may occur in conjunction with other psychiatric and physical disorders. There is no confirmed association between dementia and severe violence. There are also no specific offences associated with dementia, although there is some association.

Head Trauma

Depending upon severity and localization, violence is associated with brain injury. Brain damage from head injury, even in the absence of significant cognitive impairment, may produce a profound alteration in personality, resulting in excessive aggression, for example, to a partner, who may then find it impossible to continue to live with the individual. A cool and docile person changing into a highly volatile and angry person is a common manifestation in such a condition. Brain damage also reduces alcohol tolerance, which in turn may predispose to further head injuries.[46] Frontal lobe trauma leads to dysexecutive syndrome resulting into:
- Disinhibition
- Impulsive behavior
- Increased agitation
- Cognitive impairment.

Huntington's Chorea

Huntington's disease may present in the early stages with psychopathic behavior. Activities as a manifestation of Huntington's disease are, at times, likely to come in conflict with the law of the land.[47]

Epilepsy

A possible relationship between epilepsy and violence has been debated for over a century. The debate has taken on new importance because of the increasing use of the "epilepsy defense" in criminal cases. Those with epilepsy are up to twice as likely to offend than members of the general population, but this appears to be due to premorbid factors, such as head injury and organic brain damage (e.g. due to child physical abuse), personality, or the perceived stigma of having epilepsy. Ictal violence is very rare. The previously described overrepresentation of those with epilepsy among the prisoners no longer seems to be evident. Prevalence of epilepsy in general population is 0.5-1%. 1-2% prisoners suffer from epilepsy. Its prevalence in forensic psychiatry patients is around 5%. About 20-30% patients with epilepsy have comorbid psychiatric disorders of which 2-9% suffer from psychosis, 20-60% from depression and 20-40% from substance abuse.

Epilepsy can be associated with complex behavior which may occasionally result in violence. Violence in persons with epilepsy is usually due to other risk factors which are responsible for violence in epilepsy. In epilepsy, violent behavior may occur during seizures (ictal violence) or in between the seizures (interictal violence).[2] The relationship between aggressive or violent behavior and epilepsy has been extensively debated. A longstanding belief that patients with epilepsy exhibit increased aggression and are prone to violence was proposed by a number of early studies including studies noting an increased incidence of epilepsy in prisoner populations.[1] The description of bizarre though stereotyped behaviors during some seizures, particularly of frontal lobe origin[2] and the not infrequent use of epilepsy as a courtroom defense strategy for violent crime,[3] continue to perpetuate this belief. While the association between epilepsy and aggression remains in question, it continues to contribute to public perception and amplifies the stigma associated with the disease.[3]

While it is unclear that patients with epilepsy exhibit increased aggression, aggressive acts have been seen in association with seizures themselves. Most commonly, aggression may occur in the postictal state and can be seen even hours to days after initial periods of confusion.[4] In particular, directed, postictal violent behavior may be seen in association with postictal psychosis.[5] Rarely violent behavior may be part of the seizure itself, and when aggressive behavior occurs, typical characteristics of seizures must also be present.

Ictal violence (violence committed during a seizure) is rare. It is likely to occur in complex partial seizure than in generalized tonic-clonic seizures. It is likely that most offending occurs in the postictal or interictal period, often when there is also some external influence (pressure from other person).

Abnormality of temporal lobe which may cause complex partial seizures may itself directly cause violence. Temporal lobe abnormalities are associated with controversial diagnosis of *episodic dyscontrol syndrome*, in which there is apparent lack of memory for explosive episodes of sudden uncontrolled violence.

Assessment of association between violence and epilepsy
A neurologist should be involved. Assessment of an epileptic alleged to have committed violence should be done as follows:
- Diagnosis of epilepsy should be confirmed with an electroencephalography (EEG).
- Epileptic automatism should be established with clinical history and closed circuit TV-EEG monitoring.
- Aggression should be observed by closed circuit TV-EEG monitoring.
- The violent act should be characteristic of patient's usual seizures.
- Any obvious motive, planning or premedication should be considered.
- Concealment of the offence.
- Whether the offence is senseless or out of character.

Sleep Disorders

Sleep disorders are rarely associated with violence. Relationship between forensic psychiatry, epilepsy and parasomnias is historically based on their association with clinical phenomenon of automatism and consequent inexplicable crime. In deep sleep (stage 4) or in context of abnormal sleep after brain damage (during REM), sleep such a behavioral abnormality may erupt.[46] About 2–25% of the general population suffer from all types of parasomnias.

Sleep disturbance is a common feature of many psychiatric disorders, but it is distinct from sleep walking and other parasominas such as sleep terror disorder, and nightmare disorder. These disorders are more common in children.

Sleep disturbance and violence
Violence is observed in male adults who had history of parasomnias and nocturnal enuresis during their childhood.

Sleep terror disorder and sleep walking often overlap and may be present in the same episode. A period of sleep deprivation, alcohol, marijuana, and caffeine have been reported as being associated with provoking sleep walking. Victims of crime associated with sleep are usually known to the perpetrator. The sleep walkers may not appear to hear any cries of the victims or recognize their victims.

Whether the episode occurs in REM (Rapid eye movement) sleep or non-REM sleep may be significant. The notion that an individual in REM sleep is paralyzed and, therefore, cannot be violent is no longer accepted. The possibility of nocturnal epilepsy can further confuse the assessment, and may need to be considered as an alternative diagnosis.

Assessment of association between violence and sleep disturbance: The following points should be considered while making an assessment:
- Is there a history of childhood parasomnias?
- Was the violence preceded by a period of sleep by the perpetrator?
- Did the arousal from sleep occur soon after the sleep onset?

- Is there any evidence of complex, goal-directed behavior?
- Is the victim well known and loved?
- Was there any evidence of recognition of the victim?
- Was there any period of confusion after the attack?
- Is there amnesia for the event?
- Was there any obvious motive, planning or premedication?
- Was there any concealment of offence?
- Was the offence sensational or out of character?
- Was the violence preceded by a period of poor sleep?

Psychiatric Disorders

Schizophrenia

Most individuals with schizophrenia are not convicted of criminal offenses, but overall schizophrenia is often overrepresented among offenders, especially when compared with affective psychosis. Most convictions are secondary to minor offenses and are related to the associated deterioration in the individual's personality and social functioning, rather than due to delusions and hallucinations. Schizophrenia, especially paranoid schizophrenia, can, on occasion, lead to dangerous offending and may result in planned assaults, including homicide, without apparent motive.[48] Victims are, however, more likely to be known to the individual with schizophrenia than to be strangers. Relatives are particularly at risk, as they are the individuals in most emotional contact with the subject. Antisocial behavior can present in the prodromal phase of schizophrenia, when the clinical picture may be referred to as *pseudopsychopathic schizophrenia*. Schizophrenia may cause distortion in perceptions, thought, judgment, and voluntary control of actions.[49] Matricide (the killing of one's mother) is frequently, but not invariably, associated with schizophrenia.

Delusional Disorders

People suffering from delusional disorders are likely to commit crime under the influence of their delusions. Subjects suffered from morbid delusional sexual jealousy (Othello's syndrome), which may itself frequently lead to severe aggression toward, and the killing of, a sexual partner about whom delusions of sexual infidelity are held. Jealousy itself is a risk factor for violence. In erotomania (de Clérambault's syndrome), the subject under the influence of delusion, believes another person (often of higher social status) loves the subject (usually female) intensely. Only some sufferers of this disorder cause disruptive or antisocial behavior—such as phone calls, letter writing, following the victim, and stalking—but repeated rebuttals may on occasion lead to hatred and dangerous behavior, especially in the presence of a premorbid antisocial personality and a history of past multiple subjects of such delusional beliefs.[50]

Mood Disorders

Overall, people with mood disorders are underrepresented in forensic psychiatric populations. Depressive disorder is more generally associated with the risk of suicide, but on occasion it is associated with homicide, for example, the "altruistic" homicide of a family where the individual, usually the father, feels that the family may be better off out of this "wicked" world. Homicides associated with depressive disorder are more likely to occur in the morning and usually involve family members. Puerperal psychosis or postnatal depression can also rarely lead to homicide of infants and other children. An early study conducted by Shoplifting has historically been associated with depression, particularly in middle-aged women of previously good record who may shoplift as a cry for help to bring attention to their mental state. However, most shoplifters are not depressed or otherwise mentally ill. Hypomania or manic episodes are often associated with dis-inhibited behavior, irritability, intolerance, and increased sexual drive. This may lead to convictions for breach of the peace, road-traffic offenses, impulsive violence, and sexual offending such as rape. Such patients spend money excessively, often due to their grandiosed belief that they will soon make this up, but their actions can also lead to fraud.[46] Mania is predisposed to violence and other offending behavior because of its symptoms such as:

- Elation
- Agitation
- Impaired judgment
- Impulsivity
- Associated psychosis

Depression is known for violence against self due to

- Hopelessness
- Enhanced perception of criticism by others
- Reduced threshold to loss of control.

Neurotic and Stress-related Disorders

While neurotic symptoms are common in those with personality disorder and among those in prison and forensic psychiatric facilities, forensic psychiatrists have tended to focus more on the presence or otherwise of psychosis (especially schizophrenia) or personality disorder in their assessments and psychiatric reports and recommendations, including for treatment.[51] Those with neurotic disorders are generally considered responsible for their actions. Post-traumatic stress disorder (PTSD) can lead to violence as a result of symptoms of hypervigilance, hyperarousal, increased impulsivity, anger, flashbacks, and nightmares. Offending itself may lead to PTSD requiring treatment. Those with dissociative disorder may have experienced or witnessed severe violence, and dissociation in those who have been violent is said to indicate an increased likelihood of further such offending. Dissociative amnesia, a psychogenic reaction to stress, may be associated with offenses committed in a state of high emotional arousal. Dissociative amnesia for the circumstances of an offense may be seen. Usually the amnesia is patchy (episodic) and with purposeful travel may also occur. A psychiatrist may be required to distinguish dissociative and conversion disorders, where the motivation is theoretically unconscious, from conscious malingering. However, these conditions can in practice be seen as on a continuum from a fully unconscious to a fully conscious motivation.

Some offenders describe experiencing depersonalization and derealization at the time of an offense, which may similarly reflect high emotional arousal.[52] PTSD, though, has no direct link to violence, its symptoms such as irritability, aggressiveness and substance misuse, can lead to violent actions. More symptoms could be:
- Anxiety and arousal
- Irritability, impulsivity and anger
- Hypervigilance
- Misinterpretation of objective threats
- Triggering from flashbacks, nightmare.

Personality Disorder

Personality disorder amounts to a developmental disorder. Cluster B (DSM-V) personality disorder is associated with criminal behavior (antisocial, borderline, narcissistic) characterized by impulsivity, disordered relationships, and rule breaking. Adult personality disorders are a common diagnosis among offenders, however the clear cut-off boundary between psychiatrically "normal" individuals who are offenders and individuals with personality disorders is not delineated. In some individuals a diagnosis of personality disorder is made only on the grounds of committing an offence. Personality traits associated with offending include impulsivity, lack of empathy, paranoid attitudes (often related to low self-esteem), difficulty relating to others, and a low tolerance of stress with a liability to intemperate outbursts of anger and violence. The cluster B personality disorders—such as histrionic, narcissistic, and antisocial personality disorders—are particularly associated with violence. People with personality disorder who are offenders usually are frequently seen abusing alcohol or drugs, or may be dependent on them, and may have comorbid chronic neurotic and stress-related disorders as well.[18] In the community, personality disorder is strongly associated with offending including violence.[46] In prisons 50-70% inmates have personality disorder particularly exhibiting callous and unemotional traits. Violence often occurs due to:
- Transient psychosis
  - Paranoid cognition
  - Impaired regulation of emotions including anger
  - High levels of agitation
  - Impaired empathy
  - Need for risk taking
  - Substance misuse.

Substance/Alcohol Abuse

People who abuse alcohol and drugs may offend due to the associated disinhibiting effects on behavior. In addition, substance abuse may directly lead to offending due to the effect of intoxication or withdrawal or substance-induced mental illness, or as an indirect result to fund such substance abuse. Possession and supply of illegal drugs alone may result in convictions.[46,53]

Learning (Intellectual) Disabilities (Mental Retardation)

People with learning (intellectual) disabilities are three to four times overrepresented among offenders and even higher among violent offenders.[54] This finding relates to those with milder rather than severe learning disability, as the latter tend not to enter the criminal justice system and may be because they lack understanding of the nature of their behavior and its legal consequences, they are more suggestible, and they are easier to catch. Learning disabilities may also lead to feelings of frustration, which in turn may lead to violence and even homicide. Also, in panic or frustration, such people may commit arson or sexual offenses that relate to their difficulty initiating and sustaining interpersonal and sexual relationships. This leads to their overrepresentation among arsonists and sexual offenders in studies on secure hospital populations of UK.[46,54]

Autistic Spectrum Disorders

Autistic spectrum disorders have become increasingly recognized. Asperger's syndrome and autism are found to be associated with offending in an increased rate, especially violence and criminal damage but also, due to defects in social reciprocity and theory of mind, stalking and, due to restricted, repetitive interests, computer crime.[46] Following manifestations may be relevant to violent offending:
- Lack of concern for social norms
- Lack of awareness of the consequences
- Lack of empathy
- Lack of understanding of others' behavior
- Lack of understanding of what is wrong.

In *Asperger's syndrome* offending is particularly related to:
1. *Theory of mind deficit:* There is a tendency to egocentricity which results in lack of awareness of impact on victim, and of what is 'wrong' in social and emotional terms.
2. *Deficits in social reciprocity:* Predisposes an individual to sexual offences in particular, i.e. the individual wanting sexual contact, without appreciating the complex reciprocal interactions, essential between two potential partners in order for consensual sexual activity to take place.
3. *Restricted, repetitive interests:* Include, fire-setting or other crimes which may be bizarre or persistent without any apparent or understandable motive—'motive' is merely repetition of act.

Offending behavior in *Asperger's syndrome* may also be revenge for persistent bullying, change in routine, exploitation, and coerced involvement in criminal activity. Such offences can be extremely violent, even homicidal.

Attention Deficit Hyperactivity Disorder

Attention deficit hyperactivity disorder (ADHD), hyperactivity disorder, hyperkinetic syndrome are some of the terms used for a syndrome characterized by—persistent overactivity, impulsivity and difficulty in sustaining attention. The occurrence of symptoms both within and outside the home, the presence of both inattention and overactivity, and the presence of conduct disorder (CD) are all associated with a more serious condition that is less responsive to treatment and has a poorer outcome. There is an overlap between ADHD and CD but they are different clinical entities.

Inattentive and overactive subtypes of ADHD have distinct profiles. Those with the hyperactive-impulsive subtype of ASDHD are characterized by extreme overactivity, with oppositional aggressive behavior. Conduct problems are their most prevalent, school-based difficulties and they have high rates of school suspension and special educational placements. Children with the hyperactive-impulsive profile are at risk of long-term antisocial behavior problems and poor school adjustment.

Prevalence of ADHD: About 5–10% children during school and 2.5% individuals during adulthood in the general population suffer from ADHD. However, there is no data for its prevalence *among the psychiatric patients.* About 30% of the young offenders in the prisons suffer from ADHD. The prevalence rates are further higher in males than females.

ADHD symptoms and risk of violence: Impulsivity, hyperactivity and inattention in school can result in school failure, which can be a risk factor for offending. Impulsivity may reflect deficits in executive functioning of the brain, located in the frontal lobe. The individuals suffering from these neuro-psychological deficits will tend to commit offences because they have poor control over the behavior, a poor ability to consider the consequences of their actions and a tendency to focus on immediate gratification. Children with ADHD have learning difficulties.

ADHD symptoms are a common feature among individuals with early onset, persistent antisocial behavior and the prognosis for antisocial individuals with ADHD symptoms is especially poor. Some are diagnosed in adulthood with antisocial personality disorder. In either case, the long-term risk of offending behavior is high.

Other harms associated with ADHD: Impulsivity is the most crucial personality dimension that predicts offending. Children with ADHD display a greater degree of difficulty, with aggression, oppositional and defiant behavior; and conduct problems. The most common conduct problems are lying, stealing, truancy, and physical aggression. The symptoms of ADHD correlate with later violent behavior and criminality.

Comorbidity with other mental disorders: Comorbid conditions commonly occur with ADHD are ODD, CD, mood disorder, anxiety disorder and learning disorders.

What is the risk?
1. Hyperactivity at 11–13 years significantly predicts arrest for violence up to 22 years of age especially among boys who have been the subjects of delivery complications.
2. Problem of attention and restlessness at age 5 more than double the risk for delinquency.
3. Each comorbid condition further increases the risk for delinquency or offending.

Conduct Disorder and Oppositional-defiant Disorder

Conduct disorder (CD) is characterized by the persistent failure to control behavior within the socially defined rules. Conduct problem involves three overlapping domains of behavior:
- Defiance of the will of someone in authority
- Aggressiveness
- Antisocial behavior that violates other people's rights.

Oppositional defiance disorder (ODD) refers to a pattern of conduct problem characterized mainly by tantrums and conduct problems (typically occur in preschool years). ODD is distinct from CD and is less pervasive but is recognized as a possible developmental precursor of CD.

Prevalence of CD and ODD: Lifetime prevalence in general population of ODD is 10% and CD, 7% in males and 3% in females.

Impact of symptoms on risk of violence and offending:

Antisocial behavior increases the risk of juvenile and adult offending. About 40% children of CD will go on to become young offenders (90% of young offenders had CD in childhood). Whereas ODD is not particularly associated with offending behavior.

Parental risk factors for CD:
- Low monitoring
- High conflict
- Inconsistent and harsh discipline
- *Individual risk factors:*
- Soft neurological signs
- Impulsivity
- ADHD.

Aggressive children have low levels of pro-social skills which make them socially isolated (this is a risk factor for offending). Because of social isolation they cannot establish supportive relationships with the non-deviant peers. Disruptive and aggressive adolescents are often rejected by their peers and they tend to associate with deviant peer groups during adolescence, which increases the risk of maintaining antisocial behavior.

Individuals with conduct disorder exhibit hostile attributional biases. They interpret ambiguous social situation as threatening. They are often hypervigilant, become aggressive in response to any fear stimulus and interpret others with fear.

Association with offending behaviour: There are several explanations as to why traumatic brain injury increases the risk of perpetration of violent behavior:
- Cognitive impairment affecting recognition of legal boundaries and motivation to adhere to laws.
- Impulsive control deficit.
- Increased aggression, irritability or personality changes.
- Poor social judgment.
- Increased vulnerability to involvement in criminal activities.
- Comorbid antisocial personality disorder (PD)/psychopathy.
- Disinhibition.

Fire-setting

Pyromania is a disorder of impulse control which is characterized by a pattern of fire setting for pleasure, gratification, or relief of tension.

Diagnostic criteria:
1. Deliberate fire-setting and on purpose on more than one occasion (multiple episodes involved)
2. Feels a tension or affective arousal before setting the fire
3. Fascination, interest, attraction and/or curiosity for fire making paraphernalia, fire fighting equipment or any fire-related topic
4. Pleasure, gratification, or relief may be felt:
   - when setting fires
   - while witnessing a fire
   - when participating in the aftermath

Exclusion criteria: The fire setting cannot be better explained by another disorder (mania, antisocial personality conduct disorder, other).

The fire setting is not done (1) for monetary gain–insurance, etc. (2) to express a sociopolitical ideology, (3) to conceal a criminal act, (4) as a conscious expression of anger or vengeance, (5) to improve one's living circumstances, (6) in response to a delusion or hallucination, (7) due to superstitious belief, and (8) as a result of impaired judgment due to delusion or intoxication.

ARE THE PUBLIC AT RISK?

Both serious mental illness and serious violence are uncommon events. Since the family members are the frequent victims of violence by mentally ill, McArthur Risk Assessment[55] study found that 87% victims were family members and friends. Hospital discharged patients were less likely to attack strangers (10.7%) than the community treated patients (22.2%). Reasons of violence against family members were studied in a social network project.[56] The reasons were:
- When family relationships were characterized by mutual threat
- Financial dependence
- Concurrent substance abuse in the mentally ill
- Infrequent use of mental health services.

According to various epidemiological studies[45], only 4.3% violence was attributable to major mental disorders. Mental illness comorbid with substance abuse cause contributed 5% of all violence. A Canadian study[46] in a survey of 1151 newly detained criminal offenders—3% of violent criminal offenders suffered from mental illness such as schizophrenia, and depression. An additional 7% of violent crime was attributable to offenders with primary substance abuse.

CRIME IN SOCIAL CONTEXT

Magnitude of crime in a given society reflects a picture of criminal rule breaking behavior. The most common rule breaking is 'theft' and other types of acquisitive offences like burglary. About 20% of all crimes involve physical violence and only very few of those involve serious physical harm. It is a matter of debate whether violence is a normal and integral component of human behavior under certain circumstances or whether it represents an essentially abnormal behavior indicator of some unusual mental state. Whichever view is correct, mental disorder do place an individual at risk for violence by creating circumstances for violence or precipitating unusual mental state.

The increase of crime over the years, has led to various assumptions on the causes of rapid escalating crime. Experts including psychiatrists have been engaged in search of this increase and measurement of the crime. Several methods can be employed for measuring the prevalence of crime in a given society. Public surveys are sometimes carried out to estimate the magnitude of crime which are reported to police. Such surveys are carry some reliability for assessing trend of various criminal activities. However, they come with their own set of limitations and generally the statistics are not useful enough for local crime prevention. They often ignore offenses against children and do not count offenders brought before the criminal justice system. Rates of crime differ in different countries and even at the same place at different times. To determine the magnitude of crime, court records and rates of conviction and imprisonment data can be useful, but the most commonly cited and reliable measures of crime are national and international police records of crime and household surveys of victimization. But the police records only reflect crimes that are reported, recorded, and not subsequently cancelled. There always remains a possibility of false reporting which is likely to give spurious results. Law enforcement agencies in certain countries offer compilations of statistics for various types of crime which provides reliable information about the nature of crime in that country. Less frequent crimes such as intentional homicide and armed robbery generally have more reliable reporting, but suffer from under-recording.[1] Since laws and practices vary between different jurisdictions, comparison of crime statistics between and even within countries can be unreliable: typically only violent deaths (homicide or manslaughter) can reliably be compared, due to consistent and high reporting and relative clear definition. Thanks to the increased public awareness and assertiveness in relation to their rights, reporting of crimes, particularly of the sexual offences like rape has become more transparent *in India*.[6]

Sources of Comparative Crime Statistics
- National Crime Records Bureau of India
- British Crime Survey (BCS)
- US National Crime Survey
- European Sourcebook of Crime and Criminal Justice Statistics
- Home Office Research Development & Statistics (RDS) Publication
- UN International Crime Victims Survey (ICVS)
- US Department of Justice
- World Fact Book of Criminal Justice Systems.

Prevalence
Comparative prevalence figures for different countries are expressed in numbers per hundred thousand per year. Research employing a series of surveys done on victims, in 18 countries

of the European Union, funded by the European Commission, has shown (2005) that the level of crime in Europe is back to those seen in 1990. Declining trends in level of common crime was noted in the US, Canada, Australia and other industrialized nations as well. Demographic change has been identified as the main cause for this changing international trend by European researchers. A rise in homicide and robbery rates in the US was seen in the 1980s, however by the end of the century they had come down by 40%. European research has also suggested that "increased use of crime prevention measures may indeed be the common factor behind the near universal decrease in overall levels of crime in the Western world", since decreases have been most pronounced in property crime with limited decrease in contact crimes.[1]

While comparing the crime rates of 1953 and 2006, the *National Crime Records Bureau* (NCRB) of India highlighted that burglary in India fell steadily over a period of 53 years by 79.84% (39.3/100,000 in 1953 to 7.9/100,000 in 2006). The same report has noted increase in the rate of murders by 7.39%. *Kidnapping* increased by 47.80%, with decline in robbery by 28.85% and rioting by 10.58%.[6]

The recently released report of NCRB on 2016's crime graph in India notes the increasing trend. The report says that India suffered crimes 233/100,000 population in 2016. Child rape has increased by 82% in 2016 compared to 2015. 19900 children were raped in 2016 compared to 10934 in 2015. Juvenile crime has also increased during 2016 by 7.2%. Juvenile rapes in 2015 were 1688 which rose to 1903 in 2016 with 13% increase. 9932 juveniles held guilty of crime were released on probation while another 10019 were sent back home after admonition and warning. 111569 children were reported missing in 2016 of 60% were girls; 50% of the missing children were found and restored to their parents. 338954 cases of crime against women have been reported during the year.[6,7]

Dowry deaths are a crime which are unique only to India. They occur when young women, unable to bear the harassment and torture, commit suicides. Most of these suicides are by means of hanging, poisoning or by fire. Bride burning-women killed by setting fire on them, and is usually disguised as suicide or accident are also frequently reported. Research has shown that there are proportionately more spousal murders in the United States, but "dowry" gets implicated in India as a cultural crime due to persistent colonial narratives.[57,58] In 2012, 8,233 dowry-related death cases were reported across India. Dowry issues caused 1.4 deaths per year per 100,000 women in India.[59]

Location also plays a significant role in crimes in India. In 2012, Kerala reported highest cognizable crime rate of 455.8 among the states of India while Nagaland reported the lowest rates. In 2016, Uttar Pradesh (UP) had the largest share of all crimes in the country—9.5% crimes occurred in UP alone. Delhi had the highest rate of crime 974/100,000 against the national crime rate of 233/100,000.[7]

Almost all offenders have psychological motives for crime which had fueled psychoanalytical interest ever since the time of Sigmund Freud. However, despite this interest no psychological treatment was seen to be successful and effective treatment for offenders in general. Crime is increasingly being seen as a sociological phenomenon which is better explained by sociological theories than by individual psychological theories. Psychiatric explanations for an offense may provide better understanding of the offender, but is neither an excuse nor does it remove legal responsibility. Psychiatrists are trained in detecting the presence or absence of mental illness; they lack the necessary skills to assess a defendant's responsibility for his actions, which is a legal concept.[8] It does well for academic interest to know whether an individual is acting of complete free will: our response to events is a factor of our genes, previous experiences, and ongoing stresses in life. The legal system strives to clarify whether an individual offender is either "unstable," and therefore in need of psychiatric intervention, or "bad," and therefore in need of retribution. While the multifactorial psychiatric explanations of offending behavior is not a characteristic for any mental disorder, and may be secondary to a combination of mental illness, premorbid personality difficulties, and current circumstances. The judiciary generally has a commiserating view of mental illness as a cause of offence and offers psychiatric treatment as an alternative approach than custodial sentences which are known to be of limited effectiveness but guarantee that an individual will not offend for the period of sentence. Court may sometimes dismiss psychiatric evidence, especially when established on the history obtained from the individual. Courts and juries have been observed to be more dismissive of psychiatric evidence when there evident lack of sympathy for the accused, for instance, in a notorious case, and a wish to discipline and vengeance for what the offender has done.[48]

Gender and Offending Rates

The number of men who are convicted is usually more than women in most of the societies. This excess may be attributed to the strength of males in general for repetitive violence (women tend to commit only isolated offenses of violence), opportunity at work (e.g., fraud, although this is an area where women are also increasingly being convicted), the psychology of the men as breadwinner, and women being generally more conforming in behavior. A female offender is likely to come from a more damaged background with more psychological and behavioral disturbance than a male offender who has committed the same offense. Hence, women in prison are more likely to be behaviorally and psychiatrically disturbed than their male counterparts. After an offense has been committed, a mentally abnormal individual may be arrested and detained in a hospital under the civil provisions of the country's mental health act, be cautioned by police, or be charged. An individual must normally be charged within 3 days of arrest in the United Kingdom. If charged, the individual may be remanded on bail or in custody (e.g., in prison) until the court case is heard.[1]

Multifactorial Nature of Offending

It is of significance to keep in mind that no psychiatric disorder is specifically characterized by offending, when assessing an offender. An offense should be viewed as the combined result of the offender, the victim, and the situation/environment. In situations where one has psychiatric disorder other than depression, young and male have increased chances of committing an offense. Those with chronic mentally illness are more prone to commit offenses than those who are acutely ill. People whose mental illness has relapsed and who are not compliant to treatment are also have high chances to commit offenses. The motivation for crime may be the similar to those not mentally ill (e.g. as a reaction to rejection), or secondary to delusions or hallucinations, or as a consequence of a deterioration in social functioning and personality as a result of mental illness. Such individuals are more impulsive and have a lower stress tolerance (e.g. in schizophrenia or depressive disorder). People with paranoid schizophrenia may have isolated paranoid delusions about particular individuals, which may go unnoticed, and they may be functioning adequately in daily life. Hence, they may be more efficient in planning attacks and their execution compared to individuals with other types of schizophrenia. Specific body parts, such as the eyes, are more likely to be target of such patients. The victim is often a family member with whom the individual lives in close proximity. This stands true for victims of both mentally disordered people and apparently "normal" individuals. Most conflicts in such case occur within the family circle. While the role of the victim should not be overrated, the victim can accidentally provoke an attack, especially if he or she is physically or mentally ill or has been abusing alcohol or drugs. The victim may fail to appreciate the amount of stress that a potential assailant is dealing with. Battered children are more likely to be temperamentally more difficult to manage than those not subject to such abuse. Circumstances may also play an important role, e.g. in a pub, where both victim and offender are intoxicated. Mentally ill individual is also more at risk to commit offense of criminal nature against public property, and in situations where they are likely to be apprehended. The availability or absence of weapons is also play a role.

SOCIAL FACTORS IN CRIME

There are some criminology schools which explain the genesis of crime on underlying social factors. Crime is often linked with various social factors such as urbanization, rapid economic growth, mass political upheaval, violent conflicts and inadequate or inappropriate policy. Poverty, unequal distribution of resources, rising expectations and a sense of moral outrage at some members of the society preferentially growing rich, have allegedly led to the higher and growing levels of crime.

This explanation has been politically controversial, especially through some right-wing politicians being unwilling to accept any kind of causative link between social factors and crime for the fear that it would undermine the presumption that individuals are responsible for their own crimes. However, most studies on social factors and crime found strong association between the two. Commonly identified factors include:

Economic and Health Factors
- Poverty
- Unemployment
- Chronic physical/mental illness.

Familial Factors
- Parental inadequacy (i.e. poor role-model, erratic discipline, inadequate supervision) leading to inadequate child socialization.

- Parental criminality
- Intrafamily violence
- Large family
- Child abuse and neglect.

Peer Factors
- Antisocial/delinquent peers
- Gang membership.

School Factors
- Low educational ability
- Low academic achievement
- Lack of parental involvement.

Societal Factors
- Unequal distribution of social standing, power, discrimination, deprivation
- Poor access to, or low perceived value of, education
- Prejudice, poverty
- Lack of community cohesion or leadership.

Delinquency

It is antisocial and criminal behavior in children and teenagers. It is frequently cited as a critical predictor of adult criminality. Family break-down and poor parenting are often cited as the causative factors. Despite this, parental attitude and behavior, while still predictive, are less good predictors of future delinquency than family income and deprivation.

The peak age for manifestation of crime across lifespan is 14–15 years. Such crime is typically a social phenomenon, with peers, or through interaction with peers. Some adolescents commit a serious offence. Those who show signs of delinquency earliest commit most acts over the longest period.

SOCIAL FACTORS IN CRIME PREVENTION

The essential focus of all governments remains how to minimize the rate of crime during their tenure. They concentrate on tackling the social and economic problems with the hope this will lead people who might otherwise have committed crime to engage in more prosocial behavior, such as obtaining a job and paying taxes.

The governments have, therefore, directed resources towards improving public housing, increasing access to education, expanding social services, and improving local health services, among others. Though some studies have found reduction in crime with these efforts the situation is complex. The effect of public spending directed this way may be impossible to disentangle from simultaneous changes in other socioeconomic factors, such as an economic boom or bust, or increased rates of mobile phone possession amongst school-age children.

FORENSIC PSYCHIATRY AND CRIME

In the United Kingdom, men to women ratio in prison is 30 to 1, but female prisoners have higher prevalence of mental and physical disorders. Mentally abnormal offenders are usually secondary to petty and minor offenses. In fact, it is highly debatable that mentally disordered people break the law more frequently than nonmentally disordered people. Studies exploring the relationship between mental disorder and crime need to be carefully interpreted, e.g. regarding whether an offence occurred at a time before the subject's mental disorder was treated or at a time the subject was in receipt of treatment, and whether offending rates are based on official recording of offenses or are based on self-reports or third-person reports. Around 40% of routine psychiatric hospital admissions are following threatened or actual aggression, but in majority of these cases, it is not ordinarily considered profitable for these individuals to be charged with their offenses.[39]

In India too, specific populations such as prisoners stand fairly greater chances of having mental health problems. Estimates suggest that 1–3% of all offenders and up to one-third of those in Indian prison have some kind of mental abnormality.[60] Other estimates place the prevalence at even higher percentages. Most of these individuals are diagnosed with personality disorder/psychopathy or alcohol and drug-related problems. Nevertheless, learning (intellectual) disabilities and both functional and organic mental illnesses are overrepresented in prison population. Imprisonment may also act as precipitating factor in mental illness. A study of mentally ill offenders convicted of murder found that most were males (80%). About 50% of all offenders had the diagnosis of schizophrenia, 40% suffered from mood disorders and the remaining 10% were diagnosed as personality disorder.[25] Another study on insanity-related homicide reveals that out of all the mentally ill prisoners charged with murder, 47% had diagnosis of schizophrenia, while 20% had alcohol and drug-related problems. Remaining had bipolar disorder, and epilepsy and mental retardation.[9] Similar prison-based study showed high prevalence of personality disorder especially antisocial personality disorder, alcohol and substance use disorders, with low prevalence of serious mental disorders like schizophrenia. This can be attributed to nonreferral of the criminals with personality disorder for psychiatric evaluation by the prison authorities.[26]

The association between offending behavior and mental illness is of background relevance. What is crucial, in particular to the courts, is description of how, in the defendant, his disorder is likely to have led to offending—including in terms of both an apparent association in the past, in him, between given symptoms and offending within his own biography of offending and formulation of his offending.

REFERENCES

1. Eastman N, Adshead G, Fox S, et al. Forensic Psychiatry. Oxford Specialists Handbooks. London: Oxford University Press/Forensic Psychiatry Oxford University Press, 2017.

2. Anderson, Craig A, Bushman, et al. Human aggression. Annual review of Psychology. 2002;53:27-51.
3. Berkowitz L. Aggression: The causes, consequences and control. New York. McGraw-Hill, 1993.
4. Buss AH. The psychology of aggression. Hoboken NJ, John Wiley, 1961.
5. Afifi TO, Henriksen CA, Asmundson GJG, et al. Victimization and perpetration of intimate partner violence and substance use disorders in a nationally representative sample. J Nerv Ment Dis. 2012;200:684-91.
6. Snapshot between 1953 and 2006. The National Crime Records Bureau. The Times of India, 2017.
7. Crime in India. NCRB, Government of India. 2012. p. 206.
8. Drug-related crime—Factsheet, Drug Facts. Whitehousedrugpolicy.gov. Retrieved on 19.1.2018.
9. Drug Trafficking. United Nations Office on Drugs and Crime. Retrieved on 20.1.2018.
10. Dennis B, Kean L. People of the Opiate: Myanmar's Dictatorship. The Nature. 1996;263(20):11-20.
11. Hanes William Trans. The Opium War: The addiction of one empire and the corruption of another. Source Books inc.p36.
12. India Information and Technology Act 2000, Government of India Publication, New Delhi.
13. Jason F. Competition on the NADSAQ and the growth of electronic communication network. J Bank Fin. 2006;30(9).
14. Stafford J. Equity marketing and promotion analysis. Jom Wiley and Songs, 2014.
15. Embassy of India Washington. website: https://www.indianembassy.org/visited on 22.1.2018
16. Davis, James W, Parks, et al. Victims of Domestic Violence on the Trauma Service: Unrecognized and Underreported. Journal of Trauma and Acute Care Surgery. 2003;54(2):352-5.
17. Crime Statistics Agency Victoria, 2016, https://www.crimestatistics.vic.gov.au/crime-statistics/latest-crime-data/family-incidents-0">https://www.crimestatistics.vic.gov.au/crime-statistics/latest-crime-data/family-incidents-0">https://www.crimestatistics.vic.gov.au/crime-statistics/latest-crime-data/family-incidents-0, 2016.
18. Farrington DP. The Twelfth Jack Tizard Memorial Lecture: The development of offending and antisocial behaviour from childhood; key findings from the Cambridge Study in Delinquent Development. Journal of Child Psychology and Psychiatry and Allied Disciplines. 1995;36:929-64.
19. Krishnaram. Mentally ill offenders: A study of fifteen convicts of murder. Proceedings of 21st Annual Conference of Indian Psychiatric Society (SZ), Tiruchirapalli, 1988.
20. Anderson AD, Oquendo MA, Parsey RV, Milak MS, Campbell C, Mann JJ. Regional brain responses to serotonin in major depressive disorder. J Affect Disord. 2004;82:411-7.
21. Jenniing B, Thompson S. Fundamentals of media effect. New York McGraw-Hills. Humanities/social Sciences/Languages, 2001.
22. Nietzsche Beyond Good and Evil (1886). Translated by Walter Kauffman. Vintage Books, New York, 1996.
23. Libet Benjamin. Unconscious central initiative and role of conscious will in voluntary action. Behavioural and Brain Sciences. 1985;8:529-66.
24. Grigorenko EL, Sternberg RJ. The Nature Nurture Issue. In: Slater and G Brammer (Eds). An introduction to developmental psychology. Maiden MA. Blackwekk, 2014.
25. Bernstein WM. A basic Theory of Neuropsychoanalysis. Kamac Books, 2011.
26. Trinberger N. The Herring Gull's World. Collins London, 1953.
27. Bandura A. Social learning theory. Englework Cliffs NJ. Prentice Hall, 1977.
28. Autor SM. The strength of conditioned reinforcers as a function of frequency and probability of reinforcement. Harvard Univ.; Cambridge, MA: 1960. PhD thesis.
29. Freud S. In: AA Bril (Ed). The Basic Writings of Sigmund Freud. New York: Modern Library, 1938.
30. The public's view of the competence, dangerousness, and need for legal coercion of persons with mental health problems. Am J Public Health. 1999;89:1339-45.

31. A disease like any other?" A decade of change in public reactions to schizophrenia, depression, and alcohol dependence. Am J Psychiatry. 2010;167:1321-30.
32. The predictive value of risk categorization in schizophrenia. Harv Law Rev. 2011;19:25-33.
33. Perpetration of violence, violent victimization, and severe mental illness: balancing public health outcomes. Psychiatr Serv. 2008;59:153-64.
34. Applebaum PS, Robbins PC, Monahan J. Violence and delusions: Data from the MacArthur Violence Risk Assessment Study. American Journal of Psychiatry. 2000;157:566-72.
35. Somasundaram O. Guilty But Insane: Some Aspects of Psychotic Crimes. Indian J Psychiatry. 1960;805.
36. Rowlands MW. Psychiatric and legal aspects of persistent litigation. British Journal of Psychiatry. 1988;153:317-23.
37. Mullen PE. Schizophrenia and violence: From correlations to preventative strategies. Advances in Psychiatric Treatment. 2006;12:239-48.
38. Humphrey MS, Johnstone EC, MacMillan JF, et al. Dangerous behaviour preceding first admission for schizophrenia. Br J Psychiatry. 1992;161: 501-5.
39. Taylor PJ, Hodgins S. Violence and Psychosis: Critical Timings. Criminal Behavior and Mental Health. 1994;4(4):266-89.
40. Link BG, Stueve A, Phelan J. Psychotic Symptoms and Violent Behaviors, Probing the Components of "threat/control-override" Symptoms. Social Psychiatry and Psychiatric Epidemiology. 1998;33(Suppl): S55–S60.
41. Rath NM. A study of insanity related homicide. Indian J Psychiatry. 1990;32(1):69-71.
42. Dickey B, Azeni H, Weiss R, et al. Schizophrenia, substance use disorders and medical co-morbidity. J Ment Health Policy Econ. 2000;3:27-33.
43. Kavanagh DJ, McGrath J, Saunders JB, et al. Substance misuse in patients with schizophrenia. Drugs. 2002;62:743-55.
44. Unk BG, Stueve A. Psychotic symptoms and the violent/Illegal behaviour of mental patients compared to community controls. In: Monahan J, Steadman HJ. Violence and Mental Disorder. Developments in Risk Assessment Chicago. IL: University of Chicago Press. 1994. pp. 137-59.
45. Swanson JN, Holzer CE, Ganju VIC, et al. Violence and psychiatric disorder in the community: Evidence from epidemiologic catchment area survey. Hospitals and Community Psychiatry. 1990;41:761-70.
46. Eastman N, Krljes S, Latham R, et al. Handbook of Forensic Psychiatric Practice in Capital Cases, 2nd Edn. The Death Penalty Project. Forensic Psychiatry Chambers. London, 2018.
47. Oliver JE. Huntington's chorea in Northampton shire. Br J Psychiatry. 1970;116:241-53.
48. Kvaraceus W. Dangerous Youth. Columbus, OH: Columbus Press, 1966.
49. Steadman HJ, Mulvey EP, Monahan J, et al. Violence by people discharged from acute psychiatric inpatient facilities and others in the same neighbourhoods. Archives of General Psychiatry. 1998;55:393-401.
50. Brockman F, Maguire M. Reducing Homicide: Summary of a Review of the Possibilities. RDS occasional paper No. 84. London: Home Office, 2003.
51. Monahan J, Steadman HJ. Violence and mental disorder: Developments in risk assessment. Chicago, IL, US: University of Chicago Press, 1994. pp.324.
52. Douglas KS, Hart SD, Webster CD, et al. HCR-20V3: Assessing Risk of Violence: User Guide. Burnaby, Canada, Simon Fraser University, Mental Health, Law, and Policy Institute, 2013.
53. Taft CT, Creech SK, Kachadourain L. Assessment and treatment of posttraumatic anger and aggression: A review. Journal of Rehabilitation Research & Development. 2012;49:777-788. doi: 10.1682/JRRD.2011.09.0156.

54. Hodgins S. Mental disorder, intellectual deficiency, and crime: Evidence from a birth cohort. Archives of General Psychiatry. 1992;49:476-83.
55. Torrey EF, Stanley J, Monahan J, et al; MacArthur Study Group. The MacArthur Violence Risk Assessment Study revisited: two views ten years after its initial publication. Psychiatr Serv. 2008;59(2):147-52.
56. Morland LA, LoveAE, Mackintosh MA. Treating anger and aggression in military populations: Research updates and clinical implications. Clinical Psychology: Science and Practice. 2012;19:305-22.
57. Srinivasan, Padma, Gary R Lee. "The Dowry System in Northern India: Women's Attitudes and Social Change". Journal of Marriage and Family. 2004;66(5):1108-17.
58. Teays, Wanda. "The Burning Bride: The Dowry Problem in India". Journal of Feminist Studies in Religion. 1991;7(2):29-52.
59. Bloch, Francis, Vijayendra R. "Terror as a Bargaining Instrument: A Case Study of Dowry Violence in Rural India". The American Economic Review. 2002; 92(4):1029-43.
60. Chadda RK, Amarjeet. Clinical profile of patients attending a prison psychiatric clinic. Indian J Psychiatry. 1998;40:2605.

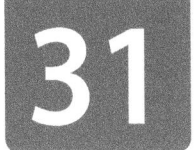

Homicide and Mental Disorders

> **LEARNING OBJECTIVES**
> - Culpable homicide
> - Mental disorders and homicide
> - Infanticide and related behaviors
> - Honor killing
> - Murder-suicide
> - Nonfatal assaults
> - Neurobiology of criminal behavior
> - Crime and violence from developmental perspective

Homicide is the killing of one human being by another. When it amounts to murder, it is conventionally regarded as the most heinous offence; and yet at the same time it can be legally sanctioned, such as in wartime or in self-defense.

CULPABLE HOMICIDE

To be culpable is to deserve blame for an act. The Indian law provides for a definition of culpable homicide. According to the Section 299 of Indian Penal Code (IPC), whosoever causes death by doing an act with the intention of causing death, or with the intention of causing such bodily injury as is likely to cause death, or with the knowledge that he is likely by such act to cause death, commits the offence of culpable homicide.[1] Culpable homicide is broadly put into two categories:
a. Act done with the intention to kill
b. *Act done with the knowledge that it would kill.*

Essential Features of Culpable Homicide
- That death of a human being was caused
- The act that resulted in death was carried out with the intention of causing death, or
- It was carried out with the intention of causing such bodily injury as is likely to cause death, or
- It was carried out with the knowledge that the act was likely to cause death.

Without one or the other of these features an act, though it may be in its nature criminal and may occasion death, will not amount to the offence of culpable homicide.

Types of Culpable Homicide
- Culpable homicide amounting to murder
- Culpable homicide not amounting to murder.

Culpable Homicides not Amounting to Murder
All murders are culpable homicides but not vice-versa. The culpable homicides not amounting to murder are:
- Due to provocation
- Right of private defense
- Public servant exceeding his power
- Sudden fight
- Consent.

Bombay High Court offered relief to a woman who had killed her minor daughter's alleged rapist—a relative. The High Court held her guilty of less grave culpable homicide not amounting to murder.

MENTAL DISORDERS AND HOMICIDE
Certain mental disorders such as schizophrenia, and other psychotic conditions are associated with an increased risk of serious assault or homicide, but personality disorders, particularly antisocial personality disorder (ASPD) and psychopathy, and substance misuse are very much greater risk factors, and a significant proportion of homicides are committed by people with no mental illness.[2]

- About 5% of the persons suffering from schizophrenia commit homicide while prevalence of schizophrenia in the general population is around 1%.
- In Europe, between 1980 and 2004 the number of homicides committed by the people with mental illness fell from 120 to 20 per year and also fell significantly as a proportion of homicide.
- In a study from Sweden, 9% of the homicide offenders had schizophrenia, 12% other psychoses, 54% a principal or secondary diagnosis of personality disorder.
- About 10% people convicted of homicide have some form of abnormal mental state at the time of committing the offence (mania, hypomania, psychotic symptoms) of which two-third have psychosis.
- About 10% of the homicides are committed by people who have had some contact with mental health services during the past one year.

Murder rates in India have declined over time. With the rate of 4.6 murders per 100,000 people in 1992, homicide rate has come down to 2.6 per 100,000 people in 2015. 32,127 persons were killed by homicide (88 persons every day) in 2015.[3] As per data from South Asia Terrorism Portal, 34,691 civilians and security men were killed in terror attacks in India from 1994 to 2016. United Nations Office on Drugs and Crime (UNODC) reveals that murder rate in India in 2012 was (3.5) almost half compared to the world average (6.2). However, there is no data on how many of those committed murder had psychiatric illness.

Victims of Homicide

Victims of homicide committed by mentally ill are more likely to be acquaintances than strangers. Mentally ill women who commit homicide are more likely to kill family members. Timely treatment for the mentally ill has been repeatedly emphasized as a way to prevent such violence. Untreated mentally ill are at a risk for higher rates of murder compared to the treated mentally ill individuals. More than 1000 homicides in US are committed by untreated severely mentally ill every year.[4] Though mentally ill are considered potential perpetrators, in truth they are also victims of such heinous violence. A new study suggests that having a mental illness increases the risk of being a victim of murder nearly five fold.[5]

INFANTICIDE AND RELATED BEHAVIORS

The intentional killing of an infant (up to 12 months of age) by its mother is conventionally regarded as separate from other homicides in many cultures, because of the effect of childbirth and stresses of early child-rearing are believed to have on the mother's mind. There is separate infanticide offence in some jurisdictions.

Infanticide and Associated Causes

- Maternal depression
- Maternal postpartum psychosis
- Maternal childhood sexual abuse.

Neonaticide is the killing of a newborn baby which may not be typically associated with a maternal mental disorder.

Filicide is the killing of a child (of any age) by a parent. One proposition for categorization of filicide is:
- Altruistic
- Psychotic
- Accidental
- Unwanted child
- Spousal revenge
- Female child.

About 50% of the women who kill their children have some kind of mental illness.

Feticide

Female feticide continues to be a major problem in India. MacPherson estimates that 100,000 abortions every year continue to be performed in India solely because the fetus is female.[6] A son is often preferred as an "asset" since he can earn and support the family, due to still-prevailing rigid gender roles in the Indian society. A daughter is considered a "liability", especially with the culture of dowry still prevailing despite its criminalization, and the prevailing social standards that frown upon women's employment and financial independence.

The Medical Termination of Pregnancy (MTP) Act of 1971[7] made abortion legal in for medical risk to mother and in rape cases. With increasing availability of sex screening technologies in India through the 1980s, and its misuse, Pre-natal Diagnostic Techniques Act (PNDT) in 1994[8] came which was further amended into the Pre-Conception and Pre-Natal Diagnostic Techniques (Regulation and Prevention of Misuse) (PCPNDT) Act in 2004[9] to deter and punish prenatal sex screening and female feticide. Initiative (locally called *Laadli scheme*), which initial data suggests may be lowering the birth sex ratio in the state.

HONOR KILLING

Honor killing is defined as the murder of a woman by her family due to the presumed loss of honor of the family resulting from her choice of a partner. Such a death is awarded to a woman of the family for marrying against the parents' wishes, having extramarital and premarital relationships, marrying within the same gotra or outside one's caste or marrying a cousin from a different caste. Honor killing is different from the dowry deaths in which case there is harassment from the in-laws and the victim commits suicide if not killed.

The historical origin of honor killings can be traced to the pre-Islamic tribal culture of Baluchistan and the Northwest frontier province. Migrating tribes from Baluchistan carried their tribal code across the border into upper Sindh and southern Punjab and Haryana where the practice of honor killing, rooted in ancient custom, continues to this day.[10] Even in their rule, the British did attempt, with only moderate success, to stop this practice of unlawful killing.[11] In fact, the banning led to an increase in the incidence of female suicides being reported from many villages across the province. British law levied a fine on the entire village where a suicide happened (as it was suspected to be killing masked as female suicide), and all of the relatives of the dead woman's family were, forcibly banished to exile in Karachi.[12] In fact, according to historical narratives and anthropological studies, the killing of women to restore male honor and maintain patriarchal structures has been taking place for centuries in lands that were the cradles of world civilizations in agrarian societies, in tribal societies, in some parts of Southern Europe as well as in countries across the Atlantic.[13]

This tradition was first viewed in its most horrible form in India during the partition of the country in between the years 1947 and 1950 when many women, most of them being victims of other forms of abuse including sexual abuse, were killed so that family honor could be preserved. The partition years was the beginning of the tradition of honor killing on a large scale.

Why Honor Killing?

Why should parents kill their daughter to preserve their family honor? The most evident reason for this practice to continue in India, is because of the caste system with its endogamous characteristics which are deeply ingrained in its social fabric. It is an assault on the dignity and honor of the entire membership of a high caste if someone, especially a woman, already at a social disadvantage compared to a man, marries someone from a lower caste. According to this belief system, if a daughter chooses someone 'unacceptable' by their standards to marry, it would bring dishonor to the family and would be a threat to their social status. This threat, in their view, is deserving of punishment by death. Sociologists believe that the reason honor killings have continued to occur is the continued rigidity of the caste system. The fear of losing their caste status through which they gain many social benefits makes them commit this heinous crime in the name of honor.

Because of the prevailing sociocultural norms, certain communities force their women into an early marriage, impose restrictions in their daily social life and in the most extreme form, forced suicide or murder. Honor killing is a ghastly custom that makes seemingly sane people kill their own daughters, to whom they have given birth and have spent many years parenting and nurturing in the name of reputation.[14] From an evolutionary standpoint, the concept of honor killing makes little sense as, from a post-Darwinist view, human beings are least likely to kill people with whom they share a genetic commonality.[15]

Theories of Honor Killing

Psychological theorists link honor killing to an extreme form of status anxiety—where there exists a fear of losing one's status and the desire to salvage it.[16] Pathological insecurity has been noted in the regions where honor killing occurs along with a constant pressure to adhere to strict social norms and rules with a fear of losing face, and being ostracized by the community. Disobeying social convention carries a risk of losing one's position in a particular social group. Just like war, honor killing stems from a sense of existential vulnerability and incompleteness and this sense of vacuum creates the need for status and saving face along with the paranoid fear of losing the same.[15]

In many cases of honor killing reported, it is triggered by a rumor, suspicion or heresay about the alleged shameful behavior. Honor killings are often planned. Usually it is the social pressure which expects to happen.[17,18] Researchers have found that the acceptability of violence was higher amongst fathers who had lower occupational status and mothers who had a lower educational status.[19] Being witness to violent acts in the past increased the acceptability of honor killings. Forced marriages of underage children under social pressure from the community often occur as a direct result of the family's beliefs of preventing honor-related stigma befalling them.[20] Refusing to stay within these restrictions, to marry a partner of their own choice, refusal to marry or escaping a forced marriage, was found to bring shame upon family.

The ambit of honor killings is not restricted to women chosing their partners. Women can be killed for a variety of behaviors, including talking to unrelated males, consensual sexual relations outside marriage, being a victim of rape, seeking a divorce, or refusing to marry the man chosen by the family members. Even suspicion of transgression may result in a killing. Women may also be assaulted physically, without an actual murder.[21] No research till date is available on the neurobiological basis or pathways that may lead to honor killing. It is definitely an area for future research.

There are psychological theories coupled with cultural and religious determinants, which explain honor killing. This explanation is intertwined with social pressure, soaked in rituals and community norms. Masculine dominance and exposure to such violence at an early age may be propelling factors towards the crime. No research on the genetic or epigenetic contributions to honor killing are available which could explain why people kill their own kids to satisfy their ego.

MURDER-SUICIDE

People charged with homicide may require assessment. Therefore, suicide by the perpetrator directly after the murder is not common but does occur, particularly in intimate relationships and in crimes that are perpetrated by men. Substance misuse and a past history of crime are of less significance than with other homicides. Depression is found more commonly in perpetrators of murder-suicide when compared to other homicides. Clinical issues, specific legal and practical issues should be taken into account.

NONFATAL ASSAULTS

Injuries sustained during the assaults include bruises, black eyes and minor cuts. Distribution of assaults in a particular society could be possibly as follows:
- Most serious violence in the community are around 2% (including homicide)
- Less serious wounding 45%
- Assault without injury 23%
- Harassment 25%
- Others 5%

In English Common Law a person is guilty of assault if he intentionally or recklessly causes other person to apprehend the application of immediate unlawful force, which include:
- Being put in fear of violence
- Psychological assault
- Stalking behavior
- Reckless or intentional application of unlawful force to the body of other person.

Consent

Assault is defined as the presence or threat of unlawful force. Force is defined as "unlawful" if there is an absence of consent; and if the force is not justified in terms of self-defense, necessary or the reasonable discipline of a child. Theoretically, it is possible for people to consent to the use of force against them; although it remains legally contentious where certain type of injury results.

It is the gaining of consent that protects doctors from charges of battery; although in practice failure to gain consent results in civil actions not criminal because of the lack of malicious intent.

NEUROBIOLOGY OF CRIMINAL BEHAVIOR

Biological explanation of criminal behavior in general and homicidal violence in particular has fascinated researchers for centuries. Recent findings in neurobiological research have renewed the interest in the field, with the hope that murderous behavior and criminal rule-breaking can be explained biologically. The current research may not be in position to explain individual crimes such as honor killing, findings of research so far give the glimpse of associations, not yet any biological explanation for something as complex as human volition.

Could violent behavior be explained directly by biology or biology could only explain psychologically defined phenotypes (i.e. psychopathology), which in turn explain behavior? Many studies purport to correlate psychological and biological descriptions.

Functional Neuroimaging Studies

Several studies have concluded that individuals with significant antisocial personality traits have dysfunction of frontal and temporal lobes. Positive emission tomography (PET) studies have demonstrated association between reduced metabolism in frontal cortex and aggression, violence and murder. Single photon emission computed tomography (SPECT) studies have shown association between reduced frontal lobe perfusion and antisocial behavior.

Abnormalities in activation of areas of frontal lobe have been found on functional magnetic resonance imaging (fMRI) scans during the processing of emotional stimuli by antisocial and psychopathic individuals, and in response inhibition tests in which the subject has to withhold his usual response to a stimulus.

Several studies have linked damage to frontal lobe (traumatic brain injury), especially damage to prefrontal cortex, to personality change and social disinhibition.

Genetic and Neuroendocrine Studies

Around 40% of variability in antisocial behavior between individuals is explained by genetic factors. This was found in meta-analysis of twin and adoption studies. There is increasing evidence that environmental and genetic factors interact with respect to antisocial behavior, some type of antisocial behavior is more heritable than other [e.g. children with callous-unemotional traits (CU)]. Genetically mediated deficiencies in monoamine oxidase type A [MAOA] activity have been associated with increased levels of violence and aggression, leading to at least one successful claim that an alleged murderer should be acquitted on the grounds of his low levels of MAOA. MAOA activity seems to mediate experiences of childhood abuse and maltreatment, such that children with high MAOA levels are less likely to display antisocial behavior.

In mice, target disruption of certain genes has been associated with aggressive behavior; many such genes have role in brain development and the function of neurotransmitter systems implicated in aggression (e.g. neuronal nitric oxide synthase and the serotonergic system). The evidence from human studies suggests that testosterone has a role in social dominance but less clear in its role in aggression.

Callous-Unemotional Traits and Psychopathy

Children with significant CU traits and adults with psychopathy are less able to recognize facial emotional expressions, especially fearful emotional expressions; and they have reduced physiological and behavioral responses to such expressions observed in others.

The deficit may be partly attentional: Children with CU traits fail to concentrate on eyes when looking at faces, and telling them to look into eyes before responding improves their accuracy.

Amygdala is known to be involved in processing emotional stimuli particularly stimuli-inducing fear and submission and adults with psychopathy show reduced amygdala activation to facial recognition stimuli compared to controls. It is also involved in stimuli reinforcement learning, and impairment in this function may explain why adults exhibiting psychopathy find it difficult to learn from punishment or other negative outcomes. Structural abnormality in main white matter tract connecting the amygdala with the orbito-frontal cortex, the uncinate fasciculus, have also been associated with psychopathy.

People with CU traits also show endocrine abnormalities, including persistently low levels of cortisol. Low cortisol and decreased cortisol response to stress, appear to be related to cold, unemotional violence, whereas serotonergic dysfunction appears to be associated with emotional, explosive violence.

CRIME AND VIOLENCE FROM DEVELOPMENTAL PERSPECTIVE

There is considerable continuity of aggression and violence across the life-span. Childhood aggression is highly predictive of future aggression and violence. Aggressive behavior in the classroom is the predictor of delinquency, and aggression in middle childhood predicts conduct problems in adolescence. Predictive relationships have been shown across different cultures.

There are two distinct trajectories in relation to antisocial behavior, the result of individual combinations of risk and resilience factors. With the adolescence limited trajectory, violence and antisocial behavior start in early adolescence, around age 15–16, and disappears almost entirely around age 21. In the lifecourse-persistent trajectory, instead of peaking around age 15, the rate of violence and antisocial behavior keeps increasing steadily until the mid-twenties, after which it declines slowly, falling to a low level only in mid-forties.

With the lifecourse-persistent group, a subgroup has callous and unemotional traits, which are linked with later emergence of psychopathology; remainder have higher levels of anxiety and lower levels of IQs and are likely to develop antisocial personality disorder (ASPD).

Offending during Adolescence

In UK, only a small percentage of children before the age of 12 get into conflict with law. The antisocial behavior rises to the peak at age 15 for the girls and age 18 for the boys. During adolescence, more than 50% boys and about 33% girls commit an offence, though they may not be prosecuted for it. These offences often include under-age sex and truancy. By the time the boys reach 21 and the girls 17, this offending behavior almost ceases. As the age progresses, there is a typing progression of offence type—during 12-13, they tend to commit criminal damage, and minor assaults, at 15-16 they commit theft and other property offences and those aged 18-21 commonly commit drug offences and vehicle theft for joy riding.[1]

Risk Factors for Persistence of Violence

A number of childhood risk factors have been identified in various longitudinal studies, which predict later violence during adolescence and adulthood. These risk factors include:
- Low intelligence
    - Poor problem-solving skills
    - Low empathy
    - Impulsivity
    - Risk taking
- Family environment
    - Parental conflict
    - Harsh and inconsistent discipline
    - Low supervision and monitoring
    - Parental criminality and unemployment
    - Large family size
- Peer factors
    - Antisocial delinquent peers
    - Gang membership
- School factors
    - Low attainment
    - Exclusion
    - Truancy
    - Lack of parental involvement
- Community factors
    - Socioeconomic deprivation
    - High crime neighborhood
    - Protective factors against persistence of crime:
        - First born
        - Small family size
        - Being an active and affectionate child
        - Resilient temperament
        - High IQ
        - Positive disposition
        - Adequate attention from parents
        - Social bonding such as healthy relations with parents, peers and children.

More the presence of risk factors during the childhood, greater are the chances of later violent offending. Socioeconomic and child-rearing factors are more important for the female children and parental characteristics are more predictive of offences in males.

The earlier the onset of offending behavior, the more likely it is that the person will commit more offences and will have a longer criminal career.

Do Mentally Ill Cause Violence?

It is highly debatable issue. Among the professionals, in 1980s, there was a dominant view that violence among mentally ill is no different than in general population and they are unnecessarily stigmatized with the blame of being more violent. They also held the view that after completion of treatment, the patients should be permitted to live freely in the community. From 1990s onwards, as a result of accumulating evidence, it became a dominant view that some patients were inherently dangerous, substantially more likely to become violent than rest of the population, and should be detained on the grounds of risk to the public even after treatment. This shift in view resulted chiefly from several high profile incidents of violence by patients and accumulation of some scientific evidence.

The Scientific Evidence

From mid-1980s onwards, evidence became to accumulate of greater than average frequency of violence among persons with mental illness. Incidence of mental illness in criminal population was studies. Offending behavior was also studied in mentally ill. These studies showed:

- Psychosis was found to be more common in prisoners implicated in a violent offence than in those prisoners incarcerated for nonviolent offences.
- About 10% patients with schizophrenia in the community reported a violent act in the previous 12 months compared to 2% in people without schizophrenia. The rate of violence was 12 times higher in alcohol dependent patients, and 16 times higher in those with drug dependence in USA and Sweden.
- Rates of arrests and self-reported violence were higher in patients than non-patients.
- Comorbid personality disorder doubled the risk of violent behavior.
- About 70% persons with psychopathy in Canada re-offended within 5 years after release from prison—three times more than the persons without psychopathy.
- Prevalence of schizophrenia in perpetrators of homicide in the UK was 5% as compared to 1% in the general population.
- UK, the population attributable risk of violence was 2% for psychosis, 20% for antisocial personality disorder, 33% for all personality disorders, 55% for alcohol dependence, and 21% for drug dependence.
- In Sweden, 9% homicide offenders had schizophrenia, 12% had other psychoses and 5% had personality disorder.

REFERENCES

1. The Indian Penal Code (Act No. XLV) 1860. Allahabad: Ram Narayan Lal, Beni Prasad, Law Publishers.

2. Eastman N, Adshead G, Fox S, et al. Forensic Psychiatry. Oxford Specialists Handbooks. London: Oxford University Press; 2017.
3. Murder rate declining in India. The Hindu, 2018.
4. Dawsom JM, Langan PA. Murder in families. UD Department of Justice, 1994.
5. Miao Szalavitz. Mental illness increases risk of being homicide victim. Time, March 7, 2013.
6. MacPherson Y. Images and icons: harnessing the power of media to reduce sex-selective abortion in India. Gender and Development. 2007;15(2):413-23.
7. Medical Termination of Pregnancy (MTP) Act, 1971. Ministry of Health and Family Welfare, Government of India Publication, New Delhi.
8. Pre-natal Diagnostic Techniques Act (PNDT), 1994. Ministry of Health and Family Welfare, Government of India Publication, New Delhi.
9. Pre-Conception and Pre-Natal Diagnostic Techniques (Regulation and Prevention of Misuse) (PCPNDT) Act in 2004. Ministry of Health and Family Welfare, Government of India Publication, New Delhi.
10. Sreenivasa Murthy HV. A History of India. Lucknow: Eastern Book Company; 1993.
11. Jasam S. Honour, Shame and Resistance. Lahore: ASR Publications; 2001.
12. Ali R. The Dark Side of Honour : Women Victims in Pakistan. Lahore: Shrikat Gah Women Resource Centre Pakistan; 2001.
13. Mogadham VM. Patriarchy and politics of gender in modern societies: Iran, Pakistan and Afghanistan. Int Sociol. 1992;7(1):35-53.
14. Feldman S. Shame and honour: the violence of gender norms under conditions of a global crisis. Wom Stud Int Forum. 2010;33(4):305-15.
15. Husseini R. Murder in the Name of Honour. Oxford: One World Publications; 2011.
16. Meetoo V, Mirza H. There is nothing honourable about honour killing : gender, violence and the limits of multiculturalism. Wom Stud Int Forum. 2007;30(3):187-200.
17. Gill A, Brah A. Interrogating cultural narratives about honour based violence. Eur J Wom Stud. 2014;21(1):79-93.
18. Thiara R, Gill A. Violence Against South Asian Women : Issues for Policy and Prevention. London: Jessica Kingsley Publishers; 2010.
19. Araji SK, Carlson J. Family violence including crimes of honour in Jordan. Viol Against Wom 2001;7(5):586-621.
20. Kulwicki AD. The practice of honour crimes : a glimpse of domestic violence in the Arab world. Iss Ment Health Nurs. 2002;23(1):77-87.
21. Rao M, Gangolli G, Gill A. Violence between female in laws in India. Int J Wom Stud. 2013;14(1):147-60.

CHAPTER 32

Medicolegal Responsibilities in Management of Victims of Domestic Violence

> **LEARNING OBJECTIVES**
> - Prevalence
> - Dynamics of violence
> - Domestic violence: Impact on health
> - Mental illness and increased vulnerability
> - Risk factors for domestic violence
> - Identification of domestic violence experienced by psychiatric patients
> - Intervention for psychiatric patients experiencing domestic violence

Domestic violence is defined as any incident of threatening behavior, violence or abuse (psychological, physical, sexual, financial or emotional) between adults who are or have been intimate partners or family members, regardless of gender or sexuality'.[1]

This definition of perpetrators of domestic violence applies to all adult family members (above 17 years old). There is no international consensus on what constitutes domestic violence. Some believe that the term is misleading because 'domestic' implies that the violence always occurs at home. Some authors use the term 'intimate partner violence', but this implies an intimacy that partners may not share. It also limits the experience of violence as being perpetrated only by the partner when other family members may be involved. The term domestic violence is used throughout this chapter, but will specify where studies refer to non-heterosexual partner violence or other family members.

Domestic violence encompasses traditional cultural practices, including forced marriage, honor crimes and female genital mutilation, in addition to partner violence. However, most research has been confined to partner violence.

There are several domestic violence laws in India. The earliest law was the Dowry Prohibition Act, 1961, which made the acts of both giving as well as receiving dowry a crime. In order to have more stringent implications of the act, two new sanctions were introduced in the Indian Penal Code: Sections 498A and Section 304B. The most recent legislation is the Protection of Women from Domestic Violence Act (PWDVA) 2005. The PWDVA, a civil law, includes all physical, emotional, sexual, verbal, and economic abuse as domestic violence.

■ PREVALENCE

According to the National Family Health Survey (NFHS) in 2005, total lifetime prevalence of domestic violence was 33.5%, and 8.5% respectively for physical and sexual violence among women aged 15-49 years.[2-5] The 2012 National Crime Records Bureau report of India states a reported crime rate of 46 per 100,000, rape rate of 2 per 100,000, dowry homicide rate of 0.7 per 100,000 and the rate of domestic cruelty by husband or his relatives as 5.9 per 100,000.[6] These reported rates are significantly smaller than the reported intimate partner domestic violence rates in many countries, such as the United States (590 per 100,000) and reported homicide (6.2 per 100,000 globally), crime and rape incidence rates per 100,000 women for most nations tracked by the United Nations.[7-9]

Domestic violence is common and it is universally seen that women are at greater risk of repeated coercive, sexual or severe physical violence.[10] For example, the British Crime Survey for England and Wales estimated that, in 2001, 89% of people who experienced four or more domestic violence assaults were women. The same survey estimated that 45% of women and 26% of men aged 16-59 years had experienced at least one episode of interpersonal violence; when financial or emotional abuse were excluded, then 21% of women and 10% of men had experienced domestic violence since the age of 16 years.[11]

Most of the prevalence studies have focused on female populations, owing to the higher risk of serious morbidity for female victims.[12] A multi-country study conducted by the World Health Organization reported that lifetime prevalence of physical or sexual partner violence, or both, varied from 15% to 71% globally, with two sites having a prevalence of less than 25%, seven between 25% and 50% and six between 50% and 75%.[13] This study also found that between 4% and 54% of respondents reported physical or sexual partner violence, or both, in the past year. In all but one setting, women were at far greater risk of physical or sexual violence by a partner than from violence by other people. Another study conducted a systematic review of 134 international studies (published between 1995 and 2006) measuring the prevalence of domestic violence among women (although they excluded pregnant women and those with disabilities). Mean lifetime prevalence rates for adulthood physical and sexual violence were found to be highest in studies conducted in healthcare settings, including psychiatric and obstetric/gynecology settings.[14]

The National Family Health Survey of India in 2006 estimated the lifetime prevalence of sexual violence among women aged 15-49 years, including instances of marital rape, which is still not recognized as a criminal offence in India. The study included in its definition of "sexual violence" all instances of a woman experiencing her husband "physically forcing her to have sexual intercourse with him even when she did not want to; and, forcing her to perform any sexual acts she did not want to".[14] The study sampled 83,703 women nationwide, and determined that 8.5% of women in the 15-49 years of age group had experienced sexual violence in their lifetime.[14] This figure includes all forms of forced sexual activity by husband on wife, during their married life, but not recognized as marital rape by Indian law.

The 2006 NFHS study reported sexual violence to be lowest against women in the 15-19 years of age group, and urban women reporting 6% lifetime prevalence rate of sexual violence, while 10% of rural women reported experiencing sexual violence in their lifetime.[14] Women with ten years of education experienced sharply less sexual violence, compared to women with less education.[15] of some 83703 women took part and of 67426 Hindu women who took part in it 22453, that is equal to 33.3% respondents said yes to being physically abused at their home, similar is the case of Buddhist women where 40% women said yes to being physically abused. The high prevalence of violence may be explained by a greater cultural acceptance of violence in the domestic setting. According to UNICEF's *Global Report Card on Adolescents 2012*, 57% of boys and 53% of girls in India think a husband is justified in hitting or beating his wife.[16]

DYNAMICS OF VIOLENCE

Patriarchal Social Structure

There are three main aspects of the patriarchal household structure in India that affect women's agency: marriage, active discrimination by abuse, and diminished economic agency and limited opportunity for independence.[17] In all these dimensions, there is a clear relationship between strong patriarchal familial structures and limited capabilities and agency for women. These limited capabilities are strongly correlated with causal factors for domestic violence in findings such as gender disparities in nutritional deprivation and a lack of women's role in reproductive decisions.[18]

Dowry System

Domestic violence often happens in India as a result of dowry demands.[19] Dowry payments are another manifestation of the prevailing patriarchy. There are strong associations between domestic violence and the practice of dowry, a cultural practice deeply rooted in many Indian communities. Dowry is a practice in which money, goods, or property the woman/woman's family brings to a marriage become the assets of the husband. This leads to unreasonable demands of money often placed on the woman's family from the husband's family, and in cases where these demands are not met, violence against the woman ensues. This practice continues even today in India although banned by law since 1961, and in recent years dowry amounts have risen dramatically.[26]

Repeated Victimization

Victims of one form of domestic violence are often also victims of other forms of domestic violence: around half of women experiencing domestic violence face more than one type of violence.[20] Findings also suggest a greater burden of repeated victimization among women: male victims experience up to 7 instances of repeated victimization, whereas female victims an average of 20 incidents.[3] Among all violent crimes, domestic violence has the highest rate of repeated victimization.[2] The psychological consequences of this repeated trauma are discussed below.

Homosexual Relationships

Less is known about gender differences in male compared with female homosexual relationships, but a US survey found that rates of emotional and physical violence experienced by urban men in homosexual relationships were substantially higher than reported among heterosexual men—34% reported psychological violence, 22% physical violence, and 5% sexual violence.[21] Studies from the USA increasingly suggest that prevalence of domestic violence may be similar across same-sex and heterosexual relationships and what makes these populations different are help-seeking behaviors. In a UK survey of 800 homosexual men and women, Hester reported similar rates of domestic abuse among men and women in same-sex relationships, with 38% men and 40% women respectively reporting experience of abuse. However, the main prevalence data on domestic violence worldwide are derived from surveys that do not identify individuals in same-sex relationships, so current knowledge on violence occurring in homosexual relationships in epidemiologically representative populations is limited.[22]

Domestic Violence: Impact on Health (Table 1)

Table 1: Impact of domestic violence

Impact on physical health	<ul><li>Gynecological problems</li><li>Sexually transmitted diseases (including HIV/AIDS),</li><li>Physical injuries</li><li>Functional symptoms such as headaches, irritable bowel syndrome</li><li>Chronic pelvic pain</li><li>Death</li></ul>	<ul><li>Post-traumatic stress disorder (PTSD)</li><li>Depression</li><li>Suicidal ideation</li><li>Substance misuse</li><li>Functional symptoms</li><li>Exacerbation of psychotic symptoms</li></ul>

A review of the impact of domestic violence on physical health is beyond the scope of this chapter but some of the most common sequelae include gynecological problems, sexually transmitted diseases (including HIV/AIDS), physical injuries and functional symptoms such as headaches, irritable bowel syndrome and chronic pelvic pain.[23] The most severe consequence of domestic violence is death; assessments done in England and Wales, are suggestive of murder of two women in a week by a partner or ex-partner, with risk highest in the months after leaving the partner.[24] Similar mortality rates have been found throughout the international literature. Worldwide, domestic violence is as serious a cause of death and incapacity among women aged 15–49 years as cancer.[2]

Domestic violence is associated with many mental health problems, including post-traumatic stress disorder (PTSD), depression, suicidal ideation, substance misuse, functional symptoms and exacerbation of psychotic symptoms.[25] Ludermir (2010) estimated the population attributable fraction (PAF) for domestic violence associated with postnatal depression to be 10% in a Brazilian population. Population attributable fractions of domestic violence for other mental disorders have not been assessed but these findings demonstrate that reducing the prevalence of domestic violence in our society could substantially reduce the burden of mental disorders and the great costs they impose upon health services.

Domestic violence is more hidden and potentially more psychologically harmful than stranger violence because of the nature of the relationship between the perpetrator and victim.

It has been shown to have deleterious psychological effects which extend beyond the incidents of abuse. Research conducted on Israeli women demonstrated that compared to women who had no experience of domestic violence, women who had such experiences had much greater rates of PTSD and other psychiatric symptomatology.[14] Several studies have indicated that psychological violence can be as detrimental to mental health as physical violence.[14] Findings also indicate that women who have multiple exposures to violence, or who experience more than one form of violence suffer a greater burden of mental illness and comorbidity.

Complex Post-traumatic Stress Disorder

The psychological effects of domestic violence can, in most cases, be conceptualized within a trauma framework, but some women, with exposure to excessive control and repeated assaults have more complex presentation and their experiences are better captures with the concept of complex post-traumatic stress disorder.[14] These women also have a greater probability of having experienced childhood abuse.

Complex post-traumatic stress disorder extends beyond the classic cluster of intrusive, avoidance and arousal symptoms to incorporate changes in victims' attitudes about self, the perpetrator, relationships and beliefs. Symptoms include those of post-traumatic stress disorder with additional disturbance in affect regulation and interpersonal relationships (see associated features of post-traumatic stress disorder in the DSM-IV, including: feelings of ineffectiveness, shame, despair or hopelessness; feeling permanently damaged; loss of previously sustained beliefs; hostility; social withdrawal; feeling constantly threatened; impaired relationships with others; or a change from the individual's previous personality characteristics).

MENTAL ILLNESS AND INCREASED VULNERABILITY

Mental health issues also predispose to exposure to domestic violence. Suffering from serious mental illness puts individuals at risk of being placed in unsafe environments, abusive relationships, and violent victimization.[15] Violence and mental illness follow a bidirectional relationship. Not only does the presence of mental illness put individuals at a greater risk of abuse, but being victims of abuse has also been found to lead to mental health issues, in both prospective studies as well as systematic reviews. Moreover, the cessation of violence has been associated with improvement of mental health problems. A systematic review[16] found that rates of depression declined over time once the abuse had ceased and that the severity or duration of violence was associated with the prevalence or severity of depression.

There is therefore evidence supporting a causal association between domestic violence and psychiatric disorders in both directions: psychiatric disorders can render a person more vulnerable to domestic violence, and domestic violence can damage mental health. A review found a history of severe domestic violence in at least 30% of psychiatric in-patients, with some studies reporting prevalence of more than 60%, suggesting that being a victim of domestic violence is likely to be more prevalent in psychiatric patients than in the general population. A study of women in contact with community mental health teams in south London found that

60% had experienced domestic violence from partners (about 27% during pregnancy).[17] It is not clear to what extent there are gender differences in the prevalence of domestic violence in patients with severe mental illness, but severe mental illnesses such as schizophrenia may increase the risk of being a victim of domestic violence for men as well as women.[15]

RISK FACTORS FOR DOMESTIC VIOLENCE
Risk Factors for Domestic Violence

Female gender	Poverty
Young women	Isolated communities
Those who are separated	Communities with high levels of violence
Pregnancy	Witnessing parental violence
Mental illness	History of childhood abuse

Domestic violence cuts across the barriers of social class, religion, ethnicity and geographical areas. There are identifiable risk factors associated with the experience of domestic violence. In addition to the gender differences described above, there is increasing evidence to show that the prevalence of domestic violence is higher among young women, those who are separated, or who have a history of childhood abuse or witnessing parental violence and poverty.[2] Research has shown that some domestic violence can start or get exacerbated during pregnancy.[18] In his report, The Confidential Enquiry into Maternal Deaths, Lewis in its chapter on maternal deaths resulting from domestic violence, reports on a case where a woman with severe mental illness and a history of serious domestic violence was not provided with an appropriate package of care, did not attend antenatal appointments and was killed by her known violent partner.[19] Migrant women are also at a greater risk of exposure to violence because of their disenfranchisement, isolation, and barriers in access to social support, legal aid, and medical services. In communities, domestic violence is more common in isolated communities and in those with high levels of violence, for example Palestinians exposed to political violence in the Israeli territories.[2]

IDENTIFICATION OF DOMESTIC VIOLENCE EXPERIENCED BY PSYCHIATRIC PATIENTS

There is evidence to suggest that women disclose domestic violence more readily to healthcare professionals than to police. According to some reports, women are assaulted an average of 35 times before they report domestic violence to the police.[20] However, qualitative research in primary and secondary care settings has found that women may not reveal exposure to domestic violence unless they are asked.[21,22] In the review of domestic violence assessment in mental health care services, it was found that it is under-detected in services globally. Only 10–30% of recent violence is asked about and disclosed in clinical practice. Similar findings have been reported for primary care settings.

A UK study found various common barriers to disclosure of domestic violence for psychiatric patients. The first among these is fear of the consequences such as involvement of the social services and consequent child protection proceedings; fear that disclosure would not be believed; and fear that disclosure would lead to further violence. Other barriers included the hidden nature of the violence, actions of the perpetrator (such as always being present when the victim is seen by health professionals) and feelings of shame. The main barriers professionals found in routine enquiry for domestic violence concerned role boundaries, competency and confidence. Enquiry and disclosure were facilitated by a supportive and trusting relationship between patient and professional, confirming similar findings in other healthcare settings.[23]

Routine Enquiry

There is some evidence that routine enquiry for domestic violence in mental health services improves reporting of such violence. However, improved detection does not necessarily translate to formulation of management plans based on issues surrounding domestic violence such as safety planning or trauma centered therapy. Some regions such as England, parts of the USA, and New Zealand have covered routine domestic violence enquiry in psychiatric settings under their mental health policies. Routine enquiry refers to 'asking all people within certain parameters about the experience of domestic violence, regardless of whether or not there are signs of abuse, or whether domestic violence is suspected'.

However, evidence is equivocal on improved health outcomes with routine enquiry for domestic violence. In fact, it can have adverse consequences, particularly if the perpetrator finds out about the partner's disclosure, as was found in an evaluation of routine enquiry in maternity services. Therefore, mental health professionals need competent and comprehensive training before routine enquiry is initiated in a healthcare setting. Additionally, pathways of care in case of positive reporting must be well established and known to provide safe and appropriate services.

In some countries, there are health authority guidelines in place for routine enquiry of domestic violence. In England, the Department of Health recommends that questions about both past and current exposure to violence and abuse should be asked during assessments and care program approach meetings. It is known that disclosure of domestic violence is more likely if specific behavior-based questions are used rather than open-ended questions about any exposure to violence. Open questions can be asked initially about relationships and normalization of the area of enquiry can also be helpful, but more specific questions about each type of abuse should also be asked. Such questions can only be asked if a patient is alone or with a professional interpreter (rather than a family member).

Introductory Open Questions

- Are you having any problems with your husband/partner?
- We know that one in four women (and one in five men) experience domestic violence at some time in their life so I ask everyone if that has ever happened to them. Has that happened to you?

- Some women have these symptoms when they are experiencing abuse. Are you afraid of anyone at home?
- Sometimes partners use physical force. Is this happening to you?
- Have you felt humiliated or emotionally abused by your partner (or ex-partner)?
- Has your partner ever physically threatened or hurt you? Or have you been kicked, hit, slapped or otherwise physically hurt by your partner (or ex-partner)?
- In the past year have you been forced to have any kind of sexual activity by your partner (or ex-partner)?

Questions about Psychological Abuse
- Does anyone insult you, call you names or swear at you?
- Does anyone make it difficult for you to see friends/family or leave the house?
- Does anyone act in a jealous way or keep track of where you go?
- Does anyone put you down, embarrass you or criticize you?
- Does anyone undermine your independence or try to make you feel small?
- Does anyone make you feel as if you have to walk on eggshells or as if you do nothing right?
- Does anyone order you around like a servant?
- Does anyone blame you for things that are not your fault?
- Does anyone control the money, make you ask for it or stop you earning?

Questions about Sexual Abuse
- Do you ever feel that you have to have sex even though you do not want to?
- Have you felt forced into sex because of what your partner might do?
- Has your partner made you have sex or carried on when it was painful?
- Has your partner made you have oral or anal sex when you did not want to?
- Has your partner used an object in a sexual way that you did not like?
- Has your partner made you do things or perform sexual acts that you did not like?
- Has your partner refused safe sex or to use birth control?
- Has your partner made you have sex with another person?
- Has your partner talked about sex or done things in a way you did not like?

Questions about Physical Abuse
- Has your partner shaken you or grabbed you roughly?
- Has your partner shoved you or made you fall?
- Has your partner slapped you or smacked you?
- Has your partner tried to hit you with something or used an object as a weapon?
- Has your partner punched you?
- Has your partner tried to choke you or put his hands round your throat?
- Has your partner pushed you against the wall or thrown you down?
- Has your partner pulled your hair?

- Has your partner burnt you or scalded you with something?
- Has your partner threatened you with a knife or gun?
- Has your partner hurt you while you were pregnant?

Although, there is limited research evidence in this area, good clinical practices must be followed, and these include making accurate notes, carrying out a risk assessment for immediate or urgent danger to the evaluee, prioritizing safety planning, avoiding victim-blaming and discussing available options.[24] Information about domestic violence services and legal aid should be given (e.g. the option of referral to a refuge for women at high risk of serious injury), but professionals need to check whether it is safe for the patient to take information home with them as there is an increased risk of violence if such information is seen by the perpetrator in the home-setting. Potential interventions are discussed below, and in general, information about pathways to care after disclosure of violence should be included in the care package.

INTERVENTIONS FOR PSYCHIATRIC PATIENTS EXPERIENCING DOMESTIC VIOLENCE

Psychological Interventions

The consequences of domestic violence on mental health have been discussed earlier. Research has shown that a wide range of individual psychological interventions benefit women with depression and PTSD, leading to improvement in depressive post-traumatic stress symptoms and improved self-esteem.[22] In particular, two trials reported that cognitive-behavioral therapy (CBT) helped women with PTSD who were no longer experiencing violence. The National Institute for Health and Clinical Excellence in the UK also recommends eye movement desensitization and reprocessing (EMDR) for post-traumatic stress disorder, but there has been little research into its efficacy for PTSD associated with domestic violence. There are also studies of group-based interventions for improving psychological outcomes in victims of domestic violence, although these have methodological limitations. It is possible that for people with complex PTSD, modified forms of therapy are needed, for example, CBT augmented by training in emotion regulation, which has been found to be more effective than stand-alone CBT in treating patients with a history of childhood abuse.[25]

These findings are applicable to women who are no longer in abusive relationships, and cannot be extrapolated to women who are continuously in abusive relationships, or those with severe psychiatric illness. Reviewers could only identify one small randomized controlled trial of trauma-focused CBT for patients with severe mental illness, and it provided some evidence of effectiveness in treatment of comorbid PTSD in women with a primary diagnosis of schizophrenia or mood disorder. However, the PTSD in this study was not specific to domestic violence. Research is also needed on the cost-effectiveness of domestic violence interventions and the effectiveness and cost-effectiveness of interventions focused on changing the behaviors of the perpetrator.

Despite the strong association between domestic violence and mental illnesses, mental health professionals often do not probe for domestic violence issues. Therefore, in some parts of the world, policies are being put in place to introduce screening or routine enquiry of domestic violence in mental health settings. The efficacy of such routine enquiry is not very well studied, but most available evidence indicates that these might help improve health outcomes. However, for these measures to be effective, healthcare professionals must have expertise in safe assessment of abuse, and if adequate referral pathways in liaison with the social and legal sector are in place. Changes in the overall care of domestic violence victims by the social and judicial system must be in place before any such policies are routinely implemented. Further research to increase the evidence base on interventions is needed, particularly with regard to interventions for people with severe mental illness.

REFERENCES

1. Home Office Violence: domestic violence. Home Office (2010). Available from http://webarchive.nationalarchives.gov.uk/20110218135832/http://rds.homeoffice.gov.uk/rds/violencewomen.html
2. Sandra Martin, Amy Tsui, Kuhu Maitra, et al. Domestic violence in Northern India. Am J Epidemiol; 1999:150.
3. Ellsberg M. Intimate partner violence and women's physical and mental health in the WHO multi-country study on women's health and domestic violence: An observational study. The Lancet. 371 (2008).
4. "Women's Empowerment in India" (PDF). National Family and Health Survey. Retrieved 2015.
5. Sexual violence and rape in India. The Lancet. 2014(383):865.
6. National Crimes Record Bureau, Crime in India 2012. Statistics Archived June 20, 2014, at the Wayback Machine. Government of India (May 2013).
7. Harrendorf S, Heiskanen M, Malby S. International Statistics on Crime and Justice. United Nations Office on Drugs & Crime (2012).
8. Intimate Partner Violence, 1993-2010, Bureau of Justice Statistics, US Department of Justice, table on page 10.
9. Global Study on Homicide 2013, United Nations Office on Drugs and Crime, page 12.
10. Howard LM, Trevillion K, Khalifeh H, et al. Domestic violence and severe psychiatric disorders. Prevalence and interventions. 2010a;40:881-93.
11. Garcia-Moreno C, Jansen HA, Ellsberg M, et al. Prevalence of intimate partner violence. Findings from the WHO multi-country study on women's health and domestic violence. Lancet. 2006;368:1260-9.
12. Alhabib S, Nur U, Jones R. Domestic violence among women: Systemic review of prevalence studies. J family viol. 2010;5:369-82.
13. Coleman K, Jansson K, Kaiza P, et al. Homicides, Firearm Offences and Intimate Violence 2005/2006. Supplementary Volume 1 to Crime in England and Wales 2005/2006. Home Office Statistical Bulletin 2007. Office for National Statistics.
14. National Family Health Survey 3. Domestic Violence. pp. 501.
15. Sinha K. 57% of boys, 53% of girls think wife beating is justified". New Delhi: The Times of India. Retrieved 25 April 2012.
16. Malhotra A, Vanneman R, Kishor S. Fertility, Dimensions of Patriarchy, and Development in India. Population and Development. Review 21 (1995). Retrieved 18 Mar 2013.
17. Kochi: Rajagiri College of Social Sciences. September 2005. Retrieved 25 April 2012.
18. Srinivasan S, Bedi A. "Domestic Violence and Dowry: Evidence from a South Indian Village." World Development 35 (2007). Retrieved 18 Mar 2013.

19. Hester M, Donovan C. Researching domestic violence in same-sex relationships. A feminist epistemological approach to survey development. J Lesb Stud. 2009;13:161-73.
20. Howard LM, Trevillion K, Agnew-Davies R. Domestic violence and mental health. International Review of Psychiatry. 2010b;22:525-34.
21. Howarth E, Stimpson L, Barran D, et al. Safety in Numbers: A Multi-site evaluation of independent domestic violence advisor services. Henry Smith Charity. 2009.
22. Jones L, Hughes M, Unterstaller U. Post-traumatic stress disorder (PTSD) in victims of domestic violence. A review of the research. Trauma, Violence and Abuse.2000;2: 99-119.
23. Khalifeh H, Dean K. Gender and violence against people with severe mental illness. Internat Rev Psychiat. 2010;22:535-46.
24. Lewis G. Saving Mothers' Lives. Reviewing Maternal Deaths to Make Motherhood Safer 2003–2005. The Seventh Report on Confidential Enquiries into Maternal Deaths in the United Kingdom. CEMACH, 2007.
25. Ludermir AB, Lewis G, Valongueiro SA. Violence against women by their intimate partner during pregnancy and postnatal depression. A prospective cohort study. Lancet. 2010;376:903-10.
26. Srinivasan P, Gary R. Lee. The Dowry System in Northern India: Women's Attitudes and Social Change. J Marriage and Family. 2004;66(5):1108-17. doi:10.1111/j.0022-2445.2004.00081.

CHAPTER 33

Medicolegal Responsibilities in Management of Homeless Persons with Mental Illness

LEARNING OBJECTIVES
- Concept of homelessness
- Magnitude of the problem
- Homelessness: Relationship with mental illness
- Problems faced by homeless populations with mental illness
- Laws concerning homeless persons with mental illness page 395
- Medicolegal approach to a case of Homeless Person with Mental Illness
- Strategies for community-based interventions for homeless with mental illness
- Psycho-social rehabilitation

CONCEPT OF HOMELESSNESS

Defining homelessness has long been a topic of debate, international agreement is elusive and most of the definitions of homelessness in use globally are as variable as definition of poverty and unemployment. Homelessness is a relative concept, which "acquires meaning only in relation of the housing conventions of a particular culture".[1]

Edgar, Doherty and Meert developed a conceptual model for European Typology of Homelessness and Housing Exclusion (ETHOS), they defined "adequate housing" as per following parameters:[2]

i. *Physical domain:* Having a decent dwelling (or space) adequate to meet the needs of the person and his/her family
ii. *Social domain:* Being able to maintain privacy and enjoy social relations and
iii. *Legal domain:* Having exclusive possession, security of occupation and legal title."

On basis of these, there can be four headings to classify homelessness or housing exclusion as per European Federation of National Organizations Working with Homeless (FEANTSA) classification proposed in 2007:[2]

i. *Roofless* (e.g. living on streets),
ii. *Houseless* (e.g. living in institutional shelters),
iii. *Insecure* (e.g. living in refugee camps, under constant threat) and
iv. *Inadequate accommodation.*

Above things can be conglomerated into two subsets (FEANTSA, 2007):[2]

Homelessness: Roofless and houseless;
Housing exclusion: Insecure and inadequate.

As per ETHOS and the New Zealand Definition of Homelessness, definition of homelessness includes following:[3,4]
i. Living in a place of habitation (during the reference period) that is below a minimum adequacy standard; and
ii. Lacking access to adequate (physical, legal and social domains) housing.

On basis of this, ETHOS suggested following model and situations for homelessness:[3,4]
i. *Homelessness:* Living in a place of habitation that is below a minimum adequacy standard (exclusion from two or more domains) AND lacking access to adequate housing
ii. *Housing exclusion:* Living in a place of habitation that is at or above a minimum adequacy standard but not fully adequate (exclusion from one domain) AND lacking access to adequate housing
iii. *Adequate housing:* Living in a place of habitation that satisfies all three domains.

Australian Society on the other hand, defined homelessness as 'not having access to safe, secure and adequate housing'. The Australian Bureau of Statistics[4] identifies following types of homelessness:
i. *Primary homelessness:* People without conventional accommodation such as those who 'sleep out', or use derelict buildings, cars, railway stations for shelter.
ii. *Secondary homelessness:* People who frequently move from temporary accommodation such as emergency accommodation, refuges, and temporary shelters. People may use boarding houses or family accommodation just on a temporary basis.
iii. *Tertiary homelessness:* People who live in rooming houses or boarding houses, medium or long-term, where they do not have their own bathroom and kitchen facilities and tenure is not secured by a lease.
iv. *Marginally housed:* People in housing situations close to the minimum standard.

In **India**, Census defines **'homeless' as a person not living in 'census houses' or build house**, person who do not possess a house, either self-owned or rented,[5,6] but instead:
i. Lives and sleeps at pavements, parks, railway stations, bus stations and places of worship, outside shops and factories, at constructions sites, under bridges and so on;
ii. Spend their nights at night shelters, transit homes, short stay homes, beggar homes and children homes;
iii. Lives in temporary structures without full walls and roof, such as under plastic sheets, or thatch roofs on pavements, parks and other common spaces.

Across several studies, opinions also differ regarding the reference period, frequency and persistence of homelessness to differentiate between short-term, long-term, chronic and repeated homelessness[7]. In most nations, measurement of homelessness is limited or non-existent, and the lack of an international, standard definition of homelessness means that there is no credible benchmark for governments to be held to.

Magnitude of the Problem

The homeless population presents special methodological challenges for collecting accurate epidemiological information leading to variability across studies in estimating prevalence of mental health, substance use, and co-occurring disorders varied.

Data from developed countries shows that 48–82% of homeless young people had a diagnosable mental illness and the most common disorders were mood disorders, anxiety disorders, such as post-traumatic stress disorder and substance use disorders in Australia.[8,9]

The story from India is also not different. Census of 2001 enumerated 1.94 million as homeless[5] and 2011 census mentioned 1.7 million as homeless persons that constituted 0.4% of Indian population.[10] Grossly it appeared as good news that there was an overall decline in the houseless population from the last Census though some accounts suggested it to be an under estimation. Between the two census years, not just the numbers changed; rather a new trend emerged of 28% decline of homelessness in rural India with 20% increase in urban homeless people.[10] Few studies were conducted in different parts of India to assess the prevalence of mental illness in such population. A study reported that of one hundred and forty homeless persons admitted in the department of psychiatry of a north Indian medical university nearly 90.7% had mental illness. Rates of comorbidity were very high, most (55.7%) had more than one psychiatric diagnosis, 44.3% had comorbid substance abuse and 38.6% had co morbid intellectual disability.[11] In another study carried out amongst inpatients of psychiatry center in Haryana, more than 60% patients met the criteria for at least one psychiatric disorder and at least 30% had serious mental illness.[12]

The high prevalence rates of mental health, substance use, and co-occurring disorders among homeless individuals across the globe highlights the need to screen for both mental health and substance use disorders and to screen routinely for the presence of a second disorder in presence of one disorder in homeless population. A broad range of treatment options should be available to meet the needs of people with co-occurring disorders.

Following are the possible reasons behind coexisting mental illness and homelessness **(Table 1)**:[13]

Table 1: Reasons behind coexisting homelessness and mental disorders.

Possible reasons behind coexisting mental illness and homelessness:	
1. Administrative and policy related factors	• Deinstitutionalization—sudden implementation without adequate preparedness of community mental health or social welfare resources resulted in increase in homelessness
2. Illness related factors	• Impaired ability to take care of self, due to illness • Disturbed interpersonal relationship due to illness • Cognitive deficits • Untreated mental illness • Predisposition to comorbid medical illnesses • Comorbid substance abuse
3. Factors related to service delivery	• Scarcity of appropriate mental health resources • Lag period in development in rehabilitative facilities
4. Social factors	• Stigma • Lack of political Will

Administrative and policy related factors
i. *Process of deinstitutionalization marked the beginning:* Prior to late 1950s most persons with mental illness resided in long-term state mental asylums not for therapeutic purpose per se, but more as a custodial setting. With the advent of effective treatment by late 1960s, deinstitutionalization gained momentum. Many persons with mental illness were released from institutions without a safety net of assured treatment, supportive services, or appropriate housing. What was thought to be as a transitional step, with sudden implementation without adequate preparedness lead to in increase in homelessness.[13]

Illness related factors
ii. *Impaired ability to take care of self due to illness:* Severe mental illness sometimes disrupts a person's ability to carry out essential aspects of daily life, such as self-care and household management. The most common reason for the patients' becoming homeless was not being treated adequately/timely. This was evident by the fact that research revealed that most patients developed clear symptoms of mental illness before becoming homeless.[14]
iii. *Disturbed interpersonal relationship due to illness:* Mental illnesses may also prevent people from forming and maintaining stable relationships or cause people to misinterpret others' guidance and react irrationally. This often results in pushing away caregivers and loosing important social support.
iv. *Cognitive deficits:* Increased confusion, memory problems, difficulty planning ahead not related to stress-induced symptom relapse but as part of illness can compound the problem further and can hamper maintaining compliance or link with caregivers or health care system.
v. *Untreated mental illness:* Serious mental illnesses rapidly deteriorate if effective treatment is not available to the patients. Less than a third of homeless people with mental health problems receive treatment.[15]
vi. *Predisposition to comorbid medical illnesses:* Mental illness may cause people to neglect taking the necessary precautions against disease and can lead to physical problems such as respiratory infections, skin diseases, or exposure to tuberculosis, sexually transmitted diseases, nutritional deficiencies, HIV or Hepatitis, which can further compound mental illness and reduces ability of client further to take care of self.[11]
vii. *Comorbid substance abuse:* Some mentally ill people self-medicate using street drugs, which can lead not only to addictions, but also to disease transmission. This combination of mental illness, substance abuse and poor physical health makes it very difficult for people to obtain employment and residential stability.[16]

Factors related to service delivery
viii. *Scarcity of appropriate mental health resources:* In low and middle income (LAMI) countries, there is a huge scarcity of resources to address the mental health needs of the population. Mental health services still continue to be urban-centered, confined to hospital-based facilities and are fragmented.[17]
ix. *Lag period in development in rehabilitative facilities:* Even with the advent of time therapeutic facilities developed well, but rehabilitative facilities, especially community

outreach services did not catch up well, especially in LAMI countries.[18] Many such persons with homelessness and mental illness are brought to health agencies for acute treatment, improves fairly but the rehabilitation back in community with good follow up care is not ensured; which brings these patients soon in similar state. The coordination between acute treatment and community care and liaison with social welfare agencies needs to be strengthened.[18]

Social factors

x. *Stigma:* The stigma attached to such illness has always been a serious issue. In developing countries, the families approach faith healers or alternative medicine often and earlier in comparison to the proper mental health settings.[19] Social isolation, stigma and a perception of being displaced from society make it difficult for this client group to canvas for better services.

xi. *Lack of political Will:* The negative social attitudes towards mental health, massive underestimation of the suffering of mentally ill people, lack of political empathy and the lack of mental health leadership increases the challenges in providing appropriate care in LAMI Countries.[18]

The mentally ill because of their affected condition are not only shunned but also receive no support or sympathy of any kind. They often face poor living condition, infection, inaccessibility to basic health services, premature death and so on. Streets have become home to many mentally ill due to lack of social support and care.[20] The difficulties of addressing combined substance misuse and mental illness (dual diagnosis) which exists in this group has long been acknowledged but not appropriately dealt with.

Problems faced by homeless persons with mental illness in conflict with law enforcement agencies

They get often arrested by police and are often suspected allegiance to and complicity with sex work, drug peddling and the petty crime of the streets. The Indian laws that criminalize the urban homeless include laws against vagrancy (such as the preventive Sections 109 and 151 in the Criminal Procedure Code,[21] begging (such as the Bombay prevention of Begging Act, 1959[22] and Tamil Nadu Prevention of Begging Act, 1945[23] and juvenile justice (The Juvenile Justice Act, 2006,[24] which provide for arrest, incarceration and custodialization for sleeping or loitering on the streets, for merely having 'no ostensible means of livelihood' or even for simply being a child 'in care of need and protection). In formal studies amongst homeless population, due to stigma, initially very few admit to arrest, but with time it is learnt that in fact many street youth had spent few years in brutalized detention centers and many had run away from these loveless facilities. The livelihoods of many homeless people like street vending and rickshaw pulling are also subject to continuous harassment and extortion by police and municipal authorities. But is still the threat of using these intensely antipoor legal provisions more than their actual deployment, which holds the homeless populations in cities the throes of habitual fear and submission to public authority.[25]

LEGAL PROVISIONS OF RELEVANCE TO HOMELESS PERSONS WITH MENTAL ILLNESS

I. **Relevant sections of Mental Health Act 1987 in regard of homeless persons with mental illness**

Section 23 of Mental Health Act 1978 empowers the police officer to take into custody wandering patients incapable of taking care of themselves and produced before a magistrate within 24 hours and then if magistrate is satisfied a reception order can be passed for admission in the mental health facility.

Limitation of this legal statute was that many of the of homeless persons ended up being in mental health establishments even in absence of mental health needs just to honor the judicial order and difficulties being faced in rehabilitation due to absence of government run facilities for homeless.

II. **Relevant sections of Mental Healthcare Act 2017 in regard of homeless persons with mental illness**

Chapter V, Section 18 regarding "Right to access mental healthcare" states that

- Every person shall have the **right to access entire range of mental healthcare and treatment** from mental health services run or funded by the appropriate government'
- **Homeless persons having mental illness** shall be entitled to mental health treatment and services free of charge at all mental health establishments run or funded or designated by the appropriate government.

Chapter V, Section 19 **regarding right to community living states that** every person with mental illness including homeless persons shall have a right to live in, be part of and not be segregated from society; and not continue to remain in a mental health establishment merely absence of community facilities

CHAPTER XIII, Section 100. **Duties of police officers in respect of homeless persons with mental illness found wandering in community.** In case of a person with mental illness who is homeless or found wandering in the community → A First Information Report of a missing person shall be lodged at the concerned police station and → The station house officer shall have a duty to trace the family of such person and inform the family about the whereabouts of the person → Police officer, i.e. investigating officer (IO) will inform the person about the reasons of taking him/her into protection and → IO will take the person within 24 hours to nearest public mental health establishment → The medical officer in-charge of the public health establishment shall be responsible for arranging the assessment of the person and the needs of the person in the particular circumstances → If on assessment it is found that person does not have a mental illness of a nature or degree requiring admission to the mental health establishment, IO should be informed about the same → It shall be duty of the IO to take the person to his/her residence, if found, else to a Government establishment for homeless persons.

MEDICOLEGAL APPROACH TO A CASE OF HOMELESS PERSON WITH MENTAL ILLNESS (HPMI)

Guidelines for management of homeless person with mental illness admitted in public mental health establishment as per MHCA 2017.
   (i) Thorough interview of accompanying person regarding following points:
      a. Complete identity of the accompanying person including address and telephone number.
      b. Place where found: exact location and nearby structures.
      c. Time since present at that place (approximately).
      d. State in which found: state of consciousness, appearance, behavior, co-operation of patient, belongings present, any material suggestive of substance use found, oral intake and hydration status.
      e. Any history of seizure, head injury.
   (ii) Complete physical examination including:
      a. Vitals: blood pressure, pulse rate, respiratory rate and temperature
      b. Detailed evaluation of scalp and overall body, record injury and scar marks.
      c. Presence of any injury marks, swelling, ulcer or any lesions over body, look for tongue bite.
      d. Complete systemic examination especially CNS including higher functions, cranial nerves, motor and sensory examination.
      e. Note the presence of signs of restraint, smell, hair and skin hygiene, dressing, passing urine or feces involuntarily or inappropriately.
   (iii) **Registering medicolegal case (MLC)** is a must through attending casualty medical officer (CMO). Verbal communication with the Police does not mean registering an MLC. All the communication in this regard should be written. Appropriate MLC form of hospital is to be filled by the resident doctor/CMO on duty, in duplicate and are to be handed over to the investigating officer on duty. The IO should inform the Police Station and return the form duly filled with the details of MLC, e.g. Belt no. of the Police personnel, etc. A copy of this is to be preserved in the patient's case file. In every MLC, detailed record of history, examination including general condition, level of consciousness, vital parameters and report of investigations should be mentioned.
   (iv) Take a photograph, take consent before, if cannot give, then after improvement.
   (v) In case of female rule out sexual assault, pregnancy and previous child birth, do a gynecology reference as routine in MLC. For suspected cases, urine pregnancy test can be done. If any signs suggestive of sexual assault, gynecology reference can be taken for needful. Medical examination for same should only proceed with consent of patient, if patient is not in a state to give consent and index of suspicion is high, it is desirable to seek permission from review board for the same.
   (vi) Go for urine substance detection test if suspecting substance abuse.
   (vii) In case of language barrier, try to find out the language patient is speaking and call a person expert in that language for thorough interview.

III. During course of admission:
   (i) Record everything that the patient reports about self no matter how irrelevant it is, provide a paper and pen constantly with patient.
   (ii) Repeatedly ask for whereabouts, home, relatives, marriage, and children. Any details given must be noted, and reconfirmed 3-4 times, till it is consistently given.
   (iii) Watch carefully the activities to evaluate level of intelligence, e.g. the way he/she takes food, buttons or unbuttons clothes, takes bath, handles objects, motor co-ordination, relates to people, communicates, language skills and vocabulary.
   (iv) Proper hygiene and care, if needed as per level of care needed by patient a trained hospital attendant to be provided for care.
   (v) Ensure protection of rights of homeless persons with mental illness at par with others.
   (vi) Medication under supervised environment.
   (vii) Prevention of sexual abuse.
   (viii) All relevant laboratory investigations to be sent routinely, decision for sending viral markers HIV, HBsAg, HAV, HCV and HEV to be individualized with consent of patient.
   (ix) Regular BP and pulse monitoring.
   (x) MRI brain if any neurological signs or patient is not responding to medication.
   (xi) Inform the review board on periodic basis about status report of patient.

IV. For rehabilitation:
   (i) Send postcard on any address patient is able to provide consistently, address validity can be confirmed on internet maps, address the post card to village head and police in-charge of the area, wait patiently for the reply. Try to establish contact with the local police station, send social worker if available, to the address.
   (ii) Plan to shift to government or nongovernment home for homeless if improved and no whereabouts traced.
   (iii) Include NGOs and social workers for address identification.
   (iv) If relatives are found and come to claim the patient then:
      a. Ask for relationship proof. Note the exact name, relation to patient, mobile or phone number and address provided along with the nearby police station. Inquire if complaint for missing was lodged; ask for a copy of it.
      b. Hand over the patient after informing the police, review board and hospital authority, keep a copy of papers given to the patient relatives along with photograph, if possible (take informed consent of patient and relatives), recognize the factors that led to patient becoming unknown and counsel the relatives accordingly, insist for follow up as per the diagnosis and management strategy and remain in contact from time to time.

SOME UNIQUE INITIATIVES FOR HOMELESS PERSONS WITH MENTAL ILLNESS

- *Mobile mental health unit (MMHU):* Homeless mentally ill, wandering on streets or homebound untreated patients is a deplorable situation, a sheer violation of right to health.

To address this problem, project Mobile Mental Health Unit (MMHU) was launched by IHBAS and Delhi State Health Mission (DSHM) under National Rural Health Mission (NRHM) in 2011. The two MMHU units are being run, each unit has a mobile van and a multidisciplinary team which plays an important role in identifying homeless/homebound persons with mental illness in the community and helping them engage in treatment with the help of Police and legal agencies.[26]

- *Mobile court facility for homeless persons with mental illness*: IHBAS has been providing services to homeless persons with mentally illness in Jama Masjid area since 2000 with NGO, Ashray Adhikar Abhiyan. In 2008, to address the issue of providing involuntary treatment in the community for the homeless with severe mental illness not in a state to give consent, with the help of Delhi State Legal Service Authority, a mobile court facility was added at Jama Masjid clinic for legal facilitation of such cases.[27]

Government and nongovernment organizations working for homeless mentally ill in India
Government - NGO - Corporate - Partnership is the ideal solution, for dealing with the homeless mentally ill. The government could provide shelter with security for the homeless. NGOs could provide services such as detection of illness, providing access to treatment, vocational therapy and finally rehabilitation with the help of corporate support. In mental hospitals NGOs could chip in with music therapy, dance therapy, Yoga, outings for patients, rehabilitation and so on which have a proven catalytic role for successful treatment. Besides, these therapies reduce staff burnout. There are many NGOs working for the people with mental illness, some of these which are working for homeless mentally are Hope Kolkata Foundation, Iswar Sankalpa in Kolkata, Banyan in Chennai, Pingla Ghar in Jalandhar, Aapno Ghar, Ashray Adhikar Abhiyan in Delhi, Ashadeep in Guwahati and Mariasadanam Charitable Trust in Kerala.[28]

STRATEGIES FOR COMMUNITY-BASED INTERVENTIONS FOR HOMELESS PERSONS WITH MENTAL ILLNESS

Community-based services for people with serious mental illnesses based on an underlying set of client-centered core values is the answer to complex problems being faced by homeless persons with mental illness. These values include a focus on treatment in the least restrictive setting; access empowerment and responsibility; diversity and flexibility; peer, family, other natural supports and the principles of mental health recovery. The mental health field has developed a well-established set of practices and services to provide community-based care to people with serious mental illnesses. To be effective, the individual service components must be coordinated in a comprehensive, integrated system of care.[20] Such a system may include case management, assertive community treatment, which may include the following components:

- Psychosocial rehabilitation services
- Community alternatives for crisis care
- Integrated services for co-occurring substance abuse and serious mental illness
- Consumer self-help, consumer-operated programs, consumer advocacy
- Family self-help and advocacy

- Housing programs
- Income, education, and employment
- *Health care integrated service systems:* Interventions providing coordinated treatment and support for homeless adults with mental illness and/or substance abuse usually result in greater improvements in health related outcomes than does usual care.

CONCLUSION

Mental health professionals should be aware about the bidirectional relationship between homelessness and mental illness and legal statutes of the country under which such persons can be offered medical help in legally and ethically correct way.

REFERENCES

1. Chamberlain C, MacKenzie D. Understanding contemporary homelessness: issues of definition and meaning. Aust J Soc Issues. 1992;27(4):274-97.
2. Amore K, Baker M, Chapman PH. The ETHOS definition and classification of homelessness: an analysis. Eur J Homelessness. 2011;5(2):19-37.
3. Statistical Standard for Occupied Dwelling Type. (2009b). Statistics New Zealand. Wellington: Statistics New Zealand.
4. Chamberlain C. Counting the Homeless: Implications for Policy Development. Australian Bureau of Statistics, Canberra, 1999.
5. Census of India Report, Homeless Population. Office of Registrar General and Census Commissioner, India, 2001.
6. The National Report on Homelessness for Supreme Court of India (2001). Supreme Court Commissioners WR196/2001.
7. Chamberlain C, Johnson G (2002). The development of prevention and early intervention services for homeless youth: intervening successfully (position paper), Melbourne, Australian Urban Housing Research Institute (AUHRI).
8. Chamberlain C, MacKenzie D. Youth homelessness. Youth Studies.2008;27:17-25.
9. Burt MR. Helping America's homeless. Washington DC: Urban Institute Press, 2001.
10. Ministry of Housing and Urban Poverty Alleviation Annual Report. Government of India, 2012-13.
11. Tripathi A, Nischal A, Dalal PK, et al. Sociodemographic and clinical profile of homeless mentally ill inpatients in a north Indian medical university. Asian J Psychiatry. 2013;6(5):404-9.
12. Gupta R, Nehra DK, Kumar V, et al. Psychiatric illnesses in homeless (runaway or throwaway) girl inmates: a preliminary study. Dysphrenia. 2013;4(1):31-5.
13. Kukreti P, Khanna A, Khanna P. Chronic Mental Illness and Homelessness. Chronic Mental Illness and Changing Scope of Intervention Strategies. IGI Global Publishers, USA, 2016.
14. Cisneros. Searching for Home: Mentally Ill Homeless People in America. Cityscape. 1997;155-72.
15. Bines W. The Health of Single Homeless People. York: Centre for Housing Policy, University of York, 1994.
16. Fischer PJ. Alcohol and drug abuse and mental health problems among homeless persons: a review of the literature, 1980-90. Rockville MD. National Institute of Alcohol Abuse and Alcoholism and National Institute of Mental Health, 1990.
17. Thirunavukarasu M. Closing the treatment gap. Indian J Psychiatry. 2011;53:199-201.
18. Saraceno B, Saxena S. A mental health resources in the world: results from Project Atlas of the WHO. World Psychiatry. 2002;1:40-4.

19. Trivedi JK, Jilani AQ. Pathway of psychiatric care. Indian J Psychiatry. 2011;53:97-8.
20. Anish KR. An evaluation of psychosocial rehabilitation facilities for homeless mentally ill in India. Arthra J Soc Sci. 2013;12(2):1-19.
21. Code of Criminal Procedure, 1973, India. Current Publications, 2015.
22. Bombay Prevention of Begging Act, 1959. Complete Act- Bare Act, India.
23. Tamil Nadu Prevention of Begging Act, 1945. Complete Act- Bare Act, India.
24. Juvenile Justice (Care and Protection of Children) Amendment Act, 2006 (Act No. 33 of 2006), Ministry of Law and Justice, India.
25. Rai A. Delhi City Report, 2008. In H Mander (Ed). Living Rough Surviving City Streets: A study of Homeless Population in Delhi, Chennai, Patna and Madurai (Vol 2). Planning Commission, New Delhi, India.
26. Annual Report, IHBAS 2010-11. Available at http:www.delhi.gov.in/wps//wcm/connect. Last accessed on 18.9.2017.
27. Treatment of Homeless People with Server Mental Illness. Joint Initiative of IHBAS, AAA and DLSA. Report of a Pilot Phase, 2008-10.
28. Thara R, Patel V. Role of non-governmental organizations in mental health in India. Indian J Psychiatry. 2010;52:S389-95.

CHAPTER 34

Clinical Legal and Ethical Issues Concerning Gender Dysphoria and Sex Reassignment Interventions

> **LEARNING OBJECTIVES**
> - Concepts
> - Gender dysphoria: evaluation strategies
> - Gender dysphoria: intervention strategies
> - Criteria for sex reassignment interventions
> - Role of mental health professional
> - Post-treatment ethical legal difficulties faced in India

NORMAL HUMAN SEXUALITY

Human sexuality encompasses the sexual knowledge, beliefs, attitudes, values and behaviors of individuals. It deals with the anatomy, physiology and the biochemistry of the sexual response system.[1] Sexuality is usually visualized as a narrow construct in terms of orientation and sexual activity, however, it is a much broader concept. It focuses on roles, identity and personality. It also reflects individual thoughts, feelings, behaviors and relationships. Healthy sexuality is a positive, dynamic and enriching part of being human. It is the sexual dimension of an individual's personality which underpins much of what a person is. It is the key to sexual health and sexual expression and also to an individual's overall health and wellbeing.[2] Sexual development starts from infancy and continues throughout lifespan. Different developmental stages shapes one's sexual attitude, identify and behavior.[3]

Definitions

Sex refers to a person's biological endowment for being categorized as male, female, or intersex. It includes sex chromosomes, gonads, internal reproductive organs and external genitalia as indicators of biological sex.[4]

Gender describes psychological recognition of self as well as wish to be regarded by others as fitting into the social categories of male or female. It refers to the attitudes, feelings and behaviors that a person associates with. It includes ones identity, sexual orientation and preferences.[5]

Stoller[6] first time defined ***Gender identity*** as a complex system of beliefs about onseself and a sense of one's masculinity or feminity. It refers to "one's sense of oneself as male, female or transgender.[5]

John Money[7] gave the concept of **Gender role** for the first time and defined it as a set of feelings, assertions and behaviors that identified a person as being a boy or a girl from the contrasting conclusions one could have reached merely by considering their anatomical sex only. It refers to socially and culturally role sanctioned to or expected from a particular gender. **Gender expression** refers to the "...way in which a person acts to communicate gender within a given culture; for example, in terms of clothing, communication patterns and interests. A person's gender expression may or may not be consistent with socially prescribed gender roles, and may or may not reflect his or her gender identity".[5]

Gender-normative behavior refers to gender specific behavior that is compatible with cultural expectations.[5]

Gender Dysphoria and Gender Nonconformity: Different Concepts[5]

Gender nonconformity refers to gender behaviors viewed as incompatible with cultural expectations. It includes variations from the norm, different influences, associations and trajectories but may not be associated with dysphoria in all cases.[5]

Gender dysphoria refers to experience of distress felt due to discordance between their internal sense of gender (their gender identity) and their physical sex (which generally matches the sex they were assigned at birth).[5]

Most people with gender nonconformity do not have Gender dysphoria. Although many people with gender dysphoria have gender nonconformity. Both frequently, but not always are associated with homosexual and bisexual orientation as well as mental health problems.[6]

Cisgender: Cis is a latin prefix meaning "on the same side". One is cisgender if one does not feel conflict with the gender assigned at birth. Cis people however, can still be gender non-confirming.[5]

LGBTQ is an acronym for Lesbian, Gay, Bisexual, Transgender, Queer. It refers to a population of people united by having gender identities or sexual orientations different from the heterosexual and cisgender majority.[5]

Coming out refers to the process in which one acknowledges and accepts one's own sexual orientation. It also encompasses the process in which one discloses one's sexual orientation to others. The term *closeted* refers to a state of secrecy or cautious privacy regarding one's sexual orientation.[5]

WHAT IS GENDER DYSPHORIA?

The term Gender Dysphoria describes a severe level of discomfort or distress an individual may experience when the gender that is assigned at birth is in conflict with the gender that they most closely associate with.[8] Expression of gender dysphoria may manifest as a strong belief that one's feelings are typical of the desired gender, as well as a need to be rid of one's sex characteristics (and acquire the sex characteristics of the desired gender) and a desire to be treated as a person of the other gender.

Gender Dysphoria in Children

Gender dysphoria is much more common in children than in adults. However, the majority of children seem to outgrow it.[6] In children, the salient disjunction of assigned gender is with gender expression in play, clothing, and peer preference and in some also with primary sex characteristics. In adolescents, the secondary sex characteristics acquire increasing salience. Gender dysphoria remaining through adolescence usually persists long-term. However, most childhood gender dysphoria has not persisted in various clinical samples (e.g. persistence rates of 1.5–37% by adolescence).[6,7] Instead, many gender dysphoric children become homosexual or bisexual but not transgender by adolescence/adulthood.

GENDER DYSPHORIA: NOSOLOGICAL CONSTRUCT

Diagnostic and Statistical Manual of Mental Disorders, Fifth edition (DSM-5) replaced the term "Gender Identity Disorder (GID)" with "Gender Dysphoria". The new criteria for adolescents and adults are as follows:[8]

- A marked incongruence between one's experienced/expressed gender and assigned gender, of at least six months duration, as manifested by at least two of the following:
  - A marked incongruence between one's experienced/expressed gender and primary and/or secondary sex characteristics (or in young adolescents, the anticipated secondary sex characteristics).
  - A strong desire to be rid of one's primary and/or secondary sex characteristics because of a marked incongruence with one's experienced/expressed gender (or in young adolescents, a desire to prevent the development of the anticipated secondary sex characteristics).
  - A strong desire for the primary and/or secondary sex characteristics of the other gender.
  - A strong desire to be of the other gender (or some alternative gender different from one's assigned gender).
  - A strong desire to be treated as the other gender (or some alternative gender different from one's assigned gender).
  - A strong conviction that one has the typical feelings and reactions of the other gender (or some alternative gender different from one's assigned gender).
- The condition is associated with clinically significant distress or impairment in social, occupational, or other important areas of functioning.[8]

IDENTIFYING GENDER DYSPHORIA: TOOLS AND STRATEGIES

Following guidelines and questionnaire can be utilized by clinicians for detection, interviewing and intervention guidelines while dealing with patients with gender dysphoria:

Standardized Questionnaires

- Gender Identity Interview for Children (GIIC) (Wallien, et al. 2009)[9]
- Gender Identity Questionnaire for Children (GIQC) (Johnson, et al., 2004)[10]

- Gender Identity/Gender Dysphoria Questionnaire for Adolescents and Adults (GIGDQAA) (Singh, et al., 2010).[11]

Guidelines
- Fenway LGBT Guide (Leibowitz, Adelson & Telingator).[12]
- WPATH SOC-7 (Coleman, et al., 2011).[13]
- AACAP LGBT Practice Parameter (Adelson, et al., 2012).[14]

Differentials
The course of GID is highly variable and plastic. Gender identity disorders are often the forerunner of a homosexual orientation. In adolescence, the main differential diagnoses are:[15]
- Intersex condition or disorders of sexual development [46, XX (masculinization of a female), 46, XY (undermasculinization of a male), ovotesticular, 46, XX testicular (XX sex reversal), and 46, XY complete gonadal dysgenesis (XY sex reversal) and most common (60-70%) congenital adrenal hyperplasia (CAH)],
- Sexual maturation disorder (ICD-10 F66.0),
- Rejected (repressed or denied) ego dystonic homosexual orientation (ICD-10 F66.1),
- Fetishistic transvestism (ICD-10 F65.1),
- Severe personality disorders, and
- Less commonly—psychotic disorders.

Before diagnosing the patient with gender dysphoric disorder, physical signs of intersex or endocrine status should also be carefully looked. Laboratory tests apart from complete physical examination might be necessary as a part of the physical work up to rule out above said disorders. Comorbid psychiatric conditions should be looked by mental health professionals as there is high rate of comorbid depressive and anxiety disorders. As they may not only increase the distress but also complicate the issue related to management.

The initial diagnosis must be made by a multidisciplinary team, where present, composed of a pediatric endocrinologist, geneticist, pediatric surgeon or urologist, and a psychiatrist. The timing of the disclosure of information to the patient is mostly adapted to the child's maturity and the social characteristics of the family.[15]

Intervention: General Principles
Support development, clarify identity, protect and promote health and well-being anticipatory guidance, screening and treatment for medical and mental illness is the mainstay of treatment. Long-term approach includes setting realistic expectations, monitor for and help manage stigma and psychosocial problems like abuse, homelessness and providing specific transgender health needs with appropriate consent.[16]

Sometimes unintentionally health professionals and teams end up hurting patient's feelings by repeated examinations and using the patient as a unique case for teaching and training purposes and forgetting the holistic care. Here are enlisted some general principles of care:[16,17]

- Provide **medical and surgical care when dealing with a complication.**
- Recognize that what is normal for one individual may not be what is normal for others; care providers should **not seek to force the patient into a social norm** (e.g. for phallic size or gender-typical behaviors) that may harm the patient.
- Minimize the potential for the patient and family to feel ashamed, stigmatized, or overly obsessed with genital appearance; avoid the use of stigmatizing terminology (like "pseudo-hermaphroditism") and medical photography; **promote openness (the opposite of shame) and positive connection with others,** avoid a "parade of white coats" and repetitive genital exams, especially those involving measurements of genitalia.
- Delay elective surgical and hormonal treatments until the **patient can actively participate in decision-making** about how his or her own body will look, feel, and function; when surgery and hormone treatments are considered, healthcare professionals must ask themselves whether they are truly needed for the benefit of the child or are being offered to allay parental distress; mental health professionals can help assess this.
- **Respect parents by addressing their concerns and distress** empathetically, honestly, and directly; if parents need mental healthcare, help them obtaining it.
- **Directly address the child's psychosocial distress** (if any) with the efforts of psychosocial professionals and peer support.
- Always **tell the truth** to the family and the child; answer questions promptly and honestly, which includes being open about the patient's medical history and about clinical uncertainty where it exists.

Apart from psychiatric and medical management, this diagnosis is almost uncomparable in the complexity of its social, ethical and political ramifications. Management sometimes requires fine balancing between the concerns of the family who wants to "cure" their patient, while on the other hand is the person battling through myriad of emotions.[18]

ROLE OF PSYCHIATRISTS

- Diagnosis of gender dysphoria
- To screen for mental health comorbidity
- Helping client realize his/her gender identity, informing about gender role expression and modes available
- Assessment of eligibility for hormonal or surgical therapies
- Making formal recommendations
- Documenting details, arranging for follow-ups and
- At all stages to continue screening for mental health comorbidity.

DIFFERENT TREATMENT STRATEGIES

Two treatment strategies are available:
- First phase involving reversible hormonal therapy followed by irreversible interventions.

- Irreversible hormonal therapy and surgery (sex reassignment surgery). A variety of surgical procedures may be directed at altering an individual's physical appearance and function to align with that of the desired gender (i.e. male to female or female to male). The permanency of surgical intervention necessitates that medical and psychological evaluations, behavioral trials, and medical treatment precede this final step.

ROLE OF MENTAL HEALTH PROFESSIONAL IN SEX REASSIGNMENT INTERVENTIONS

Sex reassignment intervention team consists of plastic surgeon, endocrinologist, psychiatrist and psychologist. They follow management protocols accepted internationally, WPATH (World Professional Association for Transgender Health) SOC version 7 (Standards of Care)[19] as detailed below, currently no acceptable guidelines are available for our country.

Criteria for Sex Reassignment Interventions

- Person shall be above 18 years of age
- Person shall meet criteria for the diagnosis of gender dysphoria
- Shall have the mental capacity to make fully informed decisions
- Person has demonstrated an understanding of the proposed male-to-female or female-to-male sex reassignment surgery with its attendant costs, required lengths of hospitalization, likely complications and post-surgical rehabilitation requirements of the planned surgery
- **Hormone therapy can be initiated with referral from qualified mental health professional**
- For genital surgical sex reassignment, person should have received at least 12 months of continuous hormonal sex reassignment therapy recommended by a psychiatrist and carried out by an endocrinologist (which can be simultaneous with the real-life experience), unless medically contraindicated
- **Surgical therapy** can be initiated after 1 year of continuous hormone therapy, and for genital surgery, **two referral letters from independent qualified mental health professionals** documented as written expert opinion is needed.
- Those with mental health issues should receive adequate treatment prior to surgery.
- No statute on minimum time spent in desired gender role to initiate reassignment in current guidelines. Earlier guidelines needed person to have successfully lived and worked within the desired gender role full-time for at least 12 months (so-called real-life experience), without periods of returning to the original gender
- Psychiatrists should be aware of potential psychological effects with use of hormone supplementation
- Psychotherapy (not an absolute requirement for hormonal and surgical treatments) unless the psychiatrist initial assessment leads to a recommendation for psychotherapy that specifies the goals of treatment, estimates its frequency and duration throughout the real-life experience (usually a minimum of 3 months).

COMPONENTS OF PSYCHIATRY EVALUATION

Psychiatrists working with gender identity disorders should have a degree recognized by the Medical Council of India and it is desirable to have special training in handling gender dysphoria cases.

A psychiatrist shall assess patients and has the following responsibilities:
- To accurately diagnose gender dysphoria
- To accurately diagnose any co-morbid psychiatric conditions and to ensure their appropriate treatment. Depressive disorder, anxiety disorder, adjustment disorder, substance use disorder and suicides must be screened for in persons with gender dysphoria
- To counsel the individual about the range of treatment options and their implications
- To engage in psychotherapy if needed
- To ascertain eligibility and readiness for hormone and surgical therapy
- To make formal recommendations to the endocrinologist and surgeons
- To document all relevant findings and recommend or reject the process, giving reasons
- To educate family, employers and institutions about gender identity disorders
- To be available for follow-up as prescribed.

Content of certification

To .... (referee physician/surgeon). Mr/Ms .... Age ....Gender .... Sex .... examined on .... (Date). On basis of history and examination, has been diagnosed as having gender dysphoria (and .... if comorbid psychiatric condition). Patient has completed treatment for .... (comorbid psychiatric condition) for .... duration/or is currently under treatment since .... duration and is currently stable. Client has capacity to give consent for .... (name of surgical procedure). Currently, from psychiatry point of view, patient is fit to undergo .... surgery (as requested).

Either two separate letters or one letter with two signatures is acceptable. One is from the treating psychiatrist. The other can be from a psychiatrist who does a document review of the process and does one final patient assessment and thereafter signs the form. If one of the psychiatric opinions is conflicting, then the patient shall be referred to a third psychiatrist and the majority decision shall prevail.

POST-TREATMENT ETHICAL LEGAL DIFFICULTIES FACED IN INDIA

In India, persons with gender dysphoria are often an outcast, as there are no specific guidelines for management and there is lot of ambiguity in law about their status. In 2009, Delhi High Court allowed plea of gay rights activists and legalised sexual activity among consenting adults of same sex, which was upheld by Supreme Court in 2013 raising new ethical and legal debates. In India, still no state except Tamil Nadu has legal statutory provisions in place for changing transgender people's birth name and sex in the official gazette and official identity documents either after realizing their gender identity or sex reassignment.[20] However, a recent landmark judgment by Supreme Court in April 2014 has identified transgender as the third gender and has ordered government to make suitable changes in law has set in some hopes. In 2017, Supreme

Court passes landmark ruling declaring individual privacy a guaranteed fundamental right. "Sexual orientation is an essential attribute of privacy," the court said, virtually reopening the 2013 judgment on gay rights. In January 2018, Supreme Court has referred Section 377 to a larger bench of the court, saying its 2013 judgement requires reconsideration. However, still there is a long way to go for achieving a stigma free society.[21]

The Rights of Transgender Persons Bill, 2014, was introduced as a Private Member's Bill in the Rajya Sabha by Mr. Siva. It was unanimously passed in the Upper House but was never debated in the Lok Sabha. The Union Cabinet approved the Transgender Persons (Protection of Rights) Bill 2016 for introduction in Parliament. Makes it illegal to force a transgender person to leave residence or village, force them into begging or bonded labor, or sexual assault. The highlights of bill are:[22]
- Criminalizes denying access to public place
- Guarantees OBC status to all transgenders
- Identifies transgender person the freedom to identify as any gender regardless of surgery or hormones
- Certificate of identity needs to be issued by a state level authority
- Rehab and welfare programs, information centers and sensitization programs.
- Instructs the police to provide assistance to aggrieved transgender people
- Makes sex reassignment interventions free of cost and covered under health insurance.

CONCLUSION

Psychiatrist will have to play active role in advocating the understanding about sexuality related issues across other disciplines of medicine. Instead of acting as gatekeepers in sex reassignment interventions, they should play an active role in proactive screening of clients with gender dysphoria and facilitated smooth staged transition as part of sex reassignment team in coordination with endocrinologist, urologist and plastic surgeon. Special training programs should be incorporated in mental health curriculum to sensitize mental health professionals about the same.

REFERENCES

1. Health Canada 2003. Canadian Guidelines for Sexual Health Education.www. hc- sc. gc. ca/pphb-dgspsp/publicat/cgsheldnemss/cgshe_ toc. htm.
2. Sheffield Centre for HIV & Sexual Health. Doing It Practical Strategies for Sexual Health Promotion 2003. Sheffield. www. sheffhiv. demon. co. uk.
3. DeLamater J, Friedrich WN. Human sexual development. Journal of Sex Research,2002;39(1):10-4.
4. Sense & Sexuality: A support pack for addressing the issue of sexual health with young people in youth work settings. National Youth Council of Ireland 2004.
5. Institute of Medicine (US), Committee on Lesbian, Gay, Bisexual, and Transgender Health Issues and Research Gaps and Opportunities. The Guidelines for Psychological Practice with Lesbian, Gay, and Bisexual Clients, adopted by the APA Council of Representatives, February 18-20, 2011.
6. Reynolds M, Herbenick DL, Bancroft JH. The nature of childhood sexual experiences: two studies 50 years apart. In: J Bancroft (Ed). Sexual Development in Childhood. Bloomington, IN: Indiana University Press 2003.

7. Bailey, JM, Zucker KJ. Childhood sex-typed behavior and sexual orientation: a conceptual analysis and quantitative review. Developmental Psychology.1995;31:43-55.
8. American Psychiatrist Association. Diagnostic and Statistical Manual of Mental Disorders. DSM 5. Wahington DC: APA;2014.
9. Wallien MS, Quilty LC, Steensma TD. Cross-national replication of the gender identity interview for children. J Person Assess. 2009;91:545-52.
10. Johnson LL, Bradley SJ, Birkenfeld-Adams AS. A parent-report gender identity questionnaire for children. Arch Sex Behav. 2004;33:105-16.
11. Singh D, Deogracias JJ, Johnson LL. The gender identity/gender dysphoria questionnaire for adolescents and adults: further validity evidence. J Sex Res 2010;47:49-58.
12. Leibowitz S, Adelson S, Telingator C. Gender nonconformity and gender discordance in childhood and adolescence: developmental considerations and the clinical approach. In: HJ Makadon, KH Mayer, J Potter, H Goldhammer (Eds). The Fenway Guide to Lesbian, Gay, Bisexual and Transgender Health, 2nd Edition (American College of Physicians).
13. Coleman E, Bockting W, Botzer M, et al. Standards of care for health of transexua, transgender and gender nonconforming people. World professional association for transgender health (WPATH) SOC-7 2012.
14. Adelson SL and the American Academy of Child and Adolescent Psychiatry (AACAP) Committee on Quality Issues (CQI). Walter HJ, Bukstein OG, Bellonci C, Benson RS, Chrisman A, Farchione TR, et al. Practice parameter on gay, lesbian or bisexual sexual orientation, gender-nonconformity, and gender discordance in children and adolescents. Journal of the American Academy of Child and Adolescent Psychiatry. 2012;51(9):957-74.
15. Izquierdo G, Glassberg KI. Gender assignment and gender identity in patients with ambiguous genitalia. Urology. 1993;42:232-42.
16. Stewart M. Towards a global definition of patient centred care. BMJ. 2001;322(7284):444-5. Available online at bmj.bmjjournals.com/cgi/content/full/322/7284/444.
17. American Academy of Pediatrics Committee on Bioethics. Informed consent, parental permission and assent in pediatric practice. Pediatrics. 1995;95(2):314-7. Available online at aappolicy.aappublications.org/cgi/content/abstract/pediatrics;95/2/314.
18. Kalra G. Psychiatrists role in coming out process: context and controversies post 377. Indian J Psychiatry. 2012;54:69-72.
19. Coleman E, Bockting W, Botzer M, et al. Standards of care for the health of transsexual, transgender, and gender-nonconforming people, version 7. Int J Transgenderism. 2012 Aug 1;13(4):165-232.
20. Available from http://www.undp.org/content/dam/india/docs/HIV_and _development/legal-recognition-of gender identity of transgender-people-in-in.pdf Last accessed on 20 Feb 2018.
21. http://www.bbc.com/news/world-asia-india-270131180.
22. Draft the rights of transgender person's bill 2016. Available from http: www.prsindia.org>media>draft of the rights of transgender persons bill 2016.

CHAPTER 35

Legal Responsibility of Psychiatrist in Organ Transplantation

> **LEARNING OBJECTIVES**
> - Laws and rules governing organ transplantation in India
> - Role of mental health professional in transplantation process

Transplantation medicine has emerged as a relatively new branch of modern medicine full of challenges. Donation of important solid organs like liver, heart, kidney not only saves lives but has also improved quality of life for many persons struggling with end stage organ diseases. With the advancement of technology number of transplants in the country are increasing, so, is increasing the awareness and demand in this regard, creating continued shortage or organs in need of donation.

■ LAWS AND RULES GOVERNING ORGAN TRANSPLANTATION IN INDIA

Legislation dealing with donation and transplantation of organs in our country is **Transplantation of Human Organs Act (THOA).** It was passed in 1994, amended twice in 2009 and 2011, gazette notified in 2014. Aim of the THOA is "to regulate removal, storage and transplantation of human organs for therapeutic purposes and for prevention of commercial dealings in human organs".[1] Health is a state subject in India, being, and each state makes own implementation rules for any health related law, so, highlights of central Act are being discussed below, for any variation readers can refer to individual rules of state or institute also in this regard:[1,2]

Following are the essential features of Transplantation of Human Organs Act **(THOA):**[1]
- The act mandates that organ donation has to be **for therapeutic purposes only**.
- It mandates all transplant centers to update their details periodically on government's concerned website e.g. number of transplants conducted, outcomes and cost involved.

National Human Organs and Tissues Removal and Storage Network

The act directs the central government to establish the National Human Organs and Tissues Removal and Storage Network at national and state levels. As part of this network, the government will maintain a website displaying current information about transplant activity in India and also maintain a registry of donors and recipients of transplantation to facilitate information exchange smoothly and transparently between patients, hospitals and government.[3]

Regulatory and Advisory Bodies for Licensing, Monitoring and Penalizing[1,2]

- *Appropriate Authority (AA):* Inspects and grants registration to hospitals for transplantation; regulates and enforces standards for hospitals, conducts regular inspections to ensure quality of transplant care and outcomes of donors and recipient. It may conduct investigations into complaints of breach of any provisions of the Act, has the powers of a civil court to summon any person, request documents and issue search warrants and may suspend or cancel registration of erring hospitals, and conducting investigations into complaints for breach of any provisions of the Act. A separate license is granted for each organ of transplantation which is valid for 5 years at a time and may be renewed.
- *Advisory Committee:* The advisory committee's role is to guide the government to appropriately implement the act and update the act and rules in accordance with medical progress in transplantation. The committee is chaired by the secretary to the state government and has a joint secretary representing ministry of health. Two experienced postgraduate medical experts (from different domains i.e. heart, liver, kidney, etc.), two eminent social workers, one from a women's organization, one legal expert i.e. an additional district judge are members of the advisory committee.
- *Authorization Committee (AC):* Regulates living donor transplantation by reviewing each case of transplant and ensure with reasonable certainty that the living donor is not exploited for monetary considerations and prevent commercial dealings in transplantation. Their purpose is to regulate the process of authorization to approve or reject transplants between the recipient and donors other than 'near relative'. The hospital based authorization committee consists of the medical director or medical superintendent of the hospital, two senior medical practitioners, not part of the transplant team, two members of high integrity, social standing, and credibility and secretary (Health) or nominee and Director Health Services or nominee. The state level authorization committee also consists of medical practitioner officiating as Chief Medical Officer or any other equivalent post in a main/major government hospital of the district.
- *Medical Board:* Panel of doctors responsible for brain death certification. Generally consists of a neurologist, neurosurgeon, Intensivist, anesthetist or in their absence any surgeon or physician nominated by medical administrator in-charge of the hospital.

Infrastructure, Facilities and Manpower Requirements and Processes for Institutions Involved in Transplantation

- THOA defines the facilities, infrastructure, equipment and manpower requirements for any transplant center and the process for grant of license for the same.

The Act Recognizes Two Types of Transplants and Defines Processes Associated with Each of them[1,2]

1. **Deceased donor (Cadaveric) transplant**
   - THOA recognizes brain death as a definite form of death and empowers specialists from the medical board to certify the same for the purpose of organ donation.
   - In cases of brain death, the primary medical team is required to make the family aware about the option of organ donation and request for the same.
   - The donor's own authorization, if it was done before death in presence of two witnesses, is adequate, unless the next of kin has a reason to believe that it was subsequently revoked.
   - Final authorization for organ donation after brain death may be given by the patient's next of kin. In case of minors, authorization may be given by the parents. In case of unclaimed bodies, 48 hours after death, if it still remains unclaimed, person in-charge of the hospital or person in lawful possession of the body may give authorization for organ donation. The format for obtaining consent for organ donation is outlined in the rules.
   - THOA outlines the procedure for certification of brain death and recognizes members from the medical board (medical practitioner in charge of the hospital, independent medical practitioner, a neurologist or neurosurgeon) or their alternatives, who are not members of the transplant team, are authorized to certify brain death. Brain death may be declared after two certifications by two experts each performed 6 hours apart. The format for certifying brain death is given in the rules.
   - THOA rules state the qualification and experience of transplant coordinators, doctors or technicians who are authorized to facilitate the process and surgically retrieve the organs after duly personally verifying formal brain death certification. The removal of eyes from a dead body of a donor is not governed by such an authority and can be done at other premises and does not require any licensing procedure.
   - The cost of donor management, retrieval, transportation and preservation should not be borne by the donor or their families.
   - In medico-legal cases, the process for facilitating organ donation without compromising the process for determining the cause of death, i.e. autopsy is outlined.
2. **Living donor transplantation**
   - Each living donor transplant case is permitted only after clearance by the authorization committee individually. The authorization committee reviews the documents and interviews the patient, donor and family to establish their relationship and rule out the possibility of organ trading with reasonable certainty.
   - For living donor transplantation, grandchildren, children, siblings, spouse, parents and grandparents of the patient are termed as "near relatives" and these cases may be cleared by the hospital based authorization committee. Near relatives are required to provide proof of their relationship by legal documents or genetic testing.
   - For living donors who are not "near relatives" and non-Indian nationals, approval from the state level authorization committee is required. Donors and patients are required

to appear for an interview after submission of all documents supporting the claimed relationship between the two. The Authorization Committee also evaluates the possibility of commercial transaction between the recipient by studying and probing the circumstances and reasons why the donor wishes to donate, financial status of the donor with evidence of their vocation and income for the previous three financial years, any gross disparity between the status of the two and involvement of middleman or tout. The proceedings of the interview are video recorded.
- For living donors who are not local residents of the state where transplant is planned, a "No Objection Certificate (NOC)" may be required from their local state of residence in a prescribed format. Similarly for foreign nationals, a senior Embassy official of the country of origin has to certify the relationship between the donor and the recipient.
- Donation is allowed only after detailed explanation of possible effects, complications and hazards of the operation on the donor and recipient and its long term effects.
- **Psychiatrist's clearance in such cases is deemed mandatory to certify the donor's mental condition, awareness, absence of any overt or latent psychiatric disease, and ability to give free consent.**
- Donation by an Indian citizen for transplantation of a foreign citizen is prohibited except in exceptional circumstances.
- **Living donation by** a minor (<18 years of age) or any other **person mentally or psychologically unable to give consent for the same is prohibited**.
- Swap transplantation is permitted for patients whose "near relatives" are unable to donate to their own patients because of medical reasons, but may be suitable for another patient. Two such patients can exchange their donors and both undergo a transplant.
- The Authorization Committee gives its decision in 24 hours in writing with the reason for rejecting or approving the application of the proposed donor. The decision of the Authorization Committee is displayed on the hospital notice board and website within 24 hours of the decision.

Stringent Penalties for Contravention of the Law

Stringent penalties have been defined for removal of organ without authority, initiation or negotiation for making or receiving payment for supplying human organs, falsification of documents or contravening any other provisions of the act to serve as a deterrent for such activities. The penalty for any violation may be 5–10 years of imprisonment and/or 5–20 lakh rupees fine. A medical practitioner may be penalized by cancelling their license to practice in addition to the above.

ROLE OF MENTAL HEALTH PROFESSIONAL IN TRANSPLANTATION PROCESS[4,5]

- Psychiatrist can be one of the members of authorization committee or advisory committee or medical board.

- *Dual role:* Psychiatrist plays the dual role as a transplant team member as well as assessing and serving needs of transplant patients, donors and carers. Psychiatrist should conduct detailed pre-transplant psychosocial evaluation regarding mental state, expectation and need of donors, patients and family receiving transplant. It can help in averting paid organ donations and can help better adjustment in post-transplant phase.
- *Pre-transplant psychosocial evaluation:* Patients awaiting transplantation may have high psychological distress due to end stage illness, long waiting period for transplant, lifelong medications, immunosuppressant related psychiatric problems and comorbid problem of substance use. Psychiatrists working with such individuals may have to deal with issues ranging from something as minor as anxiety about the surgical procedure to the fear of death and organ rejection. Psychiatrist should addresses such issues as risks of exacerbation or recurrence of a psychiatric illness, pharmacokinetic and pharmacodynamic considerations due to organ failure, potential drug interactions involving psychotropic and immunosuppressant medications, adequacy of support system, history of medical compliance, emotional and cognitive preparedness for transplantation, mental status findings supplemented by standardized cognitive testing and psychosocial rating instruments, and assessment of decision-making capacity for transplant. Various screening instruments such as the Transplant Evaluation Rating Scale (TERS), the Psychosocial Assessment of Candidates for Transplant (PACT), and Structured Interview for Renal Transplantation (SIRT) may be used to assist with the psychiatric evaluation.
- *Pre-transplant assessment of living donors and certification should include:*
    - Assessment of mental state: To assess for presence of psychiatric illness including substance dependence if any, higher mental function and need of treatment for same.
    - Ability to give consent
    - Understanding about transplant process, risk, benefit, consequences of living with a single or incomplete organ in future
    - Capability of weighing this information and communicating it
    - Donor's motivation and expectations
    - Consent being given free of any undue influence or coercion or commercialism
    - **It should be certified by qualified psychiatrist in Form 4 given in THOA.**
- *Pre-transplant psychosocial assessment of family:* Along with donor's assessment, it is also important to ensure that both patients and their families to have understood the process fully. Assessment of family interactions, expectations regarding outcome, concerns and relationships is desirable to understand primary support for the patient to fall back in future.
- *Post-transplant psychosocial assessment should include:*
    - Assessment of pre-existing mental illness
    - Assessment of any new mental health related issues arising due to illness or as result of medications (immunosuppressant) side effect or graft related issues
    - Treatment evaluation to look for possible drug interactions
    - Adjustment related issues after transplant following huge emotional distress during transplant process or significant lifestyle change.

Transplantation is a challenging process for patients, caregivers, and medical professionals. Currently, there are no clear guidelines regarding how to select or reject a particular donor with psychiatric illness. But, more than just presence of any mental disorder, competence based evaluation regarding transplant process should be of more concern. Holistic evaluation of patient, caregivers and donor can help achieve better outcomes.

REFERENCES

1. Transplantation of Human Organs Acts Amendment 2011. Gazette of Government of India. Ministry of Health and Family Welfare, notified on 27 March 2014. Available at: https://mohfw.gov.in/sites/default/files/THOA-Rules-2014%20%281%29.pdf. Last accessed on 07.02.18.
2. Transplantation of Human Organs and Tissues Rules 2011. Gazette of Government of India. Ministry of Health and Family Welfare, notified on 27 March 2014. Available at: https://mohfw.gov.in/sites/default/files/THOA-Amendment-2011%20%281%29.pdf. Last accessed on 07.02.18.
3. National Human Organs and Tissues Removal and Storage Network. Available at: https://mohfw.gov.in/sites/default/files/expansion%20thota.pdf. Last accessed on 07.02.18.
4. Anil Kumar BN, Mattoo SK. Organ transplant and the psychiatrist: an overview. Indian J Med Res. 2015;141(4):408-16.
5. Kalra G, Desousa A. Psychiatric aspects of organ transplantation. Int J Organ Transplant Med. 2010;2(1):9-18.

CHAPTER 36

Childhood Bullying and Forensic Psychiatry

> **LEARNING OBJECTIVES**
> - Bullying and chronic stress
> - Bullying and risk of mental illness
> - Bullying and somatic symptoms
> - Stress responses and allostatic load
> - Bullying, inflammation and metabolic dysfunction
> - Forensic aspects of bullying

Children are oft too familiar with bullies-individuals who uses intimidation to cause fear, distress, or harm to their victims. Bullying ranges from being called nasty names to being rejected or excluded from activities, and even physical aggression. Spreading rumors, have belongings snatched away, or be teased and threatened are other forms of bullying. With the advent of technology, including the internet, e-mail, and text messaging, bullying is no longer limited to the playgrounds. Bullying can have serious consequences as it is a chronic stress for the victim.

Early and chronic stress can profoundly and negatively affect neuroendocrine, inflammatory and metabolic processes via epigenetic programming to increase the risk for obesity, cardiovascular diseases, cognitive impairment and accelerated cellular aging.[1-6] Stress due to bullying harms both physical and mental health of the individual. The physiological mechanisms through which early life stress affect endocrine and inflammatory processes, also contribute to adverse physical and mental health outcomes associated with bullying.[7] Early intervention is needed to minimize long-term negative health implications.

Bullying, a form of chronic social stress is defined as a systematic abuse of power, with aggressive behavior or intentional harm-doing by peers that is carried out repeatedly.[8] Bullying can be physical (hitting, pushing), verbal (insulting), indirect and virtual (cyber-bullying).[9] Studies report that 25% children in the community suffer bullying by their peer groups and 10–14% of these children suffer from chronic victimization. Chronic peer victims suffer greater long-term psychological impact than those who experience briefer episodes of bullying.[10,11]

In an Indian study,[12] 60.4% children reported bullying. The prevalence was found to be more among boys than girls with the commonest forms being calling names and making fun of one's looks, caste background and disability. Ten percent children reported being physically abused. Only 39% parents knew that their children were being bullied. Symptoms such as headache, loose motions, fever and depression were reported more frequently in those who reported being bullied. Teachers were uninformed of the entire issue.

BULLYING AND CHRONIC STRESS

Acute stress may facilitate the body's capacity respond to the demands of the environment. The immediate reaction of "flight or fight" is activated in order to cope with the situation, and once the stress has subsided homeostasis returns. In chronic stress homeostatic mechanisms fail and the individual experiences a state of allostatic overload.[13] Chronic stress induces deleterious health consequences because of elevation of inflammatory mechanism, deficits in neurotrophic factors and metabolic adaptation that facilitate insulin desensitization and lipid storage and work together to alter stress reactivity.[14] Childhood is the periods of developmental vulnerability in which the experience of bully victimization can become biologically embedded to modify the individual's long-term health trajectory.[15]

BULLYING AND RISK OF MENTAL ILLNESS

The effect of being bullied is as severe as being maltreated during childhood.[16] Long-term studies have shown that those who bully others have behavioral, emotional and motor problems and experience family-break up during their pre-school years. Overprotective parenting behavior and adverse conditions during pregnancy increase the risk of becoming the target of bullying in children[17] possibly through the effects of stress response at the physiological and behavioral levels. Vulnerability to bullying may thus arise from risk factors inherently associated with later development of psychiatric illness. The presence of psychiatric illness during childhood is itself associated with increased incidence of bullying victimization.[18] Stress of being bullied can exacerbate the presentation of pre-existing or early presentation of psychiatric illness. In a study of 145 monozygotic twins bully victimization was found to be an environmental risk factor for psychiatric disturbances including anxiety and suicidal ideation and behavior. Another study demonstrated that being bullied had a significant environmental impact on childhood social anxiety.[19] These studies establish a clear role for exposure to bullying victimization in later development of mental illness. Retrospective and cross-sectional studies only help to identify the relationship between being bullied and psychopathology the directionality cannot be ascertained without longitudinal follow-up postvictimization studies. Retrospective and cross-sectional studies cannot determine whether individuals who developed depression or anxiety were premorbidly more sensitive to criticism and rejection, and thus were more inclined to interpret earlier interpersonal experiences as bullying victimization. Prospective follow-up studies reveal that the men who were victims of bullying during their childhood are at 18 times more risk of suicidality than the nonbullied counterparts, while female victims have nearly 27 times more risk for panic disorder.[20,21]

BULLYING AND SOMATIC SYMPTOMS

A recent meta-analysis[22] shows that bullied children and adolescents have a significantly higher risk for psychosomatic problems than nonbullied peers. Commonly reported health problems are poor subjective health status, poor appetite, sleep disturbances, headache, abdominal pain, breathing difficulties, and fatigue.[23,24] This association between bullying victimization and somatization is observed in children as early as four years old.[25] Personal resources such as self-efficacy, and social support can mitigate the impact of bullying on development of psychological and somatic complaints[26] indicating that the deleterious effects of bullying do not impact all individuals equally.[27] Peer victimization in late childhood and early adolescence impairs adaptive stress responses.[28]

STRESS RESPONSES AND ALLOSTATIC LOAD

Stress, if continued unabated, contributes to allostatic load on the brain and the body. Allostatic load provides an index of biological 'wear and tear' from cumulative exposure to stress.[29] Under chronic stress, over time, the increasing allostatic load accelerates wear and tear on the body as a result of chronic exposure to heightened neuroendocrine responses to stress. There is accumulation of health related risk factors which increase the chances of development of a disease.[30] Allostatic load is also implicated in the acceleration of psychiatric illness progression and poor treatment outcome. Last two decades of research have demonstrated how physiological stress burden and allostatic load can accelerate aging and neurodegenerative and disease processes.[31-41] The process of increasing allostatic load is one in which the body accrues damage over time, impairing its capacity to maintain and restore homeostasis in the face of future challenges. Through the process of allostatic load, the early adverse experiences like chaotic family environment, low socioeconomic status, experiences of abuse and other forms of interpersonal aggression have been associated with poor health outcomes in adolescence and childhood.[42] Inflammation and increased blood pressure during adulthood are linked with adverse stressful experiences in childhood.[43] The long-term health impact of early life stress is further mediated by the potential for early adversity to impair children's development of skill that foster resilience. Early life stresses increase the likelihood of reducing the capacity to cope with stress in future. The cumulative direct and indirect effects of early life stress work together, over time, to enhance negative impacts through increased biological vulnerability.[44]

BULLYING, INFLAMMATION AND METABOLIC DYSFUNCTION

Studies demonstrate a link between early life stress and inflammation.[43] Acute inflammatory responses are important for fighting infection and healing process and the chronic stress contributes to the development of and progression of various serious diseases including cardiovascular diseases.[45] Chronic inflammatory states are activated and maintained by environmental stressors and health risk behaviors like poor diet, lack of exercise, and sleep disturbances.[46] Childhood bullying predicts low grade systemic inflammation with increase in C-reactive protein (CRP) levels which is a marker for inflammation. The link between bullying, stress and inflammation is supported by various studies demonstrating that childhood bully victims had increased levels of CRP at mid-life. These findings are important in controlling variables such as body-mass index and psychopathology in children, and smoking, diet and exercise in adults. Central distribution of fat is found to be more prevalent in individuals who had been bullied during their childhood.[47]

FORENSIC ASPECTS OF BULLYING

Prevention

Parent can be pioneers in preventing bullying. Open communication between parents and the child is important to clarify certain assumptions of the child. Parents should explain what bullying is to their child and listen to his concerns, and answer his questions honestly. The child must be encouraged to pursue his interests. This may help him be more comfortable among his peers and help in making friends with kids who have similar interests. Child should be made aware that if he is being bullied he should take help from a trusted adult. He should be assured that confiding in an adult about the same will help prevent further bullying.

The child should not be blamed for being a victim to bullying. Parents should refrain from making assumptions that the child must have done something to provoke the bullying. It can also be an opportunity for the parents to work with the child with the intention to resolve it. Child should never be asked to ignore bullying. Parents should take assistance from the child in gathering information about the bullying. Ignore bullying only allows it to become more consequential. Adequately training the teachers is another step to tackle this problem. Bullying should always be considered as a possible causative agent for illness by treating pediatricians and appropriate interventions should be planned where needed.

Chronic peer victimization during childhood has shown significant physiological and mental health consequences. The cascading processes of the physiological stress response, including chronically elevated levels of inflammation might play an important role in development of psychopathology during the later life. Extensive research is needed to establish or refute claims of a direct cause-and-effect relationship between childhood bullying and poor long-term health outcome. The Mental Healthcare Act, 2017 fails to address cyber bullying as a contributing factor towards mental illness. Highlighting the health consequences of cyber bullying, comment on remedial measures that can be taken.

REFERENCES

1. Zhang Y, Ren J. Epigenetics and obesity cardiomyopathy: from pathophysiology to prevention and management. Pharmaco Ther, 2016.
2. Naninck EF, Hoeijmakers L, Kakava-Georgiadon N. Chronic early life stress alters developmental and adult neurogenesis and impairs cognitive function in mice. Hippocampus. 2015;25:309-28.
3. Drury SS, Shirtcliff EA, Sachet A. Growing up or growing old? Cellular aging linked with testosterone reactivity to stress in youth. Am J Med Sci. 2014;348:92-100.
4. Zhang J, Abdallah CG, Chen Y. Behavioral deficits, abnormal corticosterone, and reduced prefrontal metabolites of adolescent rats subject to early life stress. Neurosci Lett. 2013;545:132-7.
5. Morris MJ, Beilharz JE, Maniam J, et al. Why is obesity such a problem in the 21st century? The intersection of palatable food, cues and reward pathways, stress and cognition. Neurosci Biobehav Rev. 2015;15:36-45.

6. Dallman MF. Early life stress: nature and nurture. Endocrinology. 2014;155:1569-72.
7. Walker AJ, Kim Y, Price JB. Stress, inflammation and cellular vulnerability during early stages of affective disorder: biomarker strategies and opportunities for prevention and intervention. Front Psychiatry. 2014;5:34.
8. Greif JL, Furlong MJ, Morrison G. Operationally defining bullying. Arch Pediatr Adol Med. 2003;157:1134-5.
9. Biggs BK, Vernberg E, Little TD, et al. Peer victimization trajectories and their association with children's affect in late elementary school. Int J Behav Dev. 2010;34:136-46.
10. Kochenderfer-Ladd B, Wardrop JL. Chronicity and instability of children's peer victimization experiences as predictors of loneliness and social satisfaction trajectories. Child Dev. 2001;72:134-51.
11. Lereya ST, Copeland WE, Costello EJ, et al. Adult mental health consequences of peer bullying and maltreatment in childhood: two cohorts in two countries. Laqncet Psychiatry. 2015;2:524-31.
12. Ramya SG, Kulkarni ML. Bullying among school children: prevalence and association with common symptoms in childhood. Ind J Pediatr. 2011;8(3):307-10.
13. McEwen BS, Wingfield JC. What is in the name? Integrating homeostasis, allostasis and stress. Horm Behav. 2010;57:105-11.
14. McEwen. Protective and damaging effects of stress mediators. N Engl J Med. 1998;338:171-9.
15. Vaillancourt T, Hymel S, MaDaugall P. The biological underpinning of peer victimization: understanding how and why the effects of bullying can last a lifetime. Theory Pract. 2013;52:241-8.
16. Olweus D. Bullying at school. Basic facts and an effective intervention programme. Promot Educ. 1994;1:27-31.
17. Lereya ST, Wolke D. Prenatal family adversity and maternal mental health and vulnerability to peer victimization at school. J Child Psychol Psychiatry. 2013;54:644-52.
18. Mayes SD, Calhoun SI, Baweja R, et al. Maternal ratings of bullying and victimization: differences in frequency between psychiatry diagnoses in a large sample of children. Psychol Rep. 2015;116:710-22.
19. Silberg JL, Copeland W, Linker J, et al. Psychiatric outcome of bullying victimization: a study of discordant monozygotic twins. Psychol Med. 2016:1-9.
20. Copeland WE, Bulik CM, Zucker N, et al. Does childhood bullying predict eating disorder symptoms? A prospective longitudinal analysis. Int J Eating Dis. 2015;48:1141-9.
21. Copeland WE, Wolke D, Lereya ST, et al. Childhood bullying involvement predicts low grade systemic inflammation into adulthood. Proc Natl Acad Sci. 2014;111:7570-5.
22. Gini G, Pozzoli T. Association between bullying and psychosomatic problems: a meta-analysis. Pediatr. 2009;123:1059-65.
23. Sigurdson JF, Walland J, Sund AM. Is involvement in school bullying associated with general health and psychosocial adjustment outcome in adulthood? Child Abuse Negl. 2014;38:1607-17.
24. Boynton-Jarret R, Ryasn LM, Berkman LF, et al. Cumulative violence exposure and self-rated health: longitudinal study of adolescents in United States. Pediatr. 2008;122:961-70.
25. Menrath I, Prussmann M, Muller-Godeffroy E. Subjective health, school victimization, and protective factors in high-risk school sample. J Dev Behav Pediatr. 2015;36:305-12.
26. Ilola AM, Lempinen L, Huttunen J, et al. Bullying and victimization are common in four year old children and are associated with somatic symptoms and conduct and peer problems. Acta Pediatr. 2016;105:522-8.
27. Gini G, Pozzoli T, Lenzi M, et al. Bullying victimization at school and headache: a meta-analysis of observational studies. Headache. 2014;54:976-86.
28. Sansone RA, Sansone LA. Bully victims: psychological and somatic aftermaths. Psychiatry (Edgmont). 2008;5:62-4.

29. Konte SM, Koolhaas JM, Wingfield JC, et al. The Darwinian concept of stress: benefits of allostasis and costs of allostatic load and the trade-offs in health and disease. Neurosci Biobehav Rev. 2005;29:3-38.
30. McEwen BS, Stellar E. Stress and the individual. Mechanisms leading to disease. Arch Intern Med. 1993;153:2093-101.
31. Viera E, Popovic D, Rosa AR. The clinical implications of cognitive impairment and allostatic load in bipolar disorder. Eur Psychiatry. 2013;28:21-9.
32. Brietzke E, Kapczinski F, Glassi-Olievera R, et al. Insulin dysfunction and allostatic load in bipolar disorder. Expert Rev Neurother. 2011;11:1017-28.
33. Sylvia LG, Ametrano RM, Nierenberg AA. Exercise treatment for bipolar disorder: potential mechanism of action mediated through increased neurogenesis and decreased allostatic load. Psychother Psychosom. 2010;79:87-96.
34. Kapoczinski F, Vieta E, Andreazza AC. Allostatic load in bipolar disorder: implications for pathophysiology and treatment. Neurosci Biobehav Rev. 2008;32:675-92.
35. Nugent KL, Chiapelli J, Rowland LM, et al. Cumulative stress pathophysiology in schizophrenia as indexed by allostatic load. Psychoneuroendocrinology. 2015;60:120-9.
36. Misiak B, Frydecka D, Zawadzki M, et al. Refining and integrating schizophrenia pathophysiology: relevance of the allostatic load concept. Neurosci Biobehav Rev. 2014;45:183-201.
37. Lolioch M, Holyzman JN, Rago CM, et al. Neuroprogression and cognition in bipolar disorder: a systematic review of cognitive performance in euthymic patients. Vertex. 2015;26:265-75.
38. Da Costa SC, Passos IC, Lowri C, et al. Refractory bipolar disorder and neuroprogression. Prog Neuropsychopharmacol Biol Psychiatry. 2016;70:103-10.
39. Inal-Emiroglu FN, Resmi H, Karabay N. Decreased right hippocampal volume and neuroprogression markers in adolescents with bipolar disorder. Neuropsychobiology. 2015;71:140-8.
40. Stein K, Broome MR. Neuroprogression in schizophrenia: pathways and underpinning clinical staging and therapeutic corollaries. Aust NZ Psychiatry. 2015;49:183-4.
41. Budni J, Valvassori SS, Quevado J. Biological mechanisms underlying neuroprogression in bipolar disorder. Rev Bras Psiquiatr. 2013;35:1-2.
42. Felitti VJ, Anda RF, Nordenberg D. Relationship of childhood abuse and household dysfunction to many of the leading causes of death in adults. The adverse childhood experiences (ACE) study. Am J Prevent Med. 1948;14:245-58.
43. Danese A, Pariante CM, Caspi A, et al. Childhood maltreatment predicts adult inflammation in life-course study. Proc Natl Acad Sci. 2007;104:1319-24.
44. Raposa EB, Hammen CL, Brennan PA, et al. Early adversity and health outcome in young adulthood: the role of ongoing stress. Health Psychol. 2014;33:410-8.
45. Raposa EB, Bower JE, Hammen CL, et al. A developmental pathway from early life stress to inflammation: The role of negative health behavior. Psychol Sci. 2014;25:1268-75.
46. Steptoe A, Hamer M, Chida Y. The effect of acute psychological stress on circulating inflammatory factors in humans: a review and meta-analysis. Brai Behav Immun. 2009;23:887-97.
47. Takizawa R, Danese A, Maughan B, et al. Bullying victimization in childhood predicts inflammation and obesity at mid-life: a five decade birth cohort study. Psychol Med. 2015;45:2705-15.

CHAPTER 37

Forensic Psychiatry and Psychiatry Subspecialties

> **LEARNING OBJECTIVES**
> - General hospital psychiatry
> - Geriatric mental health
> - Addiction psychiatry

It is often said that all psychiatry is forensic psychiatry because impact of forensic psychiatry has all pervasive impact on the practice of clinical psychiastry. Historically, the non-medical lunatic asylums were built only for the custodial care of the lunatics who carried a criminal flavor and their admission and discharge regulated by judicial provisions. No patient could be admitted in a mental hospital (except voluntary admission) without a judicial nod. When general hospitals began to treat psychiatric patients beyond the ambit of Lunacy Acts their authority was often questioned. With the advent of improved treatment methods and introduction of community psychiatry, psychiatry was accepted as another discipline of Medicine, but the legal issues surrounding the practice of clinical psychiatry loom large even today.

GENERAL HOSPITAL PSYCHIATRY

Introduction of general hospital psychiatry units (GHPUs) across the world and India in particular during the fourth and fifth decades of twentieth century brought psychiatry under the ambit of medical discipline and with the possibility of medical treatment beyond custodial care. General hospital medical practice was not a stranger about the impact of psychological factors in medical disorders, arrival of psychiatrists in general hospitals brought the possibility of comprehensive management of the patient to the reality. 'Psychosomatic medicine, also known as consultation-liaison psychiatry, developed as a subspecialty of psychiatry that deals with the interface of medical, psychological, ethical, social, and legal issues arising in a general hospital setting'.

Mental Health Act, 1987 continued with the tradition of judicial admission without giving any cognizance to patients' rights. Though, not governed by the Mental Health Act directly, the general hospital psychiatry units worked with the same vigour ignoring patients' rights in their management. Complex nature of this area of practice, has led clinicians and ethicists to propose certain principles and models that outline the understanding, practice, and management of

these convoluted issues. In their work on bioethics, Beauchamp and Childress[1] defined four cardinal ethical principles in clinical care:
1. Nonmaleficence
2. Beneficence
3. Autonomy
4. Justice.

These principles are commonly recognized by many fields of medical practice. Lederberg[2] added depth to these principles by proposing a situational diagnostic methodology to define and address the different components of multilayered, ethically complex cases. His systematic approach to evaluating ethically important situations includes examinations of patient and family issues, such as mental illness both in the patient and key significant others, staff issues, family–staff relationships ("joint" issues), legal/institutional issues, and ethical issues. Hundert[3] has proposed a model suggesting the basic values comprising ethical dilemmas: *liberty, justice,* and *fairness,* which must be weighed for the relative importance of each value in order to take some moral action. In practice, laws in local jurisdictions and individual aspects of each clinical case can further complicate the execution of proposed ethical guidelines and principles in the treatment and management of patients in the general hospital setting. Therefore, psychosomatic medicine physicians and specialists need to be familiar with concepts related to these principles. Furthermore, practitioners must have knowledge of the laws associated with their local jurisdiction in order to make informed treatment decisions and recommendations for their patients and primary teams.

The common clinically relevant forensic and ethical questions encountered on the general hospital psychiatric service: *decision-making capacity*, which covers discussion on topics of informed consent, patient autonomy, and right to refuse treatment; and *duty to warn/ protect*, which will explore topics of patient confidentiality, safety, and criminality in the clinical setting.

Decision-making Capacity

With the introduction of Mental Healthcare Act 2017,[4] which commits to protect, promote and fulfill the rights of the persons with mental illness during the delivery of mental healthcare and services, there will be a paradigm shift in the management of the mentally ill. Capacity to make mental healthcare and treatment decision is the cardinal feature of the Act.

Consent for any treatment revolves around three cognitive pillars:
1. Provision of adequate information to patients by primary teams
2. Voluntariness
3. Decision-making capacity.

However, simply because a person has mental illness or cognitive impairment, it does not necessarily mean he lacks the capacity to make decisions. This can also be true for those who are involuntarily hospitalized in psychiatric hospitals. In the process of treatment decision making, which is likely to have tremendous impact on one's health and well-being, presence of fear, coercion, misconception, somatic disease, medications, and mental illness should always be recognized which could adversely affect judgment.

It will become necessary for the treating psychiatrists to assess decision-making capacity repeatedly and carefully during an acute care stay of the patients. It is important to know that psychiatrists are not the only physicians who can assess decision-making capacity; in fact, capacity may be assessed by any physician. Medical care providers consider the term capacity as the threshold determination for informed consent. Capacity is clinically determined, whereas *competency*, its legal equivalent, is clearly distinguished from capacity, as it requires judicial determination. However, both terms are often used interchangeably in both practice and literature.

Capacity is always presumed to be intact in a patient unless there is a specific concern indicating otherwise. There should be a compelling reason as to why a patient should indeed lack capacity to make a certain decision. If this is the case, a detailed assessment of decision-making capacity in the context of the specific task or decision in question should take place. Capacity evaluations only take place in reference to a specific decision or clinical situation, and if there are multiple decisions that need to be made, each decision requires its own capacity determination. Psychiatric evaluation for capacity is limited to medical and medically related decisions only (i.e. dispositional capacity when a patient is being discharged from the hospital), and it does not apply to decisions regarding finances, estates, and legal matters.

The legal standards for a patient's decision-making capacity may vary across jurisdictions. At most places, the following four components are taken into account[5-7]

1. The ability to communicate a choice
2. The ability to understand the risks, benefits, and alternatives to the proposed treatment
3. The ability to appreciate and apply this information to his or her medical condition;
4. The ability to reasonably manipulate this information to his choice.

When there is no urgency for the patient to make a medical decision and a patient lacks capacity to make that medical decision, a nominated representative may make the decision, often—spouse, adult children, siblings, other relatives, and even someone not related to the patient who knows the patient's values, morals, and preferences, in that order.[7] If a decision maker is not available, the mental health review board will nominate someone to make decision. This is of particular importance in situations where no nominated representative is available or the proxy has questionable cognitive ability or is suspected of ulterior motives. While fulfilling duty, the nominated representative shall consider the current/past wishes, life history, values, culture, beliefs and best interest of patient, give credence to views of patient, provide support to make treatment decision, seek information on diagnosis and treatment, access to family and home-based rehabilitation, and will be involved in discharge plan.[4]

Capacity is a point-determination in time, and consistency may need to be evaluated with repeat capacity evaluations. Because capacity can change over time, if a patient is initially determined not to have capacity, and the underlying reason for this inability to decide improves, he may regain capacity, and complex involvement of family and potentially the legal system may not be warranted. It is implicit in the psychosomatic medicine consultant's goals, to attempt to come up with safe ways of restoring capacity to their patients whenever possible. In practice, the stringency of the decision-making capacity evaluation varies directly with the seriousness of the likely consequences of the specific decision. This is referred to as the "sliding scale" approach.[8] This sliding scale is determined by the risk to benefit ratio of the treatment. A patient would thus require less capacity to make a decision about a low risk, low-benefit procedure than if he or she were deciding about a high-risk, high-benefit procedure.

A high level of complexity is often encountered in the practice of general hospital psychiatry. It is necessary to perform a thorough psychiatric evaluation despite the myriad pressures of the fast-paced environment of a busy hospital consultation, and as much as possible, minimize errors of omission. The interface between psychiatric illness and the law is one of the most complex and interesting areas of medicine. This type of work can be emotionally and intellectually challenging, and psychosomatic medicine physicians are typically the clinicians possessing the most experience to appropriately meet the complex needs at the heart of these challenges.

GERIATRIC MENTAL HEALTH

As a subspecialty field, geriatric psychiatry has made substantial contributions that address important challenges in forensic psychiatry with specific relevance to older adults in the areas of testamentary capacity and undue influence, driving safety, the guardianship and proxy decision-making at the end-of-life, elder abuse and neglect and euthanasia. An overview of these issues in reference to the forensic questions that commonly arise in geriatric health care settings, are discussed here.

Dementia is a clinical condition often seen in old age. It is the progressive loss of mental faculties leading to an inability to care for oneself. Alzheimer's disease is the most common form of dementia, followed by Lewy Body dementia, Parkinson's disease, Vascular dementia, and Fronto-temporal dementia.

There is impairment of certain cognitive processes such as memory, language, behavior or executive functions, impairing the decision-making of the individual.

Decision-making in Elderly

The prevalence of cognitive impairment is higher among older adults than any other age group. 22.2% overall prevalence of mild cognitive impairment (MCI) or cognitive impairment not dementia, is seen in general population.[9] and 13.9% elderly people over 70 years of age in the community suffer from dementia.[10] Alzheimer's disease is the most common cause of dementia with the prevalence of 3% in the people of 65–74 years age; 18.7% in 75–84; and 47.2% in those aged 85 years and older.[11] The prevalence of cognitive impairment and dementia is much higher in long-term care settings, such as old age homes. However, cognitive difficulties may occur in any age because of following reasons:
- Congenital problems
- Developmental disabilities
- Traumatic brain injury
- Stroke
- Neurodegenerative disorders

The elderly people are vulnerable to and account for most cases of neurodegenerative dementia, caused by:
- Alzheimer's disease
- Fronto-temporal lobar degeneration
- Lewy Body disease
- Parkinson disease.

These neurodegenerative diseases cause cognitive impairment with insidious onset and gradual progression. This characteristically slow decline presents unique challenges in determining the point at which a person's cognitive capacity significantly impedes independent decision-making. In clinical practice, it is required to monitor declining cognitive function and its effects on activities of daily living, including the management of finances, in order to recognize the point in time when the person requires the assistance of another person to help. In forensic practice, the gradual decline seen in many cases of dementia poses a challenge to develop thresholds for decision-making capacity, to identify those elders who are no longer able to effectively or safely function independently. Though most older adults with mild dementia can participate in medical decision-making as defined by legal standards,[12] it is important to know the older adult's ability to describe salient reasons for a specific choice, and ability to describe the implications of various choices. These are important to know because they help in determining if dementia limits the person's understanding of diagnostic and treatment information. Older adults' capacity to complete advance directives and participate in end-of-life planning is also an important subject-matter of geriatric mental health. Assessment tools have been developed for this purpose.[13] Research on dementia, particularly on the treatment of Alzheimer's disease is very much needed which often highlight ethical and legal dilemmas in decision-making capacity. Though the standards and methods for assessing the decision-making capacity of cognitively impaired older adults, specifically for the purpose of participating in dementia research have been defined.[14,15] In particular, the MacArthur Competence Assessment Tool for Clinical Research was designed to be customized to a variety of clinical trial designs,[16] and has been used to evaluate geriatric patients for Alzheimer's trials. The concept of assent has also been invoked in geriatric care and enrollment in clinical trials.[17] An elderly person lacking decision-making capacity may still communicate distress or displeasure with the treatment.[18] In such cases, the verbal or nonverbal refusal, or evidence of affective distress or behavioral resistance, is interpreted as a lack of assent, or dissent, should trump the consent given by the surrogate. Contemporaneous and retrospective determination of testamentary capacity in older adults is another area for the forensic psychiatrists to examine.[19-21] Classic case of Banks vs Goodfellow[22] established the task-specific nature of testamentary capacity versus the global mental status or cognitive functioning of the person. The criteria established in Banks vs Goodfellow include:
- Understanding the nature of a Will
- Knowledge of the nature and extent of one's assets
- Knowledge of the persons who are natural heirs or have a reasonable claim to be beneficiaries
- Understanding of the impact of the dispositive plan

- Being free of any delusions that influence the disposition of the assets
- Ability to communicate one's wishes clearly and consistently.

Of most relevance to geriatric psychiatry is the need to recognize situations in which the testator fails to meet these criteria either because of impairment in cognitive function or because of the presence of psychosis that influences and distorts decisions involved in making a Will. It is common for persons with Alzheimer's disease and other neurodegenerative disorders to have characteristic delusions of theft or infidelity. It is also common for these older adults to have delusions or visual agnosia associated with the belief that a family member or friend is an imposter. The content of such delusions is uniquely different from the content of delusional beliefs typically held by persons with conditions such as chronic schizophrenia or mood disorders with psychosis, though older adults with mood disorders commonly experience persecutory delusions.

Elder Abuse

What are an elderly person's requirements to stay protected and safe? To determine his protection requirements, who is being abused or neglected often depends upon his decision-making capacity and ability to fend for himself.[23] If he lives in a situation of abuse or neglect, it may itself influence the decisions that victim makes, including the decision to seek help or take legal action against the perpetrator. Elderly person with physical and cognitive disability may prefer to remain under the care of an abusive caregiver because he fears possible retaliation for trying to sever the relationship, or because of anxiety in the absence of a secure fallback position he require. Health care professionals should safeguard the interests of infirm elderly patients and report suspect cases of elder abuse, which are then referred to protective service agencies for older persons. In India, such facilities are lacking.

Those who are frail or have significant cognitive impairment may be particularly vulnerable to undue influence and other forms of elder abuse. Those who are disabled and dependent on others may feel obligated to submit to the expectations and demands of their caregivers, particularly in situations in which they feel vulnerable to abandonment, or do not have the financial resources to pay for the care they need. Frail older adults in such situations deserve careful clinical evaluation of both their cognitive function and the psychosocial context in which they live. It is required to determine whether or not they need to be protected from undue influence or other abuse. In conducting such evaluations, healthcare professionals must take special care to distinguish situations that require special protection of an older person from those situations in which the older person is still capable of making independent decisions, based on his own wishes and preferences. Often, in clinical practice, the situation requires careful balancing of beneficent protection versus assurance of autonomy.

Safety Risks and Vehicle Driving

When cognitive impairment poses safety risks, extends beyond the decision-making capacity to drive a vehicle, it becomes necessary to intervene. In some countries, healthcare professionals report to the concerned agencies. Even when the patient is responsible for self-reporting, the health care provider still has the moral and medical-legal responsibility for recognizing the risk and informing patients that their condition may render them unsafe to drive. Failure to do so exposes the clinician to substantial liability if the patient is subsequently found to be at fault in a motor vehicle accident.

There have been numerous attempts to develop cognitive assessment tools to assist health professionals in their prediction of driving safety[24] but virtual and actual road tests remain the most reliable tools for determining whether driving is no longer safe.[25] Given the gradual progression of most dementing illnesses, a patient may be tested and found to be safe to drive early in the course of the illness; yet there is no established metric to determine appropriate time interval for reassessment. That is because the patient may reach the point of dangerousness on the road at any time in the period before a reassessment is conducted. It has not been possible to establish a reliable time interval between neurocognitive tests or on-road assessments for determining the moment at which the patient declines to the point of dangerousness on the road. Frequent serial assessments are impractical, leaving patients vulnerable to accidents, and leaving clinicians liable if they fail to report cases of dementia in the early stages when, in fact, some patients may still be able to drive safely for a period of months or even a few years.[26]

Nursing Home Care Difficulties

Geriatric patients admitted in nursing home settings have a very high prevalence of medical-psychiatric comorbidity, often associated with cognitive impairment and decline in functional status. Epidemiological studies in US nursing homes have found the prevalence of psychiatric diagnoses between 80% and 94%.[27-31] Such nursing homes for elderly exist in India as well, though these facilities were never designed, staffed, or licensed for that purpose.[32] Nursing homes do not operate with psychiatrically trained staff nurses, nor do they have provisions typically found on acute hospital inpatient units, such as seclusion rooms or physical restraints. In fact, these nursing homes need to be less institutional and more homelike and person-centered. Even though it is now generally accepted that physical restraint use is inappropriate (except for acute emergency management), Mental Health Act, 1987, when implemented, patients' rights will be safe-guarded in a more effective manner.

DSM-V and Geriatric Psychiatry

From a practice perspective, the role of the geriatric psychiatrist as nursing home consultant includes regular discussions of goals for health and well-being, as well as clarification of risk tolerance with patients and family members or health care proxies; and assisting nursing home staff and administrators with incorporating the patients and family goals in the written plan of care. Thoughtful, guided discussions and careful documentation may reduce the risk of nursing home litigation. Forensic Implications of Evolving Criteria for the Diagnosis of Dementia The American Psychiatric Association Diagnostic and Statistical Manual of Mental Disorders, Fifth Edition[33] (DSM-V) has substituted "major neurocognitive disorder" for the DSM-IV diagnosis of "dementia," and added "mild neurocognitive disorder" as a diagnosis for patients with mild but clinically significant cognitive deficits. The DSM V furnishes operational descriptions of deficits in various cognitive domains, with emphasis that goes well beyond the DSM IV focus on impairment in memory. Of particular importance to forensic psychiatry is the evaluation of executive function in older adults with major neurocognitive disorders. Executive function is highly salient to forensic psychiatry because it includes awareness of one's situation and the ability to recognize one's needs; the ability to deliberate and choose goals; and the ability to plan, initiate and execute tasks, with adequate agency and appropriate sequencing to achieve one's goals. Thus, the change in DSM definitions for diagnosing cognitive disorders is likely to increase attention to the range of cognitive deficits that are relevant to issues in forensic psychiatry, from testamentary capacity and undue influence to driving safety to elder abuse and guardianships. It will almost certainly shift the focus of expert reports and court testimony to more comprehensive evaluations of executive function and other cognitive domains.

The field of geriatric psychiatry addresses and informs many areas of relevance to the field of forensic psychiatry, and vice versa. This reciprocal relationship results in substantial overlap in the training of subspecialists in both fields, and consequent overlap in the functions performed by practicing geriatric and forensic psychiatrists. Geriatric psychiatrists-in-training learn about assessment of cognitive capacity and competency, undue influence, guardianship, abuse, neglect, protective services and guardianship, liability, and other legal concepts related to aging and mental health. They also must hone their skills in report preparation and expert testimony in court. Similarly, forensic psychiatrists-in-training learn from the geriatric clinician about cognitive decline and dementia, dependency, and proper care and treatment of the elderly. The most challenging cases may require the expertise of subspecialists from both fields. The practice of medicine has become increasingly complex, and the availability of new medical knowledge, new assessment tools, evolving diagnostic criteria, and new regulations and laws may require increased coordination of psychiatric subspecialists working together with other medical specialists.

ADDICTION PSYCHIATRY

Under Narcotic Drugs and Psychotropic Substances Act (NDPSA), 1985, the possession and use of potentially addictive drugs are crime in India, although possession and using legal addictive substances such as alcohol and tobacco are not a crime under controlled environment. Other anti-social behavior performed in the service of seeking and using a dru, such as stealing, or homicide, are obviously serious crimes.

For the persons engaged in drug-related criminal activities who are addicts, therefore, more likely to participate in criminal acts, the question is how this status does and should affect their liability for criminal behavior referred to addiction.

Those who believe that addiction is a chronic and often relapsing brain disease or neurobiological disorder, think that seeking and using of drugs are solely the signs of the disease and that addicts have little choice about whether to seek and use.

Those who believe that addiction is a weakness of willpower and a moral shortcoming, think that addicts simply need pull themselves by their bootstraps.

Despite the claims to expand the mitigating and excusing forces of addiction based on burgeoning scientific research exists.

An addiction psychiatrist and a forensic psychiatrist fundamentally differ in their approach to deal with a patient. The addiction psychiatrist diagnoses the patient to formulate a therapeutic plan and a prognosis so that there is a general agreement about the nature of the disorder and its treatment. The forensic psychiatrist, however, diagnoses the patient to identify and describe the nature of the condition and to discuss the relevant behavioral and cognitive outcome of this condition and its relationship to the legal questions being posed. Moreover, two forensic psychiatrists examining the same patient may agree on diagnosis often differ in their opinions about the significance and relevance of their findings and their application to the legal question. The language and terminology used in forensic psychiatry and addiction psychiatry also differs, for example, a physician may think of a narcotic as an opiate-derivative drug, but legally it is any scheduled chemical that is prohibited or used in violation of government regulations. Thus, marijuana and cocaine are legally narcotics. Medically, use or abuse of a chemical is not the same thing as dependence or addiction to that same chemical. One may become dependent on a regular and unchanging amount of a scheduled medication such as the benzodiazepines, never increase the dose, and yet undergo a withdrawal period if stopped abruptly. This is not addiction, which is yet another phenomenon.

Addiction is characterized by craving; increasing use; sneaking, lying, and subterfuge; and increasing amounts of time and money devoted to obtaining the substance. Addiction is a term that is poorly defined both legally and medically, and yet the term is used all the time, leading to imprecise thinking. Alcoholism is no longer found in the diagnostic classification of diseases and the current terminology used is "Alcohol Use Disorder." Insanity is another word which has no medical meaning and yet is used all the time. Legally, however, insanity has a very precise and exact meaning. The concept of voluntariness also differs in medicine and law. In law, drinking is considered to be voluntary, with the single exception of when a person unknowingly ingests an intoxicating substance. In addiction psychiatry, the concept of voluntariness is widely rejected, and drinking or drug using is seen as the result of craving, compulsion, or even neurobiological activity in the brain. The psychiatrist who specializes in the diagnosis and treatment of addiction disorders is expected to know the effects of various intoxicants, the phenomenology of addiction, neurotransmitters, receptor sites, neuro-anatomy of the brain, treatment modalities, medical comorbidity, prevention, and approaches to populations with special characteristics. In addition, the addiction psychiatrist needs to know the basic principles of forensic psychiatry, or how medical knowledge of the field of addiction and that of forensic psychiatry are interwoven in many ways.[34]

The importance of the legal and forensic aspects of addictions are not discussed and seldom taught during the postgraduate training in psychiatry, nor do they make the subject matter of a text book. More than most areas of psychiatry, that of addictions is often concerned with behavior having legal dimensions. The element that ties these two disciplines together is that both the disciplines talk of human behavior, including knowledge of both the influence of chemicals on behavior as well as the consequences that may arise in not conforming one's behavior to the requirements of the law. Knowledge of the basic tenets of forensic psychiatry is helpful to the addiction psychiatrist, as the behavioral manifestations of addictions often lead to legal consequences, which have not been viewed traditionally as of medical concern.[2] The primary concerns of addiction psychiatrist has been physiological effects of chemicals on the body and mind, habituation and its treatment, issues of withdrawal and detoxification, the appropriate use of medication to treat overdoses and serious withdrawal states such as delirium tremens, ways to help with cravings and promote abstinence, prevention, and monitoring.[3] Long-term involvement for addiction psychiatrists using varied therapeutic modalities to achieve, maintain and preserve sobriety is of paramount significance whereas the forensic psychiatrist does not have this concern. His task is to impartially evaluate a person and the legal case and formulate an opinion in order to aid the court. Intervention by the forensic psychiatrist depicts that the examination by him confers no doctor–patient relationship and this is not a therapeutic evaluation for any kind of treatment.[35]

Although the ultimate goal is different, the addiction psychiatrist can gain much by considering the method and approach of the forensic psychiatrist, which is to carefully verify and corroborate as much as possible the history the person gives, by interviewing others, reviewing hospital and other records, and by employing standardized testing if helpful. Whereas the forensic psychiatrist does this in order to have opinions be credible in court, the addiction psychiatrist must address the patient's initial distorted clinical data and confirm the offered narrative as well. Patients treated by addiction psychiatrists face more legal consequences those treated by most other psychiatrists. Such consequences, may often motivate a person to enter therapy but also to withhold essential information about continuing problematic, and possibly illegal, behavior that might be clinically important, such as distribution or stealing. Such denials and omissions can mislead the clinician who is not alert about the potential legal issues that are almost always present. The need for objective correlation of the patient's narrative is one of the ways in which a forensic approach assists the addiction psychiatrist. An understanding of this forensic approach, which may seem to run counter to the classic therapeutic stance, will assist the addiction psychiatrist to work through the initial denial, distorted thinking, self-deception, projection, and minimization the new patient inevitably displays. The clinician must assess whether or not the patient wants to be sober or drug free, or whether he just wants to minimize or avoid the consequences of drug or alcohol use, much as the person the forensic psychiatrist evaluates seeks to avoid the possible legal consequences of criminal actions. The psychiatrist in either situation must assume that the patient is not initially forthcoming. The forensic psychiatrist depends upon corroborative and correlative account obtained from other people, records, and documents. The addiction psychiatrist will also interview concerned others at the beginning of therapy and seek previous treatment records as well as police records. The forensic psychiatrist does not have to believe what is related initially, and in fact is obligated to be skeptical of all narrative and to verify what the examinee is relating. The addiction psychiatrist must tread a narrow middle ground; tentatively accepting the patient's story knowing it is incomplete and perhaps deceptive, but requiring to interview others who may have a different point of view, as well as useful information. This should be done at the outset in order to make the point that the addiction psychiatrist is thorough but supportively skeptical, and not necessarily willing to accept everything at face value. In the long run this tentative position is helpful, as the psychiatrist will not collude with the patient in his defenses, but rather have the means and basis to challenge distortions in a helpful and therapeutic way. As with the forensic psychiatrist, it is important for the addiction psychiatrist to obtain previous treatment records, especially those from hospitals and rehabilitation services, if any, and to ask the patient to clarify discrepancies. Asking for permission to speak to previous therapists is often essential. If a patient refuses such permission, then the clinician is made aware early on that there are unknowns and secrets. This must be dealt with carefully at the beginning of therapy, as the position of the doubting therapist is a difficult one, but information is much more easily gathered while initially developing the patient's comprehensive past history. Early on, the psychiatrist can clear up missing facts and misstatements and then begin to develop the doctor–patient relationship. The patient knows then that his doctor will not be easily duped, and that his narrative may be questioned.

When the addiction psychiatrist is required to assist the attorney, he should clearly understand his role, whether he will be an expert witness, a fact witness, or no witness at all but only a consultant to the attorney and not expected to write a report or to testify. A consultant is required to possesses a great deal of knowledge about chemical dependence. The expectation is to be as an advisor about certain aspects of the case. All the clinical material will be reviewed with the attorney to see what facts are important and relevant, then advise the attorney what more materials are necessary, such as employment or school records. Hospital records will be reviewed in order to guide the attorney through important medical issues that may emerge. Suggestions may be offered to consider in light of the totality of the case, and perhaps to opine about whether it looks like there is a case to take forward at all, in light of all that has been considered. The psychiatrist might point out important aspects the attorney has not considered because he did not recognize their significance.[36]

If the addiction psychiatrist is summoned to assist in the defense of a malpractice case in which a physician has been accused of "causing a patient to become addicted," a not uncommon allegation, he has to blend medical knowledge and expertise with the legal elements and procedures the lawyer must work within.

- The allegations are reviewed along with medical history and records.
- The attorney and the physician assess the medical vulnerability of the defendant physician.
- Addiction expert helps the attorney to formulate questions for depositions and for cross-examining the witnesses at trial, to warn of medical pitfalls and to advise about the significance of facts and data.
- In order to assess the nature and extent of the claimed harm, in this instance causing an addiction, the expert must perform a thorough psychiatric evaluation, review and consider all pertinent documents and other information, ask for missing documents or call attention to those that are not available, obtain collateral information from others to corroborate facts and details, request results of all studies and tests, and suggest other measures such as psychological testing or neuroimaging if the claim warrants. It is extremely important to obtain all the medical records.
- The expert must be familiar with the needs of the attorney and the court.

- He should be familiar with writing a report, because this document is different, it is a treatment summary or to inform a colleague, or to prepare for an academic presentation. Ideally it is carefully crafted and includes a list and description of all materials considered important in the case.

Testamentary Capacity and Competency

An addiction psychiatrist can be invited in the matter of a will challenge. Here, the validity of a will is being challenged by a claim that the testator did not have the mental capacity to write the will at the time it was written. The issue here is the state of mind of the testator at the time the will was written, and whether or not the person understood the process and what the desired outcome would be. Issues of alcohol or drug addiction, intoxication, clouded thinking, or undue influence may be alleged. The addiction psychiatrist is required to apply knowledge of ways in which chemicals might have affected the decedent's thinking. Multiple collateral interviews are helpful, along with hospital records, bank records, tax records, correspondence, and, if available, newspaper articles, obituaries, e-mail, and social media, in order to assess whether or not the testator was of sound mind at or around the time the will was written. In addition, what evidence is there, if any, to support the claim of alcohol or drug dependence and to what extent did they influence or distort the testator's thinking? The addiction psychiatrist is not being asked to make a diagnosis, because a diagnosis is secondary to the issue of competency, but on the other hand can help explain the situation if incompetency or lack of capacity is determined.

Contracts Competency in Addicts

In another context, the addiction psychiatrist might be asked to offer an opinion about the validity of a contract, if signed while the person was in the throes of active alcoholism or addiction. The question to be examined is the state of mind of the signer of the document at the time he signed it. Again the collateral and corroborative material at or around the time of the signing is most helpful.

Competency to Divorce

In a divorce case the husband could not accept that his marriage was over. He persisted in the fantasy that his wife still loved him. During this time he was in the throes of a serious opiate addiction, but to casual observation he seemed to be functioning normally. One day, while he was in a beclouded condition, his wife abruptly presented him with a property settlement and demanded that he sign it. He stated that he could not accept even then that she was serious, and he further said that he believed she would never cause him any harm. Although he signed the document, later he stated he never read its contents because he trusted his ex-wife, and so did not know what it said or what he agreed to. Only later, once he was in recovery, did he realize that he had signed away his entire estate, past and future, and that he had agreed to give her absolutely everything he possessed. The addiction psychiatrist was asked to ascertain, as much as possible, the husband's state of mind at the time of signing, and how his thinking was influenced by his considerable opioid addiction, in order to assist the attorney to show the court that this was not a valid, knowing, and informed settlement contract. Again, collateral and corroborative material at or around the time of the signing was most helpful. The task of the addiction psychiatrist in this matter is a descriptive one, shedding as much light as possible on state of mind at a past event.

Dram Shop Case

Another matter in which the addiction psychiatrist may be asked to participate is in a dram shop case. Here the task of the addiction psychiatrist is to opine as accurately as possible whether or not the subject patron of the bar in question was "visibly intoxicated" at the time he was served additional alcohol, and whether or not the bartender should have refused service, thus preventing the events that precipitated the suit. The person whose condition is in question may be dead, so the psychiatrist's opinion must be based on as much other information as it is possible to glean. It can be expected that there will be conflicting narratives one must evaluate. In addition, the addiction psychiatrist can be asked to opine and describe what effect a given amount of alcohol might have on a person's thinking, reasoning, personality, motor functioning, coordination, speech, flushed skin, impulsivity, judgment, or aggressiveness.

Custody Cases

A custody dispute is another matter in which the addiction psychiatrist might be asked to participate, which can be one of the most difficult issues possible. Often each estranged and embittered parent claims that the other is an alcoholic or drug addict and therefore should be denied custody or visitation rights. In such a situation, if one decides to participate, the psychiatrist must insist on being retained by the court and not by either side. This arrangement permits the psychiatrist to examine both parents.

Criminal Matters

In criminal cases the addiction psychiatrist can be called upon to be of assistance but in a different way. Addictions, intoxication, or being under the influence of a drug or chemical, or claiming amnesia or a blackout are not complete defenses to a crime, but discussion of these phenomena may help place a criminal act in context and be useful at sentencing.

The addiction psychiatrist involved in a criminal case should know general criminal court procedure. He can be of help in informing and educating the court about the effects a given chemical may have on a person's behavior at the time of the crime, and how the ingestion of such a chemical might have influenced the defendant's judgment, perception, impulse control, or thinking. If retained by the prosecution, the addiction psychiatrist can be of assistance in helping to respond to a claim of "blackout" or alcoholic amnesia, a claim that is made by a significant number of defendants. The defendant claims no knowledge or memory for the acts the prosecution has charged, and may therefore maintain no knowledge or conscious control over what happened at the time. The absence of memory does not signify or imply a lack of cognitive functioning or an inability to act rationally at the time of the crime, nor does it suggest that the criminal act itself did not take place. A basic tenet of the legal view of alcoholism is at variance with the literature of alcoholism and addiction is that intoxication is always viewed as voluntary. Alcoholism and drug addiction are conceptualized quite differently from the legal view, bearing in mind the previous discussion that these terms have no diagnostic meaning but continue in the lexicon as useful concepts or "shorthand."

Drinking may be driven by cravings and strong urges. After the first drink the alcoholic no longer has the ability to predictably and consistently control intake or to stop drinking. Usually the drinking episode is stopped one way or another by an external event. Nevertheless, the law holds that the first drink is always voluntary and the defendant knows when drinking begins both of past inability to control the amount consumed as well as its ensuing consequences. Therefore, knowing what is likely to happen, the choice is made to drink anyway. In addition to the discussion of the phenomenology of pathologic ingestion of alcohol or chemicals of abuse, testimony concerning unanticipated reactions to drugs or medicines can be of great assistance to the court.

Criminal Behavior in an Addicted Individual

A young man presented in serious difficulty. He was a senior in high school and bound for college. He was an Eagle Scout and an exemplary model student held out to others as what one can accomplish as the only child of a single mother on extremely modest means. He did not drink, nor did he use drugs. He was devoutly religious and very conservative in clothing, activities, music, and recreation. Nevertheless, shortly before graduation, he was charged with calling his high school late at night to make terroristic bomb threats, and his voice was confirmed on tape. This was a devastating event, one that would imprison him and ruin his life, and one not easily explained. In brief, a history showed that during the time in question he had been suffering from a severe cold or flu for many days. He described that, in order to not miss school, he began to take a proprietary cold remedy. On inquiry it was ascertained that this remedy contained dextromethorphan and pseudoephedrine. He was impatient and so began to take a lot of it. On the night in question he had a fever and had not eaten. He did not know it, but he had taken enough pseudoephedrine to produce insomnia and so he was up all night. In addition, the amount of dextromethorphan he ingested produced hallucinations, delusional thinking, dissociation, and euphoria. In the morning he had no recollection of what he had done and thought he had a bad dream. When this information was presented to the prosecution, it changed the whole nature of the case. It was not possible to overlook a bomb threat, but the consequences were far less catastrophic.

An addiction psychiatrist may be called upon in a driving under the influence case, to challenge the results of breath or blood tests, or to offer alternative causes. Because a person has been found to be driving with a blood level above 0.08 mg/dL in most states, this does not necessarily mean that person has an Alcohol Use Disorder, using current terminology, even though driving had been affected and influenced. Often enough time has passed that testimony can be offered to show the court what the defendant has done to address the problematic drinking. This should be supported with documentation of participation in an appropriate regimen. This could involve an inpatient or outpatient rehab program, participation in a 12-step program, random urine monitoring, and documented meaningful and appropriate therapy. Although this testimony might be offered at the trial phase, it is more often given as mitigation at sentencing, to offer to the judge that the defendant has assumed responsibility for driving under the influence and is taking measures to remedy the situation.

Many psychiatrists fear and dread involvement with legal matters and avoid it at all costs, usually because of a lack of familiarity with the field. It should be evident that there are many valuable and meaningful ways to contribute and share expertise with their forensic colleagues. If indeed, as was noted at the beginning, psychiatry is more and more the study of behavior, then psychiatrists are obligated to have at least rudimentary knowledge of the kinds of behavior that have legal consequences, and be willing to participate in that process. Knowledge of the legal system, forensic approaches, and procedure and customs can make what might seem to be terrifying much more understandable and perhaps even a new and intriguing area of medicine.

The last few decades have witnessed an alarming rise in criminal activity associated with alcohol and substance use disorder in India. Apart from alcohol, other commonly abused drugs are opium and its derivatives and cannabis. The spectrum of crime committed by addicts is expansive. In a study it was found that 80% of the heroin or multiple drug users had the history of either conduct disorder or antisocial personality disorder.[37] This brings the addiction psychiatrists in India close to criminal behavior through their addicted patients. Addiction psychiatry and forensic psychiatry, both are in their infancy in India with only a couple of centers providing Addiction Psychiatry training and only one center has recently started with post-doctoral course in Forensic psychiatry.

REFERENCES

1. Beauchamp TL, Childress JF. Principles of biomedical ethics. New York: Oxford University Press, 1979.
2. Lederberg MS. Making a situational diagnosis. Psychiatrists at the interface of psychiatry and ethics in the consultation-liaison setting. Psychosomatics. 1997;38(4):327-38.
3. Hundert EM. A model for ethical problem solving in medicine, with practical applications. Am J Psychiat. 1987;144(7):839-46.
4. Mental Healthcare Act, 2017. Ministry of Health and Family Welfare. Government of India Publication, New Delhi.
5. Appelbaum PS, Lidz CW, Meisel A. Informed consent: Legal theory and clinical practice. New York: Oxford University Press, 1987.
6. Appelbaum PS. Clinical practice: Assessment of patients' competence to consent to treatment. N Engl J Med. 2007;357(18):1834-40.
7. Pennsylvania Medical Society. http://www.pamedsoc.org/MainMenuCategories/Government/LawsAffectingPhysicians/AdvanceDirectives/Act169facts.aspx. Accessed January 1, 2012.
8. Buchanan AE, Brock DW. Deciding for others: The ethics of surrogate decision-making. Cambridge: Cambridge University Press, 1990.

9. Plassman BL, Langa KM, Fisher GG. Prevalence of cognitive impairment without dementia in the United States. Ann Intern Med. 2008;148:42.
10. Plassman BL, Langa KM, Fisher GG, et al. Prevalence of dementia in the United States: The Aging Demographics, and Memory Study. Neuroepidemiology. 2007;29:125-32.
11. Evans DA, Funkenstein HH, Albert MS, et al. Prevalence of Alzheimer's disease in a community population of older persons: Higher than previously reported. JAMA. 1989;262:2551-6.
12. Moye J, Karel MJ, Azar AR, et al. Capacity to consent to treatment: empirical comparison of three instruments in older adults with and without dementia. Gerontologist. 2004;44:166-75.
13. Molloy DW, Silberfield M, Darzins P, et al. Measuring capacity to complete an advance directive. J Am Geriatr Soc. 2004;44:660-64.
14. Jeste DV, Palmer BW, Appelbaum PS, et al. A brief new instrument for assessing decisional capacity for clinical research. Arch Gen Psychiatry. 2007;64:966-74.
15. Jefferson AL, Lambe S, Moser DJ, et al. Decisional capacity for research participation in individuals with mild cognitive impairment. J Am Geriatr Soc. 2008;56:1236-43.
16. Appelbaum PS, Grisso T. MacArthur Competence Assessment Tool for Clinical Research (MacCAT-CR). Sarasota, FL: Professional Resource Press, 2001.
17. Overton E, Appelbaum PS, Fisher SR, et al. Alternative decision-makers' perspectives on assent and dissent for dementia research. Am J Geriatr Psychiatry. 2013;21:346-54.
18. Black BS, Wechsler M, Fogarty L. Decision making for participation in dementia research. Am J Geriatr Psychiatry. 2013;21:355-63.
19. Shulman KI, Cohen CA, Hull I. Psychiatric issues in retrospective challenges of testamentary capacity. Int J Geriatr Psychiatry. 2005;20:63-9.
20. Shulman KI, Cohen CA, Kirsh FC, et al. Assessment of testamentary capacity and vulnerability to undue influence. Am J Psychiatry. 2007;154:722-7.
21. Shulman KI, Peisah C, Jacogy R, et al. Contemporaneous assessment of testamentary capacity. Int Psychogeriatrics. 2009;21:433-9.
22. Banks v, Goodfellow. LR.5 Q.B. 1870:549.
23. O'Connor D, Hall MI, Donnelly M. Assessing capacity within the context of abuse or neglect. J Elder Abuse Negl. 2009;21:156-69.
24. Dickerson AE. Driving with dementia: evaluation, referral, and resources. Occup Ther Health Care. 2014;289:62-76.
25. Hoggarth PA, Innes CR, Dlarymmple-Alford JC, et al. Predicting on-road assessment pass and fail outcomes in older drivers with cognitive impairment using a battery of computerized sensory-motor and cognitive tests. J Am Geriatr Soc. 2013;61:2192-8.
26. Rapoport MJ, Naglie G, Herrmann N, et al. Developing physician consensus on the reporting of patients with mild cognitive impairment and mild dementia to transportation authorities in a region with mandatory reporting legislation. Am J Geriatr Psychiatry. 2014;22:1530-43.
27. Chandler JD, Chandler JE. The prevalence of neuropsychiatric disorders in a nursing homepopulation. J Geriatr Psychiatry Neurol. 1988;1:71-6.
28. Parmelee PA, Katz IR, Lawton MP. Depression among institutionalized aged: Assessment and prevalence estimation. J Gerontol, 1989;4:M22-M29.
29. Rovner BW, Kafonek S, Filipp L, et al. Prevalence of mental illness in a community nursing home. Am J Psychiatry. 1986;143:1446-9.
30. Rovner BW, German PS, Broadhead J, et al. The prevalence and management of dementia and other psychiatric disorders in nursing homes. Int Psychogeriatr. 1990;2:13-24.
31. Tariot PN, Podgorski CA, Blazina L, et al. Mental disorders in the nursing home: another perspective. Am J Psychiatry. 1993;150:1063-9.

32. Streim JE. Clinical psychiatry in the nursing home. In DG Blazer, DC Steffans (Eds). Essentials of geriatric psychiatry. Washington, DC: American Psychiatric Publishing. 2012;2:351-79.
33. American Psychiatric Association. Diagnostic and Statistical Manual of Mental Disorders. Arlington, VA: American Psychiatric Publishing, 2013.
34. American Psychiatric Association. Diagnostic and statistical manual of mental disorders. Arlington, VA: American Psychiatric Association. 2013.pp.483-589.
35. Shorter E. A history of psychiatry: From an era of the asylum to the age of Prozac. New York: John Wiley & Sons,1997.
36. Sinha R. The clinical neurobiology of drug craving. Curr Opin Neurobiol. 2013;23:649-54.
37. Nambi S. Prevalence of alcohol and substance abuse among mentally ill prisoners. Presented at the Annual National Conference of Indian Psychiatric Society, 1998.

CHAPTER

Euthanasia and Living Wills

> **LEARNING OBJECTIVES**
> - Concept of euthanasia
> - Types of euthanasia
> - Legal status globally
> - Religious views
> - Living Will
> - Passive euthanasia: Supreme Court guidelines
> - Medical treatment of terminally ill patients bill
> - Misuse in psychiatry
> - APA position statement

The word 'Euthanasia' is derived from Greek word εὐθανασία which means "good death" (εὖ, *eu*; "well" or "good" - θάνατος, *thanatos*; "death"). It is the practice of intentionally ending a life to relieve pain and suffering.[1,2]

CONCEPTUAL CONTROVERSIES

Like other terms borrowed from history, the word 'euthanasia' has been used in various contexts depending on usage. The first visible usage of the term euthanasia was by the historian Suetonius, who described the death of Emperor Augustus, "dying quickly and without suffering in the arms of his wife, Livia, experienced the 'euthanasia' he had wished for.[3] Francis Bacon in the 17th century was the first to use the word "euthanasia" in a medical context, to refer to an easy, painless, happy death, during which it was a "physician's responsibility to alleviate the 'physical sufferings' of the body." Bacon referred to an "outward euthanasia"—the term "outward" he used to distinguish from a spiritual concept—the euthanasia "which regards the preparation of the soul."[4]

Euthanasia has been broadly defined as the "painless inducement of a quick death."[5] However, this definition leaves open a number of possible actions which would meet the requirements of the definition, but would not be seen as euthanasia. For example, situations where a person kills another, painlessly, but for no reason beyond that of personal gain; or accidental deaths that are quick and painless, but not intentional.[6,7]

Another approach to define euthanasia has tried to incorporate the notion of suffering into the definition.[11] The Oxford English Dictionary defines euthanasia as "the painless killing of a patient suffering from an incurable and painful disease or in an irreversible coma."[8] Marvin Khol and Paul Kurtz tried to refine the definition as "a mode or act of inducing or permitting death painlessly as a relief from suffering".[9] However, such definitions may encompass killing a person suffering from an incurable disease for personal gain (such as to claim an inheritance), and commentators such as Tom Beauchamp and Arnold Davidson have argued that doing so would constitute "murder simpliciter" rather than euthanasia.[6]

This led to incorporation into many definitions of intentionality—the death must be intended, rather than being accidental, and the intent of the action must be a "merciful death".[6] Michael Wreen argued that "the principal thing that distinguishes euthanasia from intentional killing simpliciter is the agent's motive: it must be a good motive in sofar as the good of the person killed is concerned."[10] The importance of motive is emphasized by Heather Draper, arguing that "the motive forms a crucial part of arguments for euthanasia, because it must be in the best interests of the person on the receiving end."[7] Definitions such as that offered by the House of Lords Select Committee on Medical Ethics incorporated this when defining euthanasia as "a deliberate intervention undertaken with the express intention of ending a life, to relieve intractable suffering."[3] Beauchamp and Davidson also highlight Baruch Brody's "an act of euthanasia is one in which one person... (A) kills another person (B) for the benefit of the second person, who actually does benefit from being killed".[11]

Draper argued that any definition of euthanasia must incorporate four elements:
1. An agent and a subject
2. An intention
3. A causal proximity, such that the actions of the agent lead to the outcome
4. An outcome.

She incorporated these elements into a definition, stating that euthanasia "must be defined as death that results from the intention of one person to kill another person, using the most gentle and painless means possible, that is motivated solely by the best interests of the person who dies."[12] Beauchamp and Davidson had also offered a definition which included these elements. Their definition specifically discounts fetuses to distinguish between abortions and euthanasia.[13]

It can be argued that the death of a human being, A, is an instance of euthanasia if and only if:
1. A's death is intended by at least one other human being, B, where B is either the cause of death or a causally relevant feature of the event resulting in death (whether by action or by omission).
2. There is either sufficient current evidence for B to believe that A is acutely suffering or irreversibly comatose, or there is sufficient current evidence related to A's present condition such that one or more known causal laws supports B's belief that A will be in a condition of acute suffering or irreversible coma
3. (a) B's primary reason for intending A's death is cessation of A's (actual or predicted future) suffering or irreversible coma, where B does not intend A's death for a different primary reason, though there may be other relevant reasons.
   (b) There is sufficient current evidence for either A or B that causal means to A's death will not produce any more suffering than would be produced for A if B were not to intervene.

4. The causal means to the event of A's death are chosen by A or B to be as painless as possible, unless either A or B has an overriding reason for a more painful causal means, where the reason for choosing the latter causal means does not conflict with the evidence in 3b.
5. A is a non-fetal organism."[14]

Wreen, in part responding to Beauchamp and Davidson, offered a six-part definition: "Person A committed an act of euthanasia if and only if,

1. A killed B or let her die
2. A intended to kill B
3. The intention specified in (2) was at least partial cause of the action specified in (1)
4. The causal journey from the intention specified in (2) to the action specified in (1) is more or less in accordance with A's plan of action.
5. A's killing of B is a voluntary action.
6. The motive for the action specified in (1), the motive standing behind the intention specified in (2), is the good of the person killed."[15]
7. The good specified in (6) is, or at least includes, the avoidance of evil, although as Wreen noted in the paper, he was not convinced that the restriction was required.[21]

Wreen acknowledged the difficulty of justifying euthanasia when faced with the notion of the subject's "right to life". He argued that euthanasia has to be voluntary, and that "involuntary euthanasia is, as such, a great wrong".[16] Consent has been more directly incorporated into some definitions. According to European Association of Palliative Care (EPAC) Ethics Task Force, 2003, "Medicalized killing of a person without the person's consent, whether non-voluntary or involuntary is not euthanasia: it is murder. Hence, euthanasia can be voluntary only."[17] Although the EPAC Ethics Task Force argued that both non-voluntary and involuntary euthanasia could not be included in the definition of euthanasia, there is discussion in the literature about excluding one but not the other.[16]

The laws governing euthanasia vary in each country. The British House of Lords Select Committee on Medical Ethics defines euthanasia as "a deliberate intervention undertaken with the express intention of ending a life, to relieve intractable suffering".[18] In the Netherlands and Belgium, euthanasia is understood as "termination of life by a doctor at the request of a patient".[19] The Dutch law however, does not use the term 'euthanasia' but includes it under the broader definition of "assisted suicide and termination of life on request".[20]

Classification of Euthanasia

Based on whether a person gives informed consent or not, euthanasia may be classified into three types: [21-24]

1. Voluntary
2. Nonvoluntary
3. Involuntary

There is a ongoing debate within the medical and bioethics literature about whether or not the nonvoluntary (and by extension, involuntary) killing of patients can be regarded as euthanasia, irrespective of intent or the patient's circumstances. In the definitions offered by Beauchamp and Davidson and, later, by Wreen, consent on the part of the patient was not considered as one of their criteria, although it may have been required to justify euthanasia.[11,25] However, many others see consent as essential.

Voluntary Euthanasia

Voluntary euthanasia is carried out with the consent of the patient. Active voluntary euthanasia is legal in Belgium, Luxembourg and the Netherlands. Passive voluntary euthanasia is legal throughout the United States per *Cruzan vs. Director, Missouri Department of Health*. When the patient brings about his or her own death with the assistance of a physician, the term assisted suicide is often used instead. Assisted suicide is legal in Switzerland and the US states of California, Oregon, Washington, Montana and Vermont.

Nonvoluntary Euthanasia

Nonvoluntary euthanasia is done when the consent of the patient is not available. Examples include child euthanasia, which is illegal worldwide but decriminalized under certain specific circumstances in the Netherlands under the Groningen Protocol.

Involuntary Euthanasia

Involuntary euthanasia is administered against the Will of the patient. Involuntary euthanasia (without consent or in opposition to the patient's Will) is unlawful in all countries and is usually considered equivalent to murder.[21]

As of 2006, euthanasia is one of the vigorously researched topic in contemporary bioethics.[22] In certain countries there is a estranged public debate over the moral, ethical, and legal aspects of euthanasia.

Passive and Active Euthanasia

Voluntary, non-voluntary and involuntary types can be further divided into passive or active variants.[23] Passive euthanasia entails the withholding treatment necessary for the continuance of life.[27] Commonly known as "pulling the plug", it is legally sanctioned under some circumstances in many countries. This entails doctors to not provide, or to remove the patients from life sustaining treatment including:
- Disconnecting life-support machinery, feeding tubes, not carrying out life-saving operations, not providing life-extending drugs.
- Non-treatment is not labelled as cause of death, rather patients are understood to have died owing to underlying condition.

Active euthanasia assumes the use of lethal interventions (such as administering a lethal injection), and is the more debatable of the two. Although these terms are considered by some to be misleading and unconstructive, they are nonetheless frequently used. Certain situations such as administering increasingly necessary but noxious doses of painkillers, are controversial whether or not to be regarded as active or passive.[25]

Legal Status Globally

West's *Encyclopedia of American Law* holds that "a 'mercy killing' or euthanasia is generally considered to be a criminal homicide"[25] and is mostly used as a substitute of homicide committed at a request made by the patient.

The judicial sense of the term "homicide" includes any intervention undertaken with the express intention of ending a life, even to relieve intractable suffering.[26-28] Not all homicide are against the law. Two types of homicide that carry no criminal punishment are justifiable and excusable homicide.[29] However that's not the status of euthanasia in most countries. The word "euthanasia" is usually reserved for the active variety. The University of Washington website describes that "euthanasia generally means that the physician would act directly, for instance by giving a lethal injection, to end the patient's life".[30] Physician-assisted suicide is not labelled as euthanasia in the US State of Oregon. It is legal under the Oregon Death with Dignity Act, but inspite of its name it is not legally grouped under suicide.[31] Unlike physician-assisted suicide, withholding or withdrawing life-sustaining interventions under patient's consent (voluntary) is almost unanimously considered, at least in the United States, to be legal.[32] Similarly, the use of pain medication to alleviate suffering, at the expense of hastening death, has been upheld as legal in several court decisions.[30]

Voluntary euthanasia has been legalised by some countries in the world but majority still considers it to be criminal homicide. Countries such as Netherlands and Belgium, where euthanasia has been legalized, it still retains the status as homicide. However, it is not prosecuted and not punishable if certain legal conditions are met by the perpetrator (the doctor).[33-35]

Physician Sentiment

A 2010 survey of more than 10,000 physicians of United States found that 16.3% of physicians would consider terminating life-sustaining therapy if the family was in the favor of same, even if they thought it to be premature. Around 54.5% said they would not while the remaining 29.2% responded "it depends".[37] It was found that 45.8% of physicians were in favor of physician-assisted suicide in some cases; 40.7% did not agree at all, and the remaining 13.5% felt it was conditional.[36]

In the United Kingdom, the pro-assisted dying group Dignity in Dying cite contrasting findings on doctors' attitudes to assisted dying. A 2009 *Palliative Medicine*-published survey revealed that 64% of physicians were in favor of (34% oppose) assisted dying in cases where a patient has an incurable and painful disease. while 49% of doctors in A study published in *BMC Medical Ethics* found that 49% doctors were opposed to changing the law on assisted dying as compared to 39% in favor.[37]

RELIGIOUS VIEWS ON EUTHANASIA

Christianity is Broadly Against

The Roman Catholic Church strongly disapproves and denounces euthanasia and assisted suicide labelling it morally wrong. The Catholic Church states that, "Intentional euthanasia, whatever its forms or motives, is murder. It is gravely contrary to the dignity of the human person and to the respect due to the living God, his Creator". Hence, the practice is considered unacceptable by the Church.[38] The Orthodox Church in America, along with other Eastern Orthodox Churches, also condemned euthanasia labelling it as murder stating that, "Euthanasia is the deliberate cessation to end human life."[39]

Many non-Catholic churches in the United States take a stance against euthanasia.[40-43] Among Protestant denominations, the Episcopal Church passed a resolution in 1991 opposing euthanasia and assisted suicide stating that is "morally wrong and unacceptable to take a human life to relieve the suffering caused by incurable illnesses."[44-48]

Partially in Favor of Euthanasia

The Church of England approves passive euthanasia under limited circumstances, but has strongly condemned active euthanasia. The Church has also actively led opposition against recent attempt to legalise the same.[49] United Church of Canada also takes more or less the same stand on passive euthanasia, accepting it under some circumstances, but is in general against active euthanasia.[50]

Islam

Euthanasia is in general, considered contrary to Islamic law and holy texts. According to the Koran and Hadith, early termination of life is a crime. This includes both suicide or assisting one in committing suicide. The various viewpoints on the suspension of medical intervention are mixed and it is considered a different category of action than direct termination of life, especially in cases where the patient is suffering. Suicide and euthanasia are both considered illegal in most of the Muslim majority countries.[51]

Judaism

Euthanasia is a much debated topic in Judaic theology and ethics. Passive euthanasia was legalised by Israel's highest court under certain conditions and has gained some level of acceptance. Active euthanasia however remains illegal and the topic is actively under debate with no clear legal, ethical, theological and spiritual consensus.[52]

In a milestone verdict, expanding the Right to Life to incorporate Right to Die with dignity, the Supreme Court of India on 9th March 2018, legalised passive euthanasia. It was expanded to involve the principle of 'Living Wills' (LW) which provides terminally ill patients or those in a 'persistent and incurable vegetative state' (PVS) a dignified exit by retreating life support or cessation of life preserving treatment.[53]

The judgment paves the path for decriminalise suicide.

State's Failure

When the state is not being able to guarantee the right to healthcare for all, can the citizens be denied to die with dignity.

Stressed Finances and Facilities
Poor are forced to sell properties endangering family's future to treat terminally ill. The limited life-saving facilities are blocked by patients who would not recover.

Euthanasia was in Practice
Buddhism and Jainism allow euthanasia while Hinduism and Christianity are against it. Limited euthanasia was allowed through Medical Council Regulations 2002.

The Safeguard
Mandating provision for a double medical board, involving judicial magistrate or collector, or High Court, to implement euthanasia and Living Will.

Active Euthanasia
Active euthanasia is allowed in several Western countries, it will continue to be a crime in India.

LIVING WILL
Will expressed by a person during his life time to die with dignity when terminally ill, is Living Will.

PASSIVE EUTHANASIA: SUPREME COURT GUIDELINES ON ADVANCE DIRECTIVES

Who can Execute a Living Will?
1. It must be voluntary and without coercion or compulsion.
2. Only an adult of sound and healthy mind can execute a Living Will.
3. It must be in writing, stating when treatment may be withdrawn or no specific treatment shall be given that can delay death.

What shall it Constitute?
1. Circumstances in which to stop the treatment.
2. A mention that the individual/patient can change their mind at any time.
3. Name of the guardian or relative who, in the event of individual not in position to take decision, can consent to supporting treatment.

How should it be Recorded and Preserved?
1. It must be signed by the individual in presence of two witnesses.
2. It must be signed by relevant Judicial Magistrate First Class (JMFC).

3. Witnesses and JMFC must record that there was no coercion.
4. JMFC has to preserve a copy and forward one to the District Court.
5. JMFC must inform immediate family members if they are not present at the time of recording the Living Will.

When and by whom can it be given effect?

1. If the executor becomes terminally ill with no hope of recovery or cure treating physician must check authenticity of LW from area JMFC.
2. Doctor must inform patient, or his guardian, or close relative about nature of illness, available medical care and alternative treatment and consequences of remaining untreated.
3. Hospital to setup medical board comprising head of the treating department and at least three doctors with at least twenty years experience who, in turn visit the patient in the presence of his relatives and decide if the treatment is to be withdrawn.
4. If the medical board gives go-ahead, hospital shall inform collector.
5. Collector must immediately constitute another medical board comprising chief district medical officer and three expert doctors.
6. Board shall examine the patient and take a call.
7. It will keep JMFC informed before allowing treatment to stop.
8. JMFC must visit the patient and after examining all aspects, may permit LW be followed.

THE MEDICAL TREATMENT OF TERMINALLY ILL PATIENTS (PROTECTION OF PATIENTS AND MEDICAL PRACTITIONERS) BILL

Union Health Ministry has drafted and put it up in the public domain for consultation with stakeholders.

Key Facts

- *Living Will:* It is defined as an advance document in which a person states their desire to have or not to have extraordinary life-prolonging measures used when recovery is not possible from their terminal condition.
- Every competent patient, including minors aged above 16 years, has a right to take a decision and express the desire to the medical practitioner attending on her or him.
- Advance directive made by a competent individual will be binding on the medical practitioner. He or she has to inform the spouse, parents or any other close relative of the patient and desist from carrying out the decision for a period of three days after informing them.
- The bill provides protection to patients and doctors from any liability for withholding or withdrawing medical treatment and states that palliative care (pain management) can continue.
- The Medical Council of India has been given the authority to formulate guidelines from time to time for the guidance of medical practitioners and might review and modify the guidelines periodically.

- In case any patient is not competent enough to take a decision then his or her next of kin, including spouse, parents or sibling, can approach the High Court, which will have to take a decision within a period of one month.[54]

Although the ethical and philosophical arguments for passive euthanasia apply equally to active euthanasia, the government has made the correct decision in addressing only the former at the moment. By doing so, it has curtailed the potential for misuse of the proposed legislation. A revised bill would be a significant step towards allowing suffering individuals a measure of human dignity with adequate safeguards.

MISUSE IN PSYCHIATRY AND POSITION STATEMENT OF APA FOR PSYCHIATRISTS

In 2002, Belgium, the Netherlands, and Luxembourg removed any distinctions between "terminal" and "non-terminal" conditions, and between physical suffering and mental suffering, for legally permitted physician-assisted suicide by prescription medication or euthanasia by lethal injection (PAS/E). It opened the Pandora box undesirably for mentally ill persons too. Independent consultants had to declare their condition "untreatable," and the patient needs to declare it to be "insufferable." In the Netherlands, for example, for 'psychiatric-only' cases, at least 1 consultation is required, but 3 are suggested. At least one should be a psychiatrist but does not have to be essential. Unfortunately, this legal stand is not based solely on what physicians have to offer, but also on what the patient wishes to accept. For example, though potentially effective treatments may be offered, such as ECT, but, a "competent" patients may refuse it. That choice could make their case "untreatable." So patients can rule on both the "untreatable" and "insufferable" axes; physicians can only opine on the former.[55]

Between 2008 and 2014, it resulted in more than 200 psychiatric patients opting for euthanasia by their own request in the Netherlands (1% of all euthanasia in that country): 52% had a diagnosis of personality disorder. When asked the primary reason for seeking PAS/E, 66% cited "social isolation and loneliness."[55]

So, in December 2016, the American Psychiatric Association (APA) in concert with the American Medical Association's position on Medical Euthanasia passed an historic position statement that a psychiatrist should not prescribe or administer any intervention to a non-terminally ill person for the purpose of causing death. They maintain that the fundamental ethos of psychiatry is the prevention of suicide, both on the individual level and in its public health message. Psychiatrists are trained to help people cope with such suffering, find a path to a better future—indeed, often to help people make meaning of suffering. The APA position implies that, even where legal for the non-terminally ill, it is neither the duty of a psychiatrist to fulfill that right, nor is it ethically appropriate to do so.[55]

REFERENCES

1. Philosopher Helga Kuhse: On Euthanasia Euthanasia. Worldrtd.net. Retrieved 2018-07-0
2. Plato.stanford.edu. Retrieved 2017-07-06.
3. Philippe Letellier. History and Definition of a Word, in Euthanasia: Ethica and Human Aspects By Council of Europe, 2005.

4. Francis Bacon. The Major Works by Francis Bacon. In: Brian Vickers (Ed). 1962 .p. 630.
5. Kohl Marvin. The Morality of Killing. New York: Humanities Press; 1974 .p. 94.
6. Beauchamp, Tom L. Davidson Arnold I. The Definition of Euthanasi. Journal of Medicine and Philosophy. 1979;4(3):294-312.
7. Draper, Heather. "Euthanasia". In: Chadwick, Ruth (Eds). Encyclopedia of Applied Ethics. Academic Press, 1998.
8. Oxford Dictionaries. Oxford University Press. April 2010. Retrieved 2017.
9. Kohl Marvin, Kurtz Paul. A Plea for Beneficient Euthanasia. In: Kohl Marvin (Eds). Beneficient Euthanasia. Buffalo, New York: Prometheus Books; 1975.pp. 233-4.
10. Wreen Michael. The Definition of Euthanasia. Philosophy and Phenomenological Research.1988; 48(4):637-56.
11. Brody Baruch. Voluntary Euthanasia and the Law. In: Kohl Marvin (Ed). Beneficient Euthanasia. Buffalo, New York: Prometheus Books; 1975.p. 94.
12. Draper Heather. Euthanasia. In: Chadwick Ruth (Ed). Encyclopedia of Applied Ethics. Academic Press; 1998.p. 176.
13. Beauchamp, Tom L, Davidson, Arnold I. The Definition of Euthanasia. Journal of Medicine and Philosophy.1979;4(3):303.
14. Beauchamp, Tom L. Davidson Arnold I. "The Definition of Euthanasia". Journal of Medicine and Philosophy.1979;4(3):304. doi:10.1093/jmp/4.3.294.
15. Wreen Michael. The Definition of Euthanasia. Philosophy and Phenomenological Research.1988; 48(4):637-40. doi:10.2307/2108012.
16. Wreen Michael. The Definition of Euthanasia. Philosophy and Phenomenological Research.1988; 48(4):637-53 [645]. doi:10.2307/2108012.
17. Harris NM. The euthanasia debate. JR Army Med Corps. 2001;147(3):367-70. doi:10.1136/jramc-147-03-22.
18. Euthanasia and assisted suicide BBC. Last reviewed June 2011. Accessed 25 July 2011. Archived from the original Archived 19 July 2011 at the Wayback Machine.
19. Carr, Claudia. Unlocking Medical Law and Ethics, 2nd edn. Routledge.2014.p.374. Retrieved 2 February 2018.
20. Voluntary and involuntary euthanasia *BBC* Accessed 12 February 2012. Archived from the original Archived 5 September 2011 at the Wayback Machine.
21. Borry P, Schotsmans P, Dierickx K. Empirical research in bioethical journals. A quantitative analysis. J Med Ethics. 2006;32(4):240-45.
22. Materstvedt Lars Johan, Clark David, Ellershaw, John, et al. Physician-assisted suicide.pdf "Euthanasia and physician-assisted suicide: a view from an EAPC Ethics Task Force" Check |url= value (help) (PDF). *Palliative Medicine*. 2003;17(2):97-101.
23. Perrett RW. Buddhism, euthanasia and the sanctity of life. J Med Ethics. 1996;22(5):309-13.
24. LaFollette, Hugh. Ethics in practice: an anthology. Oxford: Blackwell.2002.pp.25-26.
25. The legal-dictionary.the freedictionary.com Last visited on 14.3.2018.
26. Carmen Tomás Y Valiente, La regulación de la eutanasia en Holanda, Anuario de Derecho Penal y Ciencias Penales – Núm. L, Enero, 1997.
27. Mohanty MK. Variants of homicide: a review. Journal of Clinical Forensic Medicine. 2004;11(4):214-8.
28. Homicide legal definition of homicide. Legal-dictionary.thefreedictionary.com. Retrieved 2017-07-06.
29. The definition of homicide. Dictionary.com. Retrieved 4 July 2017.
30. Physician-Assisted Suicide: Ethical topic in medicine. depts.washington.edu. Retrieved 4 July 2017.

31. Taylor Bill. Physician Assisted Suicide (PDF). Archived from the original (PDF) on 7 July 2017. Retrieved 7 July 2017.
32. Oluyemisi Bamgbose. Euthanasia: Another Face of Murder. International Journal of Offender Therapy and Comparative Criminology. 2004;48(1):111-21.
33. Deliens, Luc. The euthanasia law in Belgium and the Netherlands. The Lancet. 2003;362(9391):1239-40.
34. Weyers H. Euthanasia: the process of legal change in the Netherlands—the making of the "requirements of careful practice". In: Klijn A, Otlowski M, Trappenburg M (Eds). Regulating physician-negotiated death. Elsevier, s'Gravenhagen, 2001;11-27.
35. Cohen-Almagor. Belgian euthanasia law: a critical analysis. J Med Ethics. 2009;35(7):436-39.
36. Leslie Kane, MA. Exclusive Ethics Survey Results: Doctors Struggle With Tougher-Than-Ever Dilemmas. Medscape.com. Retrieved 2017-07-06.
37. Public opinion. Dignity in Dying. Retrieved 2017-07-06.
38. How to Vote Catholic: Euthanasia and Assisted Suicide. www.catholicity.com.
39. The Orthodox Christian view on Euthanasia. www.orthodoxchristian.info.
40. Assemblies of God (USA) Official Website-Medical: Euthanasia, and Extraordinary Support to Sustain Life. ag.org.
41. 21. Selected Church Policies and Guidelines. www.lds.org.
42. The Church of the Nazarene, Doctrinal and Ethical Positions. www.crivoice.org.
43. http://download.elca.org/ELCA%20Resource%20Repository/End_Life_DecisionsSM.pdf.
44. What Are Christian Perspectives on Euthanasia and Physician-Assisted Suicide? - Euthanasia - ProCon.org. euthanasia.procon.org.
45. LCMS Views - Frequently Asked Questions—The Lutheran Church—Missouri Synod. www.lcms.org.
46. General Synod Statements: Physician-Assisted Suicide—Reformed Church in America. www.rca.org.
47. The Salvation Army International—Positional Statement: Euthanasia and Assisted Suicide. www.salvationarmy.org.
48. Southern Baptist Convention "Resolution On Euthanasia And Assisted Suicide". www.sbc.net.
49. Why the Church of England Supports the Current Law on Assisted Suicide. Dr Brendan McCarthy Archbishops' Council Church House, London, 2015.
50. Submission to The Special Joint Committee on Physician-Assisted Dying. Rev. Jordan Cantwell Moderator of The United Church of Canada, 2016.
51. Islamic Perspectives, Euthanasia (Qatl al-raḥma). Abulfadl Mohsin Ebrahim. Journal of the Islamic Medical Association of North America. 2007(4).
52. Death and Euthanasia in Jewish Law: Essays and Responses. W Jacob and M. Zemer. Pitsburg and Tel Aviv. Rodef Shalom Press, 1995.
53. SC legalises passive euthanasia and living will, says right to life includes right to die. The Times of India, New Delhi, 2018.
54. The Medical Treatment of Terminally Ill Patients (Protection of Patients and Medical Practitioners) Bill. Available at www.prsindia.org/uploads/media/draft/Draft%20Passive%20Euthanansia%20Bill.pdf.
55. Komrad MS. APA Position on Medical Euthanasia: psychiatry times; 34(2):1-3. Available at: http://www.psychiatrictimes.com/suicide/apa-position-medical-euthanasia.

CHAPTER 39

Legal Issues Concerning Treatment of Foreign Nationals with Mental Health Problems

> **LEARNING OBJECTIVES**
> - Travel and mental illnesses
> - Context of presentation of foreign nationals
> - India laws governing entry, stay and exit of foreign nationals
> - Legal responsibilities for health professionals
> - Fitness for air travel

TRAVEL AND MENTAL ILLNESSES

Travel is usually a relaxing and refreshing experience but it can be stressful in certain situations and can be associated with new or breakthrough episodes of preexisting psychiatric disorders. Research shows that 11.3% travelers encounter mental health issues of some kind with almost 2.5% experiencing severe psychosis.[1] India is one of the upcoming favored destination for tourism in general as well as for medical tourism. Medical tourism is more on rise for surgical procedures and less for mental health related conditions but mental health professionals often come across the foreign national clients in need of mental health related issues often.

Reasons for Developing Psychiatric Disorders during Travel[2]

- Consumption of drugs of abuse
- Missing medications during travel
- Travel-related stress
- Time zone change
- Sleep disturbance
- Homesickness
- Culture shock
- Disrupted normal routine
- Unfamiliar surrounding
- Physical ill health during travel
- Prophylactic drugs taken for travel inducing psychiatric disorders, e.g. Mefloquine
- Drugs taken for other physical ailments inducing psychiatric disorders, e.g. a foreigner on medical visa for organ transplantation on immunosuppressants.

CONTEXT OF PRESENTATION OF FOREIGN NATIONALS

In following situations, one can come across the foreign nationals for therapeutic consultations:
1. **A person with mental illness on medical visa**
   – On medical visa for treatment of psychiatric disorders
   – On medical visa for treatment of other ailments and developed psychiatric disorder
     • Psychiatric disorder comorbid with medical illness or
     • Medications induced psychiatric disorder, e.g. immunosuppressant induced disorders during organ transplantation
2. **A person on visa other than medical visa, developing psychiatric illness**
   – Develops first episode of psychiatric disorder induced by use of drugs of abuse or
   – A known person with mental illness experiencing relapse or exacerbation due to poor compliance or induced by use of drugs of abuse

Context of health seeking by foreign nationals: A foreigner with mental health issues can seek psychiatric help in following ways:
- A person with mental health need with intact capacity for mental healthcare voluntarily seeking treatment
- A person with mental health need with impaired capacity for mental healthcare brought by relatives or friend or Embassy officials for treatment
- A person with mental health need with impaired capacity for mental healthcare brought by police officer for assessment and treatment under Section 100 of Mental Health Care Act (risk to self or others by reason of mental illness or wandering person with mental illness, incapable of taking care of self)
- A person with mental health need with impaired capacity for mental healthcare brought by police officer with magistrate order for assessment and treatment under Section 102 of Mental Health Care Act.

Thus, it is prudent to be aware about the legal sanctions associated and provide medical care without undue fear or apprehension.

INDIAN LAWS GOVERNING ENTRY, STAY AND EXIT OF FOREIGN NATIONALS

- *Entry → Passport (Entry into India) Act, 1920:* It prescribes authorization of foreign nationals on their valid travel documents/ passports for allowing entry into the country.
- *Entry, stay, departure → Foreigners Act, 1946:* It regulates the entry of foreigners into India, their presence therein and their departure therefrom.
- *Stay → Registration of Foreigners Act, 1939:* It mandates for registration of certain categories of foreign nationals whose intended stay is more than specified period.
  – *Foreigners registration in India:* All foreigners visiting India (except children less than 12 years) on long term visa (more than 180 days), Student Visa, Medical Visa, Research Visa and Employment Visa are required to get themselves registered with the Foreigners Regional Registration Officer (FRRO)/Foreigners Registration Officer (FRO) within 14 days of arrival. (Pakistan nationals are required to register within 24 hours of arrival.)[3]

CHAPTER 39: Legal Issues Concerning Treatment of Foreign Nationals with Mental Health Problems

- Medical Visa (M Visa): It is visa issued to people immigrating for purpose of receiving treatment. It is valid maximum upto one year. At maximum two attendants can be issued medical attendant visa (MX Visa) to accompany patient in one go.[3]
- As per the guidelines issued by Ministry of Home affairs (MHA) **following is the "Procedure to be adopted in case a foreigner on Tourist/ Employment/Business/ Student/Research Visa falls ill after coming to India"**[4]
  - *Minor medical condition which does not require hospitalization and prolonged treatment:* Person will be allowed to take treatment.
  - *Sudden illness requiring continuous treatment or hospitalization of period less than 180 days or the stay stipulation period prescribed on the visa:* **Obtain 'medical Permit'** from concerned FRRO/FRO by submitting a medical certificate from hospitals recognized by following:
    - Government
    - ICMR (Indian Council of Medical Research)
    - NABH (National Accreditation Board for Hospitals & Healthcare Providers)
    - MCI (Medical Council of India)
    - CGHS (Central Government Health Scheme)
- *Illness of nature requiring treatment exceeding 180 days or stay stipulation period prescribed on visa:* submit request to concern FRRO/FRO for conversion to Medical Visa. It will need following documents from concerned hospital:
  - Letter from concerned recognized hospital, where treatment is being taken along with supportive medical documents/diagnostic test reports (with tentative period of treatment).
  - Medical certificate mentioning admission details, diagnosis, tentative period of treatment on a certificate bearing applicant's photo duly attested by the Doctor.
    [Authorities concerned with registration are FRROs located at New Delhi, Mumbai, Chennai, Kolkata, Amritsar, Lucknow, Bangalore, Hyderabad, Trivandrum, Calicut, Cochin, Goa and the District Superintendents of Police in all other districts].
- Responsibility of Hospital for filling Form C: **Any** Hotel/Guest House/Dharmashala/ Individual House/University/**Hospital**/Institute/Others, etc. who provide accommodation to foreigners must submit the details of the residing foreigner in Form C online to the Registration authorities within 24 hours of the arrival of the foreigner at their premises. This will help the registration authorities in locating and tracking the foreigners.[3]

LEGAL RESPONSIBILITIES OF HEALTH PROFESSIONALS DURING TREATMENT OF FOREIGN NATIONALS

Outpatient Treatment
- One can provide treatment and treating doctor is not duty bound to inform any specific agency.
- However, the person availing treatment may request for certification of the intended treatment for obtaining 'medical permit' or 'conversion of visa to medical visa' as mentioned above to be submitted by patient in FRRO/FRO.

Inpatient Treatment

While providing treatment to any foreign national with mental health issues following should be taken care of following:

At time of admission:
- Assess for possession of valid travel documents, i.e. passport and visa
- Check for period of validity of passport and visa
- Keep copy of these documents as record
- Inform FRRO/FRO by filling FORM C within 24 hours of admission
- Inform concerned Embassy
- If language barrier, request Embassy to provide a translator for formal assessment
- If no relative or nominated representative accompanying, inform them through email or phone call
- Informing mental health review board or magistrate as per the relevant sections of admission as per Mental Healthcare Act, 2017.

At time of discharge: After improvement, at time of discharge, consider following:[2,5]
- Giving medical letter to carry on board mentioning diagnosis, medications and any other assistance needed during journey
- Certain countries and airlines have restriction on carrying narcotic and psychotropic substances, so, psychiatrist prescription is of most importance
- Ensure all medications are mentioned in generic name
- Patients should be advised to pack necessities such as medications in a carry-on bag in case checked luggage arrival is delayed.
- Contact details of phone and email of treating team to be contacted by the future mental health professional in case of need
- Anticipating travel stress, rehearsing responses to potential stressors, and practicing relaxation and breathing exercises are all helpful preparatory interventions
- Breathing exercises, regular stretches, abstinence from alcohol and plentiful fluid intake (not caffeinated) minimize the dehydrating effects of flight and avoiding drug toxicity
- Certain antipsychotic drug regimens can cause skin reactions at destinations where the sun is unaccustomedly strong 24 and such reactions can be misinterpreted in a delusional way in vulnerable persons with mental illness, cautious use of those drugs or informing client well in advance of this possibility[6]
- During flight to ensure, regular routine, medication compliance and adequate hydration/calorie intake
- Discuss with person arranging for air travel, if the concerned airlines needs a medical certificate regarding fitness for air travel and the level of assistance needed on board or liaison with the airport medical services.

■ FITNESS FOR AIR TRAVEL

Need of assessment: In a study by Matsumoto & Goebert in 2001, only 3.5% of all medical in-flight emergencies in the USA were categorized as due to psychiatric illness. In 90% of the latter, the diagnosis was that of an anxiety state, and in only 4% was it a psychotic disorder.[7]

According to a study published by World Health Organization (WHO) in 2016, three main medical illnesses are associated with air travel, cardiac problems, physical injuries and mental illnesses. Acute psychotic attacks were cause of repatriation in nearly 20% of psychiatry problems encountered in air travel.[8] Although the frequency of psychiatric emergencies is much lower than that of other medical emergencies inflight, the control of disturbed behavior in an aircraft poses much greater potential hazards than on the ground. Thus, preparedness in vulnerable clients is of utmost importance in interest of person with mental illness and public at large.

What it is: As per guidelines for medical professionals by Aviation Health Unit, UK Civil Aviation Authority, following are important considerations to assess for 'fitness to fly':[9]
- Will the condition interfere with safe conduct of flight?
- Will the flight environment exacerbate the condition?

In which situations this assessment is needed: Thus, Assessment of fitness to travel by air is advisable in following situations:[10]
- Recent illness/injury
- Recent Hospitalization/surgery
- Any acute or chronic condition where special services are required such as oxygen, use of a stretcher, or authority to carry or use accompanying medical equipment or medical escort.

Assessment and advice: A stable client is fit for travel. It is advisable to continue medicines during flight. Ensure regular routine during flight and good hydration. In case of any slightest possibility of any unexpected violent aggressive behavior, it is advisable to inform the airlines for need of travelling with a medical escort or a health professional along with necessary mouth dissolving oral or injectable medicines needed in hand bag along for such situation and verbal de-escalation techniques explained well in advance to such person. Liasioning beforehand with aviation medical services is always a better idea.

REFERENCES

1. Felkai P, Kurimay T. The most vulnerable travelers: patients with mental disorders. World Psychiatry. 2011;10(3):237.
2. Seeman MV. Travel risks for those with serious mental illness. Int J Travel Med Glob Health. 2016;4(3):76-81.
3. Bureau of Immigration (boi), Ministry of Home Affairs. Government of India. https://boi.gov.in.
4. General Policy Guidelines Relating to Indian Visa. https://mha.gov.in/PDF_Other/annexi_01022018.pdf.
5. Vermersch C, Geoffroy PA, Fovet T, et al. Travel and psychotic disorders: clinical aspects and practical recommendations. Presse Med. 2014;43(12 Pt 1):1317-24.
6. Potasman I, Beny A, Seligmann H. Neuropsychiatric problems in 2500 long-term young travelers to the tropics. J Travel Med. 2000;7(1):5-9.
7. Matsumoto K, Goeber TD. In-flight psychiatric emergencies. Aviation, Space and Environmental Medicine. 2001;72:919-23.
8. World Health Organization (WHO). International travel and health. Psychological health. General considerations. Geneva, Switzerland: WHO, 2016. http://www.who.int/ith/other_health.
9. Assessing fitness to fly. Guidelines for medical professionals by Aviation Health Unit, UK Civil Aviation Authority.
10. Gordan H, Kingham M, Goodwin T. Psychiatric Bulletin. 2004;28:295-7.

Index

A

Abortion 47
Abstinence from alcohol 458
Absurd symptomatology 123
Abuse by child, handling disclosure of 236
Access medical records, right to 76, 260
Access mental healthcare, right to 400
Access to health, right to 258
Accidental disclosure 233
Accompanying legal documents 204
Accused during stages of trial, rights of 171
Acid attack victim 292
Act
 of commission 49
 of omission 49
 of person incapable 198
 public authorities 73
Addict 278
Addiction
 expert 437
 phenomenology of 435
 psychiatrist 437
 psychiatry 434
Additional considerations 180
Additional riders in incapacity reports 187
Address child's psychosocial distress, directly 410
Adequate information, provision of 428
Adjudicative competency 181
Administration of polygraph test, guidelines for 91
Administrative and policy related factors 397, 398
Admission and Discharge Provisions of Mental Healthcare Act, 2017 267
Admission authorization 268
Admission/denial of documents 169

Adultery 47
Adulthood presentation 232
Adversarial system 170
Advertising 44
Advisory committee 416
 role 416
Affinity, relationship of 150
African admixtures 109
African-American
 adolescents, behavior of 109
 genetic heritage 109
Aggravated offences 229
Aggression 345
 psychology of 345
Agitation
 high levels of 359
 particularly level of 178
Aid of counsel 171
Air travel 459
Alcohol 287
 abuse 140
 and drugs, abuse of 250, 288
 limit and punishment in India 287
 subject of state list 287
 use 178
Alcoholic amnesia 439
Allopathic 21
Altruistic 375
Alzheimer's disease 140, 353, 354, 430-432
Amentia 4
American Academy of Psychiatry and Law 6, 5, 10, 96
American admixtures 109
American Board
 of Clinical Neuropsychology 121
 of Forensic Psychiatry 10
American Medical Association 100
American Psychiatric Association 100, 452
Amoxicillin 219
Amphetamine 48, 280, 288

Anticipated secondary sex characteristics 408
Anticipating travel stress 458
Antipsychotic
 discovery of 6
 drug regimens 458
 medication 19
Anti-rabies vaccine 99
Antisocial behavior 362
Antisocial personality disorder 374, 380
Anxiety 211, 231, 359, 422
 disorders, prevalence of 228
Anxiousness 329
Appeal in High Court 274
Appellate authority 24
Appellate powers 35
Appointment of substitute 42
Appropriate authority 416
Arousal 350, 359
Arrests and self-reported violence, rates of 382
Artificial insemination 46, 64
Asperger's syndrome 360
Assault or criminal force 211
Assessing testamentary capacity, process for 144
Assessment and advice 459
Assistant sessions judges 163
Assisted suicide 327
Associated psychosis 358
Association between violence and sleep disturbance, assessment of 356
Attack with pellet gun and knife 43
Attendance and examination 39
Attendance in court 165
Attention deficit hyperactivity disorder 353, 361
 risk of violence 361
 symptoms 361
Attestation 136
Audit and process of inquiry 257
Audit in routine course 257
Audit/inquiry, reporting of 258
Auditory hallucinations 179

Australian bureau of statistics 396
Australian legal system 182
Authorization Committee 416
Authorization, process of 416
Autistic spectrum disorders 353, 360
Autrefois acquit, principle of 171
Awareness building measures 277
Awareness of potential areas of litigation and medicolegal problems 52
Awareness of rights 312
Ayurveda, yoga and naturopathy, unani, sidha and homoeopathy (AYUSH) 250
Azithromycin 219

B

Bailable offences 166, 190
Bar of jurisdiction 275
Beast test 199
Behavior outside interview 124
Behavioral clues 141
  to undue influence 142
Behavioral consequences 115
Behavioral science consultation teams 100
Behavioral trials 411
Benchmark disabilities 292
Beneficence 94
Benzodiazepines 219, 435
Best interest of child 214
Betrayal and lack of trust 231
Betrayal through medicine 91
Biased language 116
Biological functions, record of 180
Biological psychiatry 6
Biopsychosocial model of violence 348
Biopsychosocial strategy, management 108
Bipolar disorder 140
Bisexual 407
Bizarre 123
  behavior 178
Black's law dictionary, according to 49
Blanket consent 64
Blindness 291

Blood
  pressure 87
  tests 440
Board of governors 22, 34
Body gestures 125
Body image concerns, prevalence of 228
Body-mass index 423
Bombay Prevention of Begging Act, 1959 399
Borstal or juvenile homes 164
Boundary violations 54
Brahm-hatya 18
Brain
  death, cases of 417
  electrical oscillation signature, data from 90
  fingerprinting 86, 88, 89
  injury 141
  lesions 141
  mapping 88
  mapping and brain fingerprinting 88
    drawbacks 89
    principle 89
    procedure 89
    uses 89
  neuroanatomy of 435
  neurobiological activity in 435
  signature profiling 90
  spatial representations of 88
  tumors 328
Breathing exercises 458
British crime survey 364
British house of lords 446
Buddhism and Jainism allow euthanasia 450
Bullying 423
  and chronic stress 422
  and somatic symptoms 422
Buprenorphine 280, 281
Burden of proof 51

C

Callous-unemotional traits 379, 380
Campus police 43
Cancer 328
Candidates for transplant, psychosocial assessment of 419

Cannabis 278
Capability of weighing 419
Capacity key components 59
Capacity to consent 58
  age for 58
Cardiac problems 459
Cardinal ethical principles 428
Career dissatisfaction 123
Case laws from
  Indian courts 202
  United Kingdom 182
  United States 183
Casualty medical officer 401
Categorization of filicide 375
Causing death, intention of 373
Cell block 99
Census houses 396
Central authority 75
  regulations 251
Central Bureau of Narcotics 279
Central Committee for Research on Disability 293
Central Government Health Scheme 457
Central information commission 24, 72, 74
Central Mental Health Authority 249, 251, 256
Centre for fingerprinting and diagnostics, 2007 74
Cerebral palsy 19, 24, 292
Certificate 35
  of disability
    application for 295
    issue of 296
  of identity 413
  validity of 298
Chaotic thinking 4
Charas 280
Charcot's research on hypnosis 6
Chemical examiner's report 117
Child abuse, failure to report 239
Child and family, confidentiality of 240
Child for pornographic purposes, use of 230
Child Reformation Centre 164
Child sexual abuse 227, 228, 243
  effects of 231
  epidemiology 227
  short-term effects of 231

Index

Child with benchmark disability 292
Child-friendly measures for recording statement 240
Childhood
  bullying and forensic psychiatry 421
  parasomnias, history of 356
  sexual
    abuse 232
    offences 228
Children from Sexual Offences Act, protection of 20, 27, 43, 218, 228, 234, 238
Christian Law 26
Cigarette and Tobacco Products Act, 2003 19
Cigarettes and other tobacco products 22
Cisgender 407
Civil and criminal
  cases 116
    treatment decisions in 313
  legal context, variety of 11
Civil aspects of mental health 11
Civil assessments 83
Civil cases 63
Civil negligence 50
Civil or criminal trials 101
Civil trial 169
  stages in 169
Claim of future decompensation 123
Claim professional secrecy 43
Claimed harm 437
Clinical forensic psychiatry 10
Clinical leadership, lack of 351
Clinicians assisting forensic interviewing 241
Clock-drawing test 146
Clozapine 57
CME programs 35
Cocaine 280
Code of civil procedure 169
Code of criminal procedure 170, 175
Code of medical ethics 37
  regulations, 2002 70
Code of professional secrecy 41
Codeine 278
  formulations 287
Codicil 135

Coexisting homelessness and mental disorders 397
Cognitive deficits 184, 397, 398
Cognitive distortions 140
Cognitive faculties, impairment of 203
Cognitive function
  as appropriate, assessment of 178
  assessment of 204
Cognitive impairment 146, 354, 362, 428, 431, 432
  severe 140
Cognitive pillars 428
Cognitive schemas 105
Cognitive tests 86
Cognitive-behavioral therapy 392
Collateral information 83
  and records 203
Collective violence 346
Colonial period, concept of 7
Commissioner of Food and Drugs Control Administration 283, 284
Committee on medical ethics 446
Committing crime, time of 176
Common cognitive screening tests 145
Common elements of systems 182
Common law 161
Common witness 118
Communication 59
Community
  alternatives for crisis care 403
  factors 381
  living states, right to 400
Comorbid psychiatric conditions 412
Comorbid substance abuse 397, 398
Comorbidity
  rates of 397
  with mental disorders 361
Companies Act, 1956 73
Comparative crime statistics, sources of 364
Compartmentalized confidentiality 69
Competence assessment and management issues in criminal cases 82

for standing trial for defendants with mental retardation 186
Competence to give evidence 224
Competence to stand trial 181
Competency assessment instrument 185
Competency screening test 185
Competency to stand trial-revised, evaluation of 186
Complain and redressal of grievances 48
Compromise judgment 140
Computerization of records 71
Concentration ability 177
Conceptual controversies 444
Concerning alleged crime 204
Concerning mentally ill
  challenges 247
  special issues 247
Conduct disorder 362
  and oppositional-defiant disorder 353, 362
  presence of 361
Conduct in consultation 42
Conduct money 165, 167
Conduct proper suicide risk assessment, failure to 54
Conducting forensic interview 84
Confessions, assessing
  reliability of 179
  suggestibility of 179
Confidentiality specific for mental health settings, principles of 69
Conflict rule 68
Confusion, particularly level of 178
Congenital problems 430
Consent 97, 374, 378
  and capacity assessment 56
  elements of 57
  types of 57
  waiver of 216
Constitutes basic medical record 261
Constitution of India 171
Consumer advocacy 403
Consumer Protection
  Act, 1986 19, 23, 56, 70
  rules, 1987 23
Consumer self-help 403

Consumer-operated programs 403
Content of certification 412
Content of delusional 432
Contraceptive sterilization 64
Contracts competency in addicts 438
Contravention
　of law, stringent penalties for 418
　of Provisions of Act 274
Control of Tobacco Products Act 289
Control question technique 87
Control supply of drugs 277
Controlled substance 278
Controversy, area of 73
Conversion disorders 154
Convicted by court of law 46
Cooperation, lack of 122
Cornerhouse forensic interview protocol 241
Cortical subcortical 354
Council for International Organizations of Medical Sciences 321
Country specific legal statutes 182
Course of admission 402
Course of commission of offence 213
Court of appeal 162
Court of law 43, 175
Court ordered
　evaluations 62
　examination 43
Court questions 167
Court regarding victims of sexual violence 223, 242
Courtroom behavior 119
Courts in India and judicial process 161
Covered under health insurance 413
Covers offices of public authorities 71
C-reactive protein 423
Crescendo-decrescendo of natural affects 125
Crime
　against humanity 214
　and criminal justice statistics 364
　and violence from developmental perspective 380
　in social context 363
　neighborhood, high 381
　prevention, social factors in 368
Criminal Acts 63
Criminal assessments 83
Criminal behavior
　biological explanation of 379
　in addicted individual 440
　neurobiology of 379
Criminal cases 63, 89
Criminal code of Canada 182
Criminal courts, procedures in 165
Criminal force, use of 211
Criminal justice system
　goal of 174
　world fact book of 364
Criminal law 11
　adjective 170
　Amendment Act, 2013 211, 218
　and Mental Health 20, 27
　procedural 170
　real 170
Criminal matters 439
Criminal negligence 50
Criminal offenses, cases of 162
Criminal procedure
　code 161, 215, 399
　rules of Florida 182
Criminal process
　accuracy of 175, 181
　preserving dignity of 175, 182
Criminal responsibility 95
　assessment 175
　in India 198
Criminal trial 170
　stages in 170
Criminal violence 346
Criminalizes
　consensual sexual intercourse 27
　denying access 413
Criminogenic factors 351
Crisis intervention 220
Critical Appraisal of Rights of Persons with Disabilities Act, 2016 295
　Rules, 2017 298
Cross-examination 119, 167
　by defendant 170
　by plaintiff 170
Culpability of doctor 51
Culpable homicide 373
　amounting to murder 374
　not amounting to murder 374
　types of 374
Cultural agencies 107
Cultural background 106
Cultural contexts and mental health 106
Cultural explanations 105
Cultural framework governs 107
Cultural homogeneity 103
Culture
　influences 104
　on distress, impact of 104
　shock 455
Current mental status examination 204
Custodial care 427
Custody cases 439
Cyber-bullying 421
　consequences of 424
Cybercrime 347
Cyclobarbital 288
Cyclophosphamide 288

D

Data tampering 123
de Clérambault's syndrome 357
Dead body 63
Deaf and hard of hearing 292
Death penalty 195
Debatable issues 73
Deceased donor transplant 417
Decision-making
　actively participate in 410
　capacity 428
　in elderly 430
Decree/judgment 170
Decriminalization of Suicide in Mental Healthcare Act, 2017, provision for 332
Defendant evidence 170
Defendant, appearance of 169
Defendant's faculties 204
Defensiveness 125
Delhi State Health Mission 403
Deliberate fire-setting 363

Delinquency 368
Delirium 141
Delivery
   and abortion 63
   of judgment 171
Delusional disorders 141, 353, 357
Delusions 140, 141
Dementia 4, 140, 141, 353, 354, 430
   and offending behavior 354
   diagnosis of 433
   syndrome 354
Dementing illnesses 433
Denial of symptoms 106
Depression 14, 140, 211, 232, 329
   developed 422
   prevalence of 228
   recurrent 154
Depressive patients 109
Dextromethorphan 440
   amount of 440
Diagnosing malingering, difficulty in 122
Diffuse cognitive deficits 140
Digitalized format 71
Dignity 48
Diminish auditory hallucinations 124
Diminished responsibility 201
Direct aggression 345
Directorate General of Health Services 70, 71
Disability
   Act, 1995 291
   calculation 296
   conditions of relevance for mental health 292
   covered 291
   developmental 430
   indicating period of validity, certificate of 296
   types of 291
Discharge from psychiatry hospital 193
Discharge planning 194
Disciplinary control 35, 36
Disclose professional secrets 46
Disclosure under right to information 72
Discriminatory practices for persons with mental illness 153

Disinhibition 362
Disorder
   major 152
   of reason 4
Dispense medicine, right to 47
Dispositive plan, impact of 431
Disrupted normal routine 455
Dissociative amnesia 358
Dissociative reaction 12
Distorted views about sexuality 233
Distractibility 184
Distress felt, experience of 407
District Mental Health Programme 19
District Session's Court 163
Disulfiram treatment 57
Divorce 13
   competency to 438
   concept of 151
   or judicial separation 151
Doctor-patient relationship 33, 48, 52
Doctor-state relationship 33
Doctrine of informed consent 57, 58
Documentary evidence 117
Documentation 221
   for testamentary capacity and undue influence 147
Domestic cruelty, rate of 385
Domestic violence 348, 387
   encompasses traditional cultural practices 384
   experienced, identification of 389
   impact of 387
   lifetime prevalence of 384
   prevalence of 387
   risk factors for 389
Donation of important solid organs 415
Donor management, cost of 417
Donor's mental condition, awareness 418
Donor's motivation and expectations 419
Dowry
   deaths 365
   system 386
Dram shop case 439

Drug 276
   abuse
      and crime 276
      and Indian legislation 277
      consumption of 455
   classification of 276
   controller general of India 278
   related criminal activities 434
   use 178
Drugs and Cosmetics
   Act, 1940 288
      violate provisions of 46
   Rules, 1945 288
Drunk and disorderly 46
Drunk driving 287
Duration of illness 204
Durham's test 201
Duties of doctor 37
   in consultation 41
   in general 37
   towards patients 38
   towards state 38
Duties of patient 48
Duty of confidentiality 68
Dwarfism 292
Dying declaration 117
Dynamics of violence 386
Dysphoria 407
   and sex reassignment interventions 406
Dysthymia 154

E

Eating disorders, prevalence of 228
Economic
   and health factors 367
   and physical environments 104
Educational ability, low 368
Efficiency in modern medicine, issue certificates of 46
Elder abuse 432
Electroconvulsive therapy 109, 271
   form of 19
Electrodermal reaction 87
Eligibility for hormonal therapies, assessment of 410
Eligibility for surgical therapies, assessment of 410

Emergency
- admission and treatment, procedure for 319
- case of 41
- contraception 219
- medical care 63, 218, 234
- situations 319
- treatment 271, 319
  - in Mental Healthcare Act, 2017, provision of 62

Emotional distress 179
Employers' report of behavior 83
Enactment of Protection of Human Rights Act 175
Endocrine status 409
Enjoy legal capacity 24
Enquiry stage 190
Ensure maximum privacy 84
Environment, assessment of 143
Epigenetic programming 421
Epilepsy 353, 355
- diagnosis of 356

Episodes of bullying 421
Episodic dyscontrol syndrome 356
Equality and nondiscrimination, right to 259
Erroneous conviction 177
Essential narcotic drugs 278, 282
Essentials of will making 135
Estimating prevalence of mental health, substance 396
Ethical conflicts 93
Ethical considerations 337
Ethical dilemma 93, 95, 122
- in forensic interviewing 241
- of reporting 239

Ethical guidelines for forensic psychiatry 96
Ethical issues in forensic psychiatry 93
- research 98

Ethical principles
- beneficence 214
- justice or fairness 214
- non-maleficence 214
- respect for autonomy 214

Ethical problem of free will 99
Ethical professional 116
Ethics 15
- and forensic psychiatry 95
- and psychiatry 93

in research
- committees, proactive role of 100
- involving prisoners 98
- review committee 100

Ethnicity
- culture and forensic psychiatry 102
- denotes 109
- in forensic psychiatry 109

Ethological theory 349
European commission 365
European Federation of National Organizations Working with Homeless 395
European genetic inheritance 109
European typology of homelessness and housing exclusion 395
Euthanasia 45, 444, 445, 450
- active 447, 450
- and assisted suicide labelling 448
- and living wills 444
- classification of 446
- elements 445
- passive 450

Evidence 170
- collection of 170
- of behavioral disturbances 148
- of confusion 180
- of defense 171
- of distractedness 184
- of psychomotor retardation 184
- of quick change 180
- of suggestibility 180
- of undue compliance 180
- recording of 165, 167

Evidentiary value 14
Exaggeration 125
- of actions 179
- of existing symptoms 123

Examination of person with impotence 156
Execution of decree 170
Execution of will 134, 135, 137
Executive magistrates 162, 163
Exercise equal legal capacity, right to 294
Exercise while taking consent, cautions to 63

Existential vulnerability, sense of 377
Expeditious trial 171
Expert witness 6, 118, 223
Expressed consent 57
Expressive or reactive violence 347
Eye movement desensitization and reprocessing 392

F

Facial expression 125
Fact of mental illness 155
Factitious disorder 127
Factual narration 92
Faculty Development Program 35
Fair trial
- from natural justice's perspective 175
- from rights perspective 175
- principles, violation of 177

False imputation 123
Falsely reporting 239
Familial factors 367
Family
- and caregivers of persons with mental illness, rights of 312
- concerns 239
- environment 381
- interactions, assessment of 419
- members of deceased 335
- self-help and advocacy 403
- violence 348

Farwell's brain fingerprinting 89
Fear 231
- of violence 378

Feeling of powerlessness 231
Feigning psychotic symptoms 123
Felony crimes 54
Fentanyl 278, 287
Fenway LGBT guide 409
Feticide 375
Fetishistic transvestism 409
Fiduciary duty 68
Fiduciary relationship 68, 69
- element of 67

Filing of charge sheet 170
Filing of evidence
- of affidavit by defendant 170
- of affidavit by plaintiff 170

Filing of replication 169

Filing of written statement by defendant 169
Final argument 170
 of both sides 171
Financial compensation 49
Financial decision
 capacity to make 60
 requires 314
Financial incentive 123
Financial philosophies 103
FIR, registration of 170
Fire-setting 353, 363
Fitness
 criteria for 182
 for air travel 458
 for execution, assessment of 172
 for interrogation, assessment of 82, 172, 175
 for standing trial, assessment of 82, 172, 175
 interview test 186
 situation of 178
 to plead 181
 to stand trial 113, 181
  assessment 187
Focusing on target audience 115
Food Safety and Regulation (prohibition) Act, 2011 289
Foreign medical qualifications, recognition of 35
Foreign nationals with mental health problems, treatment of 455
Foreigners Act, 1939, registration of 456
Foreigners Regional Registration Officer 456
Foreigners Registration
 in India 456
 officer 456
Forensic
 aspects of bullying 424
 assessment 96
 empathy 84
 psychiatric administration supervision 14
 science 33
Forensic interview 240
 in India 81
Forensic psychiatrist 6, 7, 11, 97
 during different stages of trial, role of 174
 fundamental 435

Forensic psychiatry 10, 14, 33, 95, 175, 178, 427
 and crime 369
 basic principles of 435
 case 85
 concept of 11
 current issues in 12
 disciplines of 95
 evaluation 81
 history of 3
 in India 13
 interview 81
  context of 81
 report 115
  quality of 81
 special investigative techniques in 87
Forensic report
 structure of 113, 115
 without clinical interview, producing 97
Form of Will 136
Formal mental health assessment, lack of 174
Formal relationship 49
Framing of charges/serving notice 170
Framing of issues 170
Free education, right to 292
Free legal aid 240
Freedom of Information Act, 2004 71
Frequent yeast infections 236
Freudian theories 350
Frontotemporal dementia 430
Frontotemporal lobar degeneration 431
Functional magnetic resonance imaging 379
Functional neuroimaging studies 379
Functional symptoms 387
Functional test of capacity 178

G

Galvanic skin response 86
Gambling Laws in India 289
Gang membership 368
Gang rape 213
Gang violence 347
Ganja 280

Gathering collateral information 180
Gay 407
Gender and offending rates 366
Gender dysphoria 407, 408
 accurately diagnose 412
 describes 407
 diagnosis of 410
 expression of 407
 identifying 408
 in children 408
 questionnaire for adolescents and adults 409
Gender dysphoric disorder 409
Gender expression 407
Gender identity 409
 disorder 408
 interview for children 408
 questionnaire for children 408
Gender nonconformity 407
Gender role, concept of 407
Gender-normative behavior 407
Gender-typical behaviors 410
General Assembly of World Psychiatric Association 305
General hospital psychiatry 427
 units 305
General principles and ethical considerations 214, 232
Generic names of drugs, use of 38
Genetic and neuroendocrine studies 379
Genetics and violence 349
Genital injuries 210
Genital surgery 156
Genitalia, measurements of 410
Genitoanal examination 217
Geriatric
 mental health 430
 psychiatrists 143
 psychiatry 433
Giving expert testimony 119
Global developmental delay 296
Global report card on adolescents 2012 386
Good medical practice, maintaining 37
Good report, characteristics of 115
Greater community participation 28
Greater cultural acceptance of violence 386

Group hostility 350
Guantanamo incidence 100
Guarantees OBC status 413
Guardians and Wards Act,1890 68
Guardianship, provision for 294
Gudjonsson compliance scale 180
Gynecological problems 387

H

Hadfield test of delusion 199
Hair samples 62
Handle child's refusal 237
Handling parent's response on disclosure 237
Harm towards, risk of 178
Hashish 280
Head injury
   cases 127
   history of 401
Head trauma 353, 354
Healers 107
Health care
   access to 104
   integrated service systems 404
   seeking
      activities 108
      stigma for 27
   services, professional treatment of 108
Health professionals 213-215, 232, 335, 339
   concerns 239
   legal responsibilities of 215, 457
   role of 213
Health seeking by foreign nationals, context of 456
Health services, quality of 104
Health, right to 214, 304
Healthcare
   service 106, 107
   setting 69
      principles for 67
Hearing impairment 292
Heart rate 87
Helping agency 108
Helping client realize 410
Hemophilia 292
Hierarchy and powers of courts in India 162
Hierarchy of courts in India 162

High court 75
Highest judicial tribunal 162
   of country 161
Hindu Marriage Act, 1955 25,151
Hindu Succession Act 1956, amendments of 134
Home and family, right to 294
Home office research development and statistics publication 364
Homeless person
   having mental illness 400
   with mental illness 400, 401
Homelessness 395, 455
   concept of 395
   measurement of 396
   persistence of 396
   primary 396
   secondary 396
   tertiary 396
   types of 396
Homicidal poisoning, case of 41
Homicide 14, 448
   and mental disorders 373
   victims of 375
Homicide-suicide 327
Homosexual relationships 386
Honesty and striving for objectivity 97
Honor killing 376
   acceptability of 377
   reported, cases of 377
   theories of 377
Hopelessness 329, 358
Hormonal therapy
   and surgery, irreversible 411
   reversible 410
Houseless 395
Housing programs 404
Human behavior 102, 435
   psychosocial development of 102
Human civilization 344
Human dignity, right to 214
Human guinea pig 99
Human macrocosm 109
Human rights 45, 303
   Act, 1993, protection of 19, 23, 303
   in India, implementation of 322

   of persons with mental illness 303
      Indian perspective of 306
Human sexuality
   encompasses 406
   normal 406
Huntington's chorea 353, 355
Huntington's disease 354
Husband's domestic 150
Husband's inability 156
Hydrocodone 278, 287
Hyperactivity disorder 361
Hyperkinetic syndrome 361
Hypervigilance 359

I

Ictal violence 355
Illegal drug trade 347
Illegal procedures, consent for 64
Illicit drug 276
Illness 346
   nature of 204
   related factors 397, 398
   response 106
   severity of 204
Immunity against capital punishment 18
Implantable cardioverter defibrillator 265
Implementation and supervision 72
Implied consent 57
Improper certificates 46
Impulsive behavior 354
Inadequate accommodation 395
Incapacity reports 114
Incarceration, process of 174
Inclusive government funded education 293
Income
   loss of 49
   low and middle 398
Independent qualified mental health professionals 411
India's constitution 303
Indian case laws 174
Indian contract
   Act states 59
   laws 20, 25
Indian Council of Medical Research 457

Index

Indian Divorce Act 1869 152
Indian Evidence Act 170, 224
Indian laws
   concerning marriage and divorce 151
   governing entry, stay and exit of foreign nationals 456
Indian legislation and policies concerning narcotic and psychotropic use 277
Indian Lunacy Act, 1912 248
Indian Lunatic Asylum Act, 1858 18
Indian Medical Association 70
Indian Medical Council Act 22, 19, 34
Indian Medical Degrees Act, 1916 34
Indian Medical Register, maintenance of 34
Indian nationals abroad 25
Indian Penal Code 13, 289
Indian Psychiatric Society guidelines 339
Indian Registration Act, 1908 134
Indian Succession Act 137, 134
Indian Trust Act,1882 68
Indicated medical specimens, collection of 217
Indirect aggression 345
Individual disability certification, guidelines for 296
Individual registered medical practitioners, guidelines for 286
Individual's physical appearance 411
Infant mortality, higher rates of 304
Infanticide
   and associated causes 375
   and related behaviors 375
Inflammation 423
Inflammatory and metabolic processes 421
Information 72
   access to 310
   and Technology Act, 2000 347
   disclosure of 409
   falsified and misleading 46
   sources of 85
   to reach on opinion, source of 114, 187
Informed consent 14, 97, 216, 233, 429
   and limitation of confidentiality 183
   for Act 53
Informed written consent 83
Injury or harm 49
Inpatient care, concepts for 271
Inpatient medical record, basic 76
Insania (disturbed judgment) 4
Insanity 176
   defense 197, 198, 204
      assessment 172, 175, 197
      criteria, evolution of 197, 199
   degree of 202
   nature and degree of 198
   recurrent attack of 155
   test of 198, 202
Instrumental violence 347
Insufferable 452
Insulin 288
Insurance claims 67
Insurance fraud 89
Insurance Regulatory Development Authority Act 1999 306
Integrate mental health 309
Integrated services for co-occurring substance abuse 403
Intellectual disability 292, 296, 299, 353, 360
   diagnosis of 296
   for children 296
Intelligence
   low 381
   quotient, relatively low 179
Interaction with judiciary 274
Intercourse 227
   attempted 227
Interdisciplinary
   fitness interview 185
   team approach 215
Interface of health systems
   and judiciary 223
   and police 223
Interface with
   legal agencies 222
   social welfare agencies 225
Interictal violence 355
International classification of disease 21
International convention
   on civil and political rights 311
   on economic, social and cultural rights, 1966 305
International covenant
   on civil and political rights 175
   on economic, social and cultural rights 305
International crime victims survey 364
Interpretive hypothesis 105
Interrogation of accused 170
Interview
   increase productivity of 177
   technique 124
Interviewer, caution for 125
Intimate partner violence 384
Intoxication, particularly level of 178
Intracavernosal injection 156
Intrafamily violence 368
Invalid consent 62
Investigating officer 400
   request of 66
Investigation and prosecution, procedure for 279
In-vitro fertilization 46
Involuntary euthanasia 447
Involuntary intoxication, defense for 198
Irresistible impulse test 199
Islam 449
Islamic regime 18
Issue false 46
Issues framed 170
Itching in genital area, complaints of 236

J

Jail medical wing, regular reporting by 196
Jail psychiatrist 98, 180
Jeopardize 109
Judaeo-Christian traditions 326
Judaism 449
Judgment 439
Judicial and administrative framework 169

Judicial determination 429
Judicial magistrate 91, 162-164
    first class 450
Judicial presumptions 170
Judicial separation 154
Judicial system 18, 99
Judicial/metropolitan magistrates 163
Juries and judges regarded 6
Justice 94, 96
    access to 294
Juvenile Courts under Children Act, 1960 164
Juvenile Justice Act 164, 399
Juvenile magistrate 164

K

Kidnapping 365
Kidney failure 328
Killing of Brahmin 18
Knowledge of accusation 171
Kraepelin's identification 6

L

Language barrier 458
Large family 368
Law
    and medical science, conflicting positions of 197
    and mental health 15
    and psychiatry in India 17
    and rules governing organ transplantation in India 415
    and testamentary capacity 143
    concerning criminal liability 27
    concerning criminal responsibility 20
    of intoxicated person 289
    concerning suicide 331
    enforcement agencies 215
    of evidence 170
    of karma, basis of 17
    of succession 133
    of torts 161
    relevant to alcohol 287
Law-breaking behavior 352
Lawful punishment 172
Lawyer, role of 187
Learning (intellectual) disabilities 353, 360

Learning disability 178
    specific 292, 297
Legal agencies 27
Legal and moral responsibility 95
Legal aspects 90
    of impotence 156
    specific to India 91
Legal assistance 114
Legal complications 156
Legal context of relevance 67
Legal domain 395
Legal guardians 68
Legal implications 91
Legal insanity 176, 198
Legal medicine 33
Legal passive euthanasia 449
Legal proceedings, types of 96
Legal psychiatry 11
Legal restrictions, evasion of 38
Legal rule 44
Legal status
    globally 448
    of attempted suicide in India 331
Legal statutes concerning
    interface of civil law 20
        and mental health 25
    medical jurisprudence 19, 22
    mental health
        establishments and de-addiction 19, 20
        professional training 20, 27
        protection 23
    substance of abuse 19, 22
Legal statutes of country 177
Legal terminology 176
Legal terms for fitness to stand trial 181, 198
Legislation
    in mental health 247
    related to addition psychiatry in India 276
    role of 322
Legislative statutes of relevance to medical records 70
Leprosy cured persons 292
Less threatening 235
Lewy body
    dementia 140, 354, 430
    disease 431
Liaison with lawyers 14
Liasioning with legal agencies 240

Licenced chemist 278
Licenced dealer 278
Licit drugs 276
Lie detector test 91
Life imprisonment 195
Lifecourse-persistent trajectory 380
Line of demarcation 93
Living donation 418
Living donor transplant case 417
Living Will 450, 451
    principle of 449
Locomotor disability 292
Locoparentis 62
Lotteries (regulation) Act, 1998 289
Low academic achievement 368
Lower life expectancy 104
Low-vision 292
Lunacy (district courts) Act, 1858 18
Lunacy (supreme courts) Act, 1858 18
Lunatic asylum superintendent 6

M

Mad doctor 7
Magistrate
    authorized admission 273
    court 162, 163
    in juvenile court 164
    of person with mental illness, report to 273
Major depression, episode of 14
Male infertility 156
Malingered psychiatry conditions 122
Malingering
    admission of 124
    concept of 122
    in psychiatry settings, assessment of 123
    negative 123
Management issues 108
Mandate of Act 228
Mandatory reporting 238
Manson points 105
Manu's essential philosophy 18
Manufacturing firms, association with 44
Marital discord 156

Marriage and divorce 25
　related
　　acts 20
　　issues 150
Marriage Laws (amendment) Act 151
Maternal childhood sexual abuse 375
Maternal depression 375
Maternal postpartum psychosis 375
McNaghten rules 204
McNaghten test 200
Media on suicide, effect of 330
Medical and surgical care 410
Medical attendant visa 457
Medical authority 297
　single 298
Medical board
　constituent of 114
　details 114, 187
　team 114
Medical certificate
　mentioning admission 457
　record maintenance 71
Medical compliance, history of 419
Medical conditions and suicide 328
Medical confidentiality 40
Medical Council of India 34, 457
Medical Council Regulations 2002 450
Medical defense procedure 53
Medical discipline 427
Medical disorder 328, 346
Medical documents 204
Medical education, continuing 35
Medical emergencies 62, 459
Medical ethics 4, 93
Medical etiquette 33
Medical euthanasia 452
Medical examination
　for legal purposes 234
　for life insurance policy 41
　of sexual assault 216
Medical health professionals 215
Medical indemnity insurance 53
Medical insanity 176, 198
Medical institution 278
Medical jurisprudence 33
　of insanity 4

Medical litigation, preventing 52
Medical maloccurrence 53
Medical malpractice 44
Medical negligence 33, 44, 49, 51
　cases 67
　requires 49
　types of 50
Medical officer
　behavior report 180
　general report 180
　in-charge of registered medical institute, responsibilities of 284
Medical profession 23
Medical qualification
　de-recognition of 35
　granted, recognition of 35
Medical record 66
　as evidence in court 67
　importance of 66
　maintenance of 37
Medical Termination of Pregnancy Act, 1971 376
Medical terminology 176
Medical treatment
　for deaddiction 279
　for de-toxification 279
　of Terminally Ill Patients Bill 451
Medical visa 457
Medical witness 118
Medical/dental practitioners 23
Medical/psychiatry review 195
Medical-psychiatric comorbidity, prevalence of 433
Medications, result of 419
Medicolegal angle 210
Medicolegal cases 49, 234, 417
　of pregnancy 63
　records concerning 66
Medicolegal contexts 125
Medicolegal examination, refusal for 216
Medicolegal injury cases 40
Medicolegal issues 14
　in suicide 325
　of relevance for mental health professionals 301
Medicolegal provisions pertaining to complete suicide in a healthcare setting 333
Medicolegal records 71

Medicolegal reports 47
Medicolegal responsibilities 195, 340
　concerning management of cases of sexual offence 207
　in management
　　of homeless persons with mental illness 395
　　of victims of domestic violence 384
Medicolegal services 213, 232
Medicolegal setting 124
Medicolegal societies 5
Mefloquine 455
Memory
　impairment, mild forms of 140
　malingering, test of 126
Mental behavioral condition 298
Mental capacity 57-59
Mental disability
　certification guidelines for 295
　mild 298
　moderate 298
　rules for 298
　severe 298
Mental disorder 11, 14, 25, 151, 153, 154, 155, 317
　and homicide 374
　and suicide 329
　certain 374
　degree of 151
　diagnosed 116
　for different legal purposes 11
　identifying evidence of 178
　in Ayurveda, forms of 18
　incurability of 153
　presence of 176
　prevalence of 28
Mental health 20, 104, 232
　Act 19, 20, 75, 306, 400, 427
　　1987, relevant sections of 400
　and criminal law, intersection of 159
　assessment 225
　　for fitness 224, 242
　authority 257
　　creation of 248
　Care Act, 2017 67, 70, 75, 193, 196, 288
　　treatment under Section 100 of 456

care and treatment related decision, capacity to make 251
Care Law 307
care, pathways into 108
establishment 194, 249, 250, 288
  categories of 256
  conditions in 311
  maintaining 256
  registration of 256
evaluation and treatment, provision for 272
high prevalence rates of 397
issues 156, 189
laws 307
  in India, history of 248
legislation 247
problems 387
  treatment of 174
professional 76, 121, 243, 251, 404
  dealing with case 335
  impact on 333
  in interrogation, participation of 100
  in jail, shortage of 174
  in sex reassignment interventions, role of 411
  in transplantation process, role of 418
  registered 254
  role of 175, 228, 241
related statues of India 176
resources, scarcity of appropriate 397, 398
review board 249, 252, 255, 256
  constitution of 255
  power and functions of 255
survey report 28
Mental healthcare 250, 256
  (rights of persons with mental illness) Rules, 2018 76
reforms in India 28
Mental Healthcare Act, 2017 19, 21, 169, 247, 248, 308, 309, 424, 428
  concordance of 315
  implications of 250
  provisions of 249
Mental ill-health 304

Mental illness 14, 76, 150, 151, 192, 249, 250, 292, 298, 369, 428
  and increased vulnerability 388
  and offence, association of 353
  and violence 350
  bullying and risk of 422
  in judicial process 275
  in past 189
  insurance for 272
  nature of person's 75
  on medical visa 456
  reason of 456
  screening for 82
  treatment of persons with 315
Mental retardation 19, 309, 360
  and Multiple Disabilities Act, 1999 24
  excludes 250
Mental state
  assessment of 419
  at time of crime 176
Mental status examination of adult victims 217
Mentally ill 194
  cause violence 382
  families and caregivers of 313
  rights of 311
Metabolic dysfunction 423
Methadone 278, 280, 287
Methamphetamine 280, 288
Methylphenidate 288
Meticulous record keeping 53
Metronidazole 219
Military psychiatrist 98
Miller forensic assessment of symptoms 86, 126
Mind deficit, theory of 360
Mind, incomplete development of 151
Mini-mental state examination 145
Ministry of Health and Family Welfare 70, 213
  guidelines for patient record retention 71
Ministry of Home Affairs 457
Ministry of Women and Child Development 227
Ministry of Women and Child Welfare 232

Minnesota multiphasic personality inventory 86, 126
Misleading certificates 46
Missing medications during travel 455
Misunderstanding 180
Mitakshara Law 134
Mobile mental health unit 402, 403
Modern civilization 98
Monitoring by mental health review board, provision of 196
Monoamine oxidase type A 379
Monopolistic rights 150
Monozygotic twins 422
Mood disorders 140, 328, 353, 358, 392, 432
Moral insanity 5
Morbidity and mortality audits 53
Morphine 278, 280
  formulations 287
Motor Accident Claims Tribunal Act 67
Motor Vehicle (amendment) Bill, 2016 288
Motor Vehicles Act, 1988 states 287
Multifactorial psychiatric explanations 366
Multiple Creutzfeldt-Jakob disease 354
Multiple disabilities 292
  Act, 1999 19
Multiple sclerosis 292
Munchausen's syndrome 127
Murder simpliciter 445
Muscular dystrophy 292
Muslim personal law 134

N

Narcotic drug 278
Narcotic Drugs and Psychotropic Substances Act, 1985 19, 20, 22, 277, 287, 434
  amendment 2014, basis for 282
  Consultative Committee 279
Narcotic of relevance to deaddiction psychiatry practice 281

Narcotics commissioner 279
Narcotics control bureau 279
National accreditation board for hospitals and healthcare providers 457
National Consumer Disputes Redressal Commission 51
National crime record bureau 385
  data, 2015 209
  of India 364, 365
National Family Health Survey 384
National fund for control of drug abuse 279
National human organs and tissues removal and storage network 415
National Human Rights Commission 23, 28, 307
National Institute for Mental Health 297
National Institute of Child Health and Human Development Protocol 241
National legal services authority 294
National Mental Health Policy 28, 308
National Mental Health Programme 19, 28, 305
National policy on narcotic drugs and psychotropic substances 277
National Rural Health Mission 403
National security 89
National trust for welfare of persons with autism 19, 24
Natural justice, principle of 170, 175
Nature and Quality of Act, knowing 176
Negligence 14
  concept of 50
  consists 49
  gross 52
  suits 43
Neo-darwinist biological determinism 349
Neurocognitive disorder 434
  mild 433
Neurocognitive tests 433

Neurodegenerative
  dementia, cases of 431
  diseases 431
  disorders 430, 432
Neuroendocrine responses 421, 423
Neurological conditions, chronic 292
Neurological disease 141
Neurological disorders 153
Neuronal nitric oxide synthase 379
Neuropsychological deficits 361
Neurotic and stress-related disorders 353, 358
Neurotransmitters 435
Neutral attitude 84
New mental health related, assessment of 419
New Mental Health Act 2017 188
Nightmares 232
No objection certificate 418
Non compos mentis 4
Nonbailable offences 190
Nonbailable warrant 166
Noncognizable offenses, cases of 164
Non-discrimination, right to 214
Nonfatal assaults 378
Non-government organizations 215
Non-Indian nationals 417
Nonmaleficence 94, 428
Nonmedical reader, descriptions for 115
Nonvoluntary euthanasia 447
Nosology 122
Nuremberg code governing research 99
Nurses, occupational therapists 335
Nursing home care difficulties 433

O

Oath taking 165
Obsessive compulsive disorders 154
Occupation and legal title, security of 395
Offence
  abetment of 230
  and penalties 279
  under NDPS Act 280, 280

and Punishment under Protection of Children from Sexual Offences Act, 2012 229
  under Railway Act, try cases of 164
Offending behavior
  association with 362
  onset of 382
One's masculinity or feminity, sense of 406
Open trial, right to 171
Operant conditioning 350
Opiophobia 281
Opposite of shame 410
Oppositional defiance disorder 362
Oral consent 57
Oral evidence 117
  types of 118
Organ donation
  option of 417
  purpose of 417
Organ transplantation on immunosuppressants 455
Organic mental disorders 353
Organization of Narcotic Drugs and Psychotropic Substances Act 277, 278
Organized violence 347
Orientation and sexual activity, terms of 406
Overcrowding 351
Oxycodone 278, 287

P

Pain during elimination 236
Pain, chronic 328
Palliative care 451
Panchayats 71
Panel of doctors responsible 416
Parade of white coats 410
Paranoid cognition 359
Paranoid delusions 141
Parental criminality 368
Parental involvement, lack of 368
Parkinson's disease 292, 354, 430, 431
Parsi Marriage and Divorce Act, 1936 26
Passport (entry into India) Act, 1920 456

Patent and copyrights 45
Patient-doctor relationship 67
Patients and Medical Practitioners Bill, protection of 451
Patriarchal social structure 386
Peer victims, chronic 421
Pejorative term 122
Pelvic inflammatory disease 210
Pelvic pain 210
   chronic 387
Pelvic surgery 156
Penal erasure 47
Penalties for offences 295
Penetrative sexual assault 229
Peno-vaginal penetration 27
Pentobarbital 288
Perpetrator dynamics, victims 231
Persistence of violence, risk factors for 381
Person to make will, competency of 136
Person with mental illness
   admission of 268
   under MHCA, 2017, admission of 269
Personal contacts and communication, right to 264
Personal information disclosure 73
Personal records 83
Personality assessment inventory 86, 126
Personality disorder 178, 351, 353, 359, 374
   severe 409
Personality inventory for youth 126
Personality, assessment of 86
Persons with disabilities 19
   Act 23, 248, 306, 308
      rights of 298
      2016, rights of 13, 20, 291, 292, 308
   Rules, 2017, rights of 295
Persons with mental illness, rights of 249, 258, 304, 321
Peyronie's disease 156
Pharmaceutical and allied health sector industry 45
Pharmacological torture 91
Philosophical debate, area of 348

Phobias 232
   social 211
Physical
   abuse 391
   domain 395
   examination, complete 401
   health, impact on 387
   ill health during travel 455
   illnesses and injuries, interventions for 219
   injuries 387
   and mental illnesses 459
   signs of intersex 409
Physical/mental illness, chronic 367
Physician sentiment 448
Physiological stress response 424
Pick's disease 354
Place of habitation 396
Plaintiff (patient) bears 51
Plaintiff evidence 170
Plastic surgeon, consists of 411
Pleasure in life, loss of 329
Police custody 41
Police transcript, assessing 180
Political phenomenon 348
Political will, lack of 397, 399
Polygraph 89
   in court, admissibility of 88
   test 87, 88, 91
Poor coping ability 329
Poor impulse control 329
Poor problem-solving skills 381
Poppy straw 280
Population attributable fractions of domestic violence 387
Positive emission tomography 379
Positive malingering 123
Post-darwinist view 377
Postexposure prophylaxis 219
Post-traumatic stress disorder 12, 211, 358, 387
   and anxiety 232
   complex 388
   prevalence of 228
   treatment for 121
Post-treatment ethical and legal difficulties faced in India 412
Post-trial
   rights 172
   stages 171, 172

Postvention guidelines 333, 340
Postvention protocols 334
Potential psychological effects, aware of 411
Potential victims 27
Potentially therapeutic 156
Poverty and unemployment 395
Powers of civil court to summon any person 416
Powers of Courts 162
Powers of Session Courts 162, 163
Powers of Supreme Court 162
Practice medicine, right to 47
Practice of clinical psychiatry 427
Prayopavesa 326
Pre-conception and Pre-natal Diagnostic Test Act, 1994 71, 376
Predisposition to comorbid medical illnesses 398
Pre-existing mental
   health condition 179
   illness, assessment of 419
Pregnancy
   and STDs in sexually abused children 234
   prophylaxis 219
   test 234
Pre-Islamic tribal culture of Baluchistan 376
Premenstrual syndrome 12
Prenatal Diagnostic Techniques Act, 1994 71, 376
Presentation of foreign nationals, context of 456
Presumption of capacity 59
Pre-transplant assessment of living donors 419
Pre-transplant psychosocial
   assessment of family 419
   evaluation 419
Pre-trial rights 171
Pre-trial stages 170, 172
Prevalent Muslim Law 26
Prism of modern legal and mental health field 204
Prisoners with mental illness 193, 273
Pritchard criteria 182
Private defense, right of 374
Process interview, ability to 177
Professional death sentence 47

Professional ethics 93
Professional jargon 115
Professional misconduct 35, 44, 45
Professional negligence, cases of 64
Profound mental disability 298
Prohibition of advertisement and regulation of trade and commerce 22
Prohibition on double jeopardy 171
Prolonged detention of mentally ill
  due to administrative lapses 174
  due to perpetual inability 174
Proper counseling and informed consent 53
Proper execution of sentence 172
Prophylactic drugs 455
Prosecution evidence, recording of 171
Protect larger public interests 75
Protection against illegal arrest 171
Protection from abuse, violence and exploitation 293
Protective privilege 44
Pseudoephedrine 440
Pseudohermaphroditism 410
Pseudopsychopathic schizophrenia 357
Psychiatric activity 10
Psychiatric disorders 139, 140, 154, 353, 357, 455
  during travel, developing 455
Psychiatric evaluation 437
Psychiatric illness 18
  developing 456
  history of 204
  presence of 419
  recurrence of 419
Psychiatric morbidity 14
Psychiatric negligence, common forms of 54
Psychiatric participation in interrogation 100
Psychiatric patients 389
  experiencing domestic violence, interventions for 392

Psychiatric social workers 215
Psychiatric symptomatology 388
Psychiatric symptoms 148, 184
Psychiatrist
  as expert witness, role of 117
  during different stages of trials, role of 172
  in insanity defense assessments, role of 203
  in organ transplantation, legal responsibility of 415
  role of 172, 410
Psychiatry 121
  assessment 81
  case records and right to access records 66
  center, inpatients of 397
  evaluation, components of 412
  hospital 194
    admission in 193
  information, nature of 76
  malpractice lawsuits 54
  misuse in 452
  problems 459
  subspecialties 427
  wing in prisons medical wing, provision of 196
Psychogenic impotence 156
Psychogenic reaction to stress 358
Psychologic testing 127
Psychological abuse 391
Psychological assault 378
Psychological assessment 180
  of malingering 125
  of personality and malingering 204
  report 266
Psychological autopsy 336
  goals of 337
  utility of 337
Psychological consequences 210
Psychological distress 105
Psychological effects
  of child sexual abuse 228
  of domestic violence 388
Psychological instruments for fitness to trial assessment 185
Psychological intervention 219, 392
Psychological milieu 148
Psychological sequelae 127

Psychological test 86, 126
  for assessment of malingering 126
  limitations of 127
  report of 114, 187
Psychologists 215
Psychologize symptoms, inability to 105
Psychometric testing 125
Psychopathic disorder 25
Psychopathological disorder 128
Psychopathy 380
Psychophysiological detection of deception 87
Psychosis, presence of 432
Psychosocial intervention 114
Psychosocial professionals, efforts of 410
Psychosocial rehabilitation services 403
Psychosomatic medicine 427
Psychotherapy 411
Psychotic
  attacks, acute 459
  disorders, classification of 6
  disorganization symptoms 184
  symptoms, exacerbation of 387
Psychotropic substance 278
Public and private school, teachers of 297
Public authorities 73
Public Gambling Act, 1867 289
Public interest litigation 28, 307
Public mental health establishments 272
Public safety and security 75
Punishment
  by death, deserving of 377
  rationale of 175
Pure malingering 123

R

Race and ethnicity 109
Rape 212
  cases of 49
  trauma syndrome 222
Reasoning, loss of 176
Receiving summons for court appearance 118
Receptive empathy 84

Recognized medical institution 278, 282
   to stock and dispense ends, process of 284
Record
   confidentiality of 221
   maintenance 70
Recovery of fees, right to 47
Refuse treatment, right to 64
Registered medical
   institute, responsibilities of 283
   practitioner 215, 278
Registering medicolegal case 401
Registration Act, under section 18 of 137
Registration numbers, display of 38
Regular stretches 458
Regulates living donor transplantation 416
Regulatory and advisory bodies for licensing, monitoring and penalizing 416
Rehabilitation 402
   and welfare programs 413
   Council of India Act 1992 20, 27
Rehabilitative facilities 398
Relapsing brain disease 434
Religious grounds sterilization, refuse on 46
Removal of organ for transplantation, consent for 63
Renal failure, chronic 156
Renal transplantation, structured interview for 419
Report writing
   for courts 187
   in forensic psychiatry 113
Reporting false information 239
Reproductive health care 234
Reproductive rights 294
Research
   consent for 63
   implications for 274
   in forensic psychiatry in India 14
Respiration 87
Rey auditory verbal learning test 127

Right against self-incrimination 172
Right to information 72, 214, 259
   Act 19, 24, 70, 71
Right to privacy 214
Rights and privileges
   of persons with mental illness 309
   of registered medical practitioners 47
Rights of persons
   violation of 174
   with disability
      convention on 250
      promotion of 19, 23
Rigorous imprisonment with hard labor 164
Rioting, cases of 164
Road side accident, case of 39
Road traffic accident cases 67
Robiological disorder 434
Rorschach test 126
Routine enquiry, evaluation of 390

S

Safe custody of will 135, 137
Safety and effective assistance, right to 214
Safety considerations 84
Safety risks and vehicle driving 432
Santhara 326
Schizophrenia 14, 109, 141, 151, 353, 357, 374
   chronic 432
   primary diagnosis of 392
   prognosis of 154
School factors 368, 381
Scientific evidence 115
Scopolamine hydrobromide 90
Seclusion and restrain, use of 271
Secobarbital 288
Secret remedies 45
Seizure, history of 401
Sensitivity about legal statutes 340
Serious assault or homicide, risk of 374
Serious injury, high risk of 392
Serious mental
   harm 76
   illness 403

Serotonergic dysfunction appears 380
Serotonergic system 379
Service delivery, factors related to 397, 398
Serving of summons, time of 167
Serving summons, procedure of 166
Session's court 163, 195
Sex determination tests 46
Sex reassignment
   intervention team 411
   surgery 411
Sexual abuse 391
   history of 234
Sexual act 209
Sexual anxiety and disorders 232
Sexual assault 210, 211, 214, 217, 229
   health consequences of 210
   reporting of 216
Sexual attitude 406
Sexual dimension of individual's personality 406
Sexual dysfunctions 210, 233
Sexual harassment 211
   of child with sexual intent 229
Sexual maturation disorder 409
Sexual offences 27, 209, 211
   cases of 62
   legal provisions concerning 211
   total 209
Sexual potency 156
Sexual relationship, consent to 225
Sexual violence 210
   adult victims of 209
   victims of 214
Sexually transmitted
   diseases 236
   infections 210, 219
Shamans 107
Sharia law 18
Sickle cell disease 292
Single photon emission computed tomography 379
Sleep disorder 353, 356
Sleep disturbance 455
   and violence 356
Sliding scale 430

Social and cultural growth of society 156
Social antecedents 351
Social learning theory 349
Social psychology theory 352
Social reciprocity, deficits in 360
Social responsibility 96
Social support agencies 215
Sociocentric society 106
Socioeconomic deprivation 381
Socioreligious rituals 5
Sodium amytal 90
Solitary imprisonment 165
Somatize 105
  depression 105
Somatoform disorder 127
Sound mind 192
Special executive magistrate 163
Special magistrate 163, 164
Special Marriage Act, 1954 25, 152
Special protection juvenile unit 238
Speech 124
  and language disability 292
Spontaneous disclosure 233
Spousal revenge 375
Stalking behavior 378
Standard medical service, maintaining 53
Standardized psychological instruments 184
State Drug Controller 283, 284
State Human Rights Commission 23
State Information Commission 72, 74
State Legislature 72
State Medical Council 35
State mental health authority 249, 251, 255, 256
States and human rights courts 23
Status fortnightly, assess 269
Statute or codified law 161
Steroids 48
Stigma 399
Stock and records, maintaining 285
Stress
  and post-traumatic stress disorder 348
  chronic 421
  reaction, acute 211
Stroke 430

Subdivisional judicial magistrate 163, 333
Subpoena 165
Subsidiary circumstances 118
Substance
  misuse 359, 387
  use disorder 233
  use or abuse 211
  use, history of 204
Substance/alcohol abuse 353, 359
Substantial disorder 250
Substantive criminal law 161, 170
Substantive law
  concerning insanity 198
  in India 204
Substitute decision-maker requires, capacity to select 314
Sudden fight 374
Suicidal behavior 211, 325
Suicidal ideation 387
Suicide 14, 328
  attempted 327
  decriminalization of 272
  effect of media 328
  foreseeability of 338
  global scenario 330
  in media, responsible reporting of 339
  Indian scenario 331
  inside healthcare establishment, complete 333
  medical conditions 328
  mental disorders 328
  methods of 330
  previous attempts and self-harm 328
  psychosocial factors 328, 329
  risk factors for 328, 328, 329
  thoughts favoring
    criminalization of 332
    decriminalization of 332
  thoughts of 232
  trigger of 330
Summons 165
  case 164
  rules of 166
  to defendant 169
Supervises and interprets law 162
Support system, adequacy of 419

Supreme Court 21, 50, 51, 52, 75, 151, 156
  decisions on management of mental hospitals 306
  guidelines 194
  rulings, recent 52
Surgical procedures, variety of 411
Surgical therapy 411
Suspected crime 42
Suspected mental illness 250
Symptom validity testing 127
Symptoms disrupt life 106
Syphilis 225
Systemic lupus erythematosus 328

T

Talaq (divorce) under Muslim Law 26
Tamil Nadu Prevention of Begging Act, 1945 399
Temporal lobe epilepsy 12
Testamentary Act 143
Testamentary capacity 13, 26, 133, 137, 143
  and competency 438
  assessment of 143
  elements of 138
  evaluation of 144
  factors affecting 139
Testamentary incapacity, symptoms of 142
Testator on Will, signature of 136
Testator's mental state 147
Thalassemia 292
Therapeutic
  care, spectrum of 232
  intervention 53
  purposes only 415
  relationship 48
  research 99
Thiopentone sodium 90
Threatening behavior, incident of 384
Tobacco consumption 14
Trained medicolegal healthcare professionals, number of 210
Training and maintenance of authorized protocol 53
Transcultural psychiatry 103

Transgender 407
Transgender Person
  (Protection of Rights) Bill,
  2016 413
  Bill, rights of 413
  identifies 413
Transient psychosis 359
Transplant evaluation rating scale
  419
Transplantation medicine 415
Transplantation of Human Organs
  Act 20, 26, 415
  aim of 415
  outlines 417
  recognizes 417
  rules state 417
Transplants conducted, number
  of 415
Traumagenic dynamics 231
Traumatic brain injury 328, 379,
  430
Traumatic sexualization 231
  result of 232
Travel allowances 167
Travel and mental illnesses 455
Travel-related stress 455
Treatment decision, capacity to
  make 59
Treatment guidelines and
  psychosocial support 218
Treatment strategies, different 410
Treatment-related decision,
  capacity for 61
Trial of cases in India
  principles of 169
  procedures of 169
Trials, types of 169

U

Undertrial prisoner 195
Undivided loyalty rule 68
Undue influence 141
Unethical conduct, exposure of 38
Unethical practice 45
United Nations Convention for
  Rights of Persons with
  Disabilities 20, 24
United Nations International
  Children Education Fund
  227
United Nations Office on Drugs
  and Crime 374
Unqualified persons, association
  with 47
Unsafe abortion 210
Unsound mind 190
Untreated mental illness 397, 398
Untruthfulness 125
Unusual injuries, repeated 236
Unwanted pregnancy 210
Urinary tract infections 210

V

Vague instructions, case of 183
Vascular cognitive impairment
  140
Vascular dementia 430
Vasoactive agent 156
Venereal disease research
  laboratory test 219
Verbal consent 57
Verbal interview 83
Vesania 4
Victim
  consent of 233
  life situation 210
  of child sexual abuse,
    management of 227
  of crimes, cases of 49
  parents 43
Victimization
  chronic 421
  repeated 386
Victoria symptom validity test 126
Video and audio recording 63
Vigilance of left over stock,
  maintaining 286
Violence 345
  against strangers 347
  biopsychosocial 348
  crime and mental disorders
    344
  manifests 346
  philosophy of 348
  psychological theories of 349
  types of 346, 386
  victims of 348
Violent behavior, risk of 382
Violent/offending behavior,
  conditions with 353
Visual
  agnosia 432
  hallucinations 124
Visuospatial ability 146
  mix of 146
Voice stress analysis 86
Voidable marriages 151
Voluntary admission 427
Voluntary and involuntary mental
  healthcare 315
Voluntary control over symptoms,
  suspicion of 123
Voluntary euthanasia 447
Voyeurism 212

W

Ward atmosphere 351
Ward behavior observation report
  204
Warrant 165
  case 164
Wild beast test 4
Will 133
  legal
    declaration 134
    document 136
  nature of 431
  person of sound mind 135
  prescribed by law 135
  secrecy of 135, 137
Wilson's disease 354
Wisconsin card sorting test 127
Witness 118
  classification 118
  examination of 170
  higher rates of malingering 121
Women from Domestic Violence
  Act, 2005, protection of 20,
  26, 384
World Health Organization 21,
  104, 209, 227, 304, 345, 459

EU GSPR Authorised Reprsentative
Logos Europe, 9 rue Nicolas Poussin
1700, La Rochelle, France
Phone: +33 (0) 6 67 93 73 78
E-mail: contact@logoseurope.eu

www.ingramcontent.com/pod-product-compliance
Ingram Content Group UK Ltd.
Pitfield, Milton Keynes, MK11 3LW, UK
UKHW050456150426

5217IPUK00025B/1705